T0335621

# Sjögren's Syndrome

# Sjögren's Syndrome
## Novel Insights in Pathogenic, Clinical and Therapeutic Aspects

*Edited by*

**Roberto Gerli**

*Co-edited by*

**Elena Bartoloni**

**Alessia Alunno**

AMSTERDAM • BOSTON • HEIDELBERG • LONDON
NEW YORK • OXFORD • PARIS • SAN DIEGO
SAN FRANCISCO • SINGAPORE • SYDNEY • TOKYO

Academic Press is an imprint of Elsevier

Academic Press is an imprint of Elsevier
125 London Wall, London EC2Y 5AS, UK
525 B Street, Suite 1800, San Diego, CA 92101-4495, USA
50 Hampshire Street, 5th Floor, Cambridge, MA 02139, USA
The Boulevard, Langford Lane, Kidlington, Oxford OX5 1GB, UK

**British Library Cataloguing-in-Publication Data**
A catalogue record for this book is available from the British Library

**Library of Congress Cataloging-in-Publication Data**
A catalog record for this book is available from the Library of Congress

ISBN: 978-0-12-803604-4

For information on all Academic Press publications
visit our website at https://www.elsevier.com/

Working together
to grow libraries in
developing countries

www.elsevier.com • www.bookaid.org

*Acquisition Editor:* Linda Versteeg-Buschman
*Editorial Project Manager:* Halima Williams
*Production Project Manager:* Karen East and Kirsty Halterman
*Designer:* Alan Studholme

Typeset by TNQ Books and Journals
www.tnq.co.in

# Dedication

**"To Monica, Michele, Veronica and Lucrezia"**

# Contents

## 10. Sjögren's Syndrome and Environmental Factors

*S. Colafrancesco, C. Perricone and Y. Shoenfeld*

## 11. Histology of Sjögren's Syndrome

*F. Barone, S. Colafrancesco and J. Campos*

## 12. Glandular Epithelium: Innocent Bystander or Leading Actor?

*E.K. Kapsogeorgou and A.G. Tzioufas*

# List of Contributors

**A. Alunno** University of Perugia, Perugia, Italy

**S. Appel** University of Bergen, Bergen, Norway

**E. Astorri** Barts and The London School of Medicine and Dentistry, London, United Kingdom

**C. Baldini** University of Pisa, Pisa, Italy

**F. Barone** University of Birmingham, Birmingham, United Kingdom

**E. Bartoloni** University of Perugia, Perugia, Italy

**M. Bombardieri** Barts and The London School of Medicine and Dentistry, London, United Kingdom

**S. Bombardieri** University of Pisa, Pisa, Italy

**S.J. Bowman** University of Birmingham, Birmingham, United Kingdom; University Hospitals Birmingham NHS Trust, Birmingham, United Kingdom

**J. Campos** University of Birmingham, Birmingham, United Kingdom

**F. Carubbi** University of L'Aquila, L'Aquila, Italy; ASL 1Avezzano-Sulmona-L'Aquila, L'Aquila, Italy

**P. Cipriani** University of L'Aquila, L'Aquila, Italy

**S. Colafrancesco** Sapienza University of Rome, Rome, Italy

**S. De Vita** Udine University Hospital, Udine, Italy

**N. Del Papa** Istituto G. Pini, Milan, Italy

**V. Devauchelle-Pensec** La Cavale Blanche University Hospital, Brest, France; University of Western Brittany (UBO), Brest, France

**R. Felten** Strasbourg University Hospital, Strasbourg, France

**B.A. Fisher** University of Birmingham, Birmingham, United Kingdom; University Hospitals Birmingham NHS Trust, Birmingham, United Kingdom

**C.M. Fox** Scripps Memorial Hospital and Research Foundation, La Jolla, CA, United States

**R.I. Fox** Scripps Memorial Hospital and Research Foundation, La Jolla, CA, United States

**S. Gandolfo** Udine University Hospital, Udine, Italy

**R. Gerli** University of Perugia, Perugia, Italy

**R. Giacomelli** University of L'Aquila, L'Aquila, Italy

**J.-E. Gottenberg** Strasbourg University Hospital, Strasbourg, France

**R. Jonsson** University of Bergen, Bergen, Norway; Haukeland University Hospital, Bergen, Norway

**E.K. Kapsogeorgou** National University of Athens, Athens, Greece

**V.C. Kyttaris** Harvard Medical School, Boston, MA, United States

**D. Lucchesi** Barts and The London School of Medicine and Dentistry, London, United Kingdom

**C. Lunardi** University of Verona, Verona, Italy

**M.N. Manoussakis** National and Kapodistrian University of Athens, Athens, Greece

**C.P. Mavragani** National and Kapodistrian University of Athens, Athens, Greece

**G. Patuzzo** University of Verona, Verona, Italy

**C. Perricone** Sapienza University of Rome, Rome, Italy

**J.-O. Pers** EA2216, INSERM ESPRI, ERI29, Université de Brest, Brest, France; LabEx IGO, Brest, France

**C. Pitzalis** Barts and The London School of Medicine and Dentistry, London, United Kingdom

**R. Priori** Sapienza University of Rome, Rome, Italy

**L. Quartuccio** Udine University Hospital, Udine, Italy

**Y. Shoenfeld** Chaim Sheba Medical Center, Tel-Hashomer, Israel; Tel Aviv University, Tel Aviv-Yafo, Israel

**J. Sibilia** Strasbourg University Hospital, Strasbourg, France

**E. Tinazzi** University of Verona, Verona, Italy

**G.C. Tsokos** Harvard Medical School, Boston, MA, United States

**A.G. Tzioufas** National University of Athens, Athens, Greece

**G. Valesini** Sapienza University of Rome, Rome, Italy

**C. Vitali** Casa di Cura of Lecco, Lecco, Italy; Istituto S. Stefano, Como, Italy

**P. Youinou** EA2216, INSERM ESPRI, ERI29, Université de Brest, Brest, France; LabEx IGO, Brest, France

# Preface

Although Sjögren's syndrome (SS) is usually thought of as a minor and uncommon disease characterized by dry eyes and mouth associated with joint pain, it is actually a common and often debilitating illness that can seriously impair patients' quality of life. In addition, the disease may be characterized by a systemic involvement that may negatively and heavily affect its long-term prognosis. However, little is known as yet on its pathogenesis. Recent unmasking of novel pathogenic mechanisms and identification of clinical and serological features associated with different subsets and possible different outcomes of the disease not only allowed us to increase our knowledge of the disease, but also to provide the rationale for possible targeted therapies, as already occurs in other rheumatic disorders such as rheumatoid arthritis and systemic lupus erythematosus.

*Sjögren's Syndrome: Novel Insights in Pathogenic, Clinical and Therapeutic Aspects* is a comprehensive and exhaustive overview of current knowledge on SS and provides the most up-to-date information available on the disorder. It summarizes a huge amount of recent literature concerning advances on genetics, background, pathogenesis, clinical picture, and treatment approaches of this disorder. It also integrates concepts of basic immunology with clinical features and pharmacological issues. This book is an invaluable resource to physicians and health care professionals, offering everything they need to improve their knowledge of the disease.

Key Features:

- Discusses heterogeneity (of topics and audience): from basic immunology to clinical aspects and therapeutics
- Provides novel lines of investigation and supports the management of patients requiring novel therapeutic approaches
- Presents a deeper knowledge of SS clinical management as well as immunological aspects, possibly leading to new lines of investigation
- Offers a bridge between the clinician and the scientist, and vice versa
- Provides the reader with most recent and relevant updates due to the novelty of topics

**Edited by: Roberto Gerli**
**Co-Edited by: Elena Bartoloni and Alessia Alunno**

Chapter 1

# Introduction: History of Sjögren's Syndrome

C. Baldini, S. Bombardieri
*University of Pisa, Pisa, Italy*

## 1. INTRODUCTION

Sjögren's syndrome (SS) is a complex disorder characterized by both organ-specific and systemic manifestations, potentially expanding to lymphoproliferative complications.[1] In addition to occurring as a primary or secondary disease, SS can occur in association with organ-specific autoimmune diseases, as well as in overlapping complex entities with the major connective tissue diseases.[2,3]

SS is named after the Swedish ophthalmologist Henrik Sjögren, who presented his doctoral thesis in 1933.[4] However, the historical traces of SS can be found in a number of case reports published during the 19th century before Henrik Sjögren. Over the years, SS has been described first as an organ-specific disorder involving salivary and lachrymal glands, and then as a systemic autoimmune disease displaying significant extraglandular manifestations.[5-7]

Norman Talal has suggested that the history of SS can be subdivided into three phases[8]: firstly, the initial definition of SS through a series of reports documenting its glandular manifestations; secondly, beginning in the 1950s, the second definition of SS as an autoimmune disorder potentially involving different organs and systems; and thirdly, since the 1980s, the era of molecular biology.

### 1.1 The History of Sjögren's Syndrome Before Henrik Sjögren

In the late 1890s through the early 1900s, many cases were published describing the presence of simultaneous ocular and oral dryness, sometimes with coexistent chronic rheumatism or gout. These cases can be considered as "antecedents" to the actual SS. The most relevant reports published in the 50 years before Henrik Sjögren's doctoral thesis are described below according to their temporal appearance in the literature.

The entity "keratitis filamentosa" (filamentous keratitis) was first reported in 1882 by the ophthalmologist Thomas Leber who, in his lecture "About the Origin of the Retinal Detachment," described three patients with a dry

Sjögren's Syndrome. http://dx.doi.org/10.1016/B978-0-12-803604-4.00001-0

1

inflammation of the cornea and conjunctiva with filamentous formations. Leber thought that they were associated to a viral infection of the cornea and did not associate this entity with the dryness of the ocular surface; however, his observation played an important role in the future concepts of SS.[9]

A few years later, at the beginning of 1888, Hutchison (1828–1913) published the case of a 60-year-old woman with a severe oral dryness, severe dysphagia, and arrested salivary secretion of the glands. Hutchison hypothesized that her condition could have been the result of a chronic nervous state.[10,11] On March 9 of the same year in London, Dr. WB Hadden (1856–93) presented to the Clinical Society his own case of dry mouth. He used the neologism of xerostomia to describe the case of a 65-year-old woman with dry mouth, "nearly unable to swallow" … "her tongue was red, absolutely dry and cracked in all directions like a "crocodile's skin" … "No tears appeared when she tried to cry." The xerostomia improved if treated with pilocarpine (Jaborandi). According to Sir William Osler, in his famous text book *The Principles and Practice of Medicine* (1982), Hutchison was the first to have coined the term *xerostomia*, while Hadden was the first to have associated the condition to the "involvement of some center which controls the secretions of the salivary and buccal glands."[12]

In 1892 the Polish surgeon Dr. Johann Mikulicz-Radecki (1850–1905) reported to the Society for Scientific Medicine in Koenigsberg the case of a 42-year-old farmer with painless symmetrical enlargement of the lachrymal and salivary glands. There was no evidence of diminution in either lachrymal or salivary secretions. He died 14 months later. The histological examination of the submandibular glands showed extensive acinar atrophy and intense round cell infiltration, which today are known to be suggestive of salivary glands with mucosa-associated lymphoid tissue lymphoma.[13] Bilateral swelling of the lachrymal and salivary glands without other disease was called *Mikulicz disease* after him; when this condition was found in association with other diseases including tuberculosis, sarcoidosis, lymphoma, it was termed *Mikulicz syndrome*.[14] Later, Morgan and Castleman concluded, on the basis of pathological descriptions, that Mikulicz disease and SS were the same entity.[15]

In 1925 the dermatologist Henri Gougerot (1881–1955) described three separate cases of progressive and chronic dryness of mouth caused by atrophy of the salivary glands. Dryness of the eyes, nose, larynx, and vagina was variably involved, suggesting that a direct assault to the glands or the alteration of the sympathetic innervations of the glands may have been involved.[16]

In 1928–29 Houwer presented four patients without tear secretion. He wrote that keratitis filamentosa was bilateral and chronic; half of the patients had keratitis filamentosa in combination with arthritis. Houwer admitted that he did not know if an innervational, toxic, or trophic cause was present, including urates. None of his patients had keratomalacia or avitaminosis A.[17]

Some clinicians over time have thought that Mikulicz, Gougerot, and Houwer had published basic concepts of what later became known as SS, and that their names should be proposed as eponyms to complement the term of SS (ie, Sjögren-Mikulicz syndrome, Gougerot-Sjögren disease, or Gougerot-Houwer-Sjögren syndrome).

Among the other authors cited subsequently by Henrik Sjögren himself as having reported cases of dry eyes and dry mouth in the decades between 1889 and 1930, the following should be mentioned: Fischer, Wagenmann, Umber, Fuchs, Deutschmann, Kreiker, Schöninger, Stock, Clegg, Scheerer, Albrich, Isakowitz, Engelking, Avizonis, Betsch, Knapp, Vogt, Pillat, Duke-Elder, Hauer, and Wissmann.[5,7]

None of these authors, however, had highlighted the systemic "nature" of the disease before Henrik Sjögren.

## 1.2  The History of Sjögren's Syndrome: Henrik Sjögren

Henrik Sjögren (1899–1986) was born in Köping, a small city in central Sweden on lake Malaren. His father, Conrad Johansson, was a businessman while his mother, Emelie, worked in a bank. In 1923, for practical reasons the family legally changed its name to the mother's maiden name, Sjögren (*Sjö* = lake and *gre* = branch of tree). Henrik studied medicine in the Karolinska Institute, and in 1927 received his medical degree as a "physician." During his medical studies, he became engaged to Maria Hellgren, the daughter of a well-known oculist. After graduating, he continued working at the eye clinic of Serafimer Hospital at the Karolinska Institute. In 1929 the Royal Medical Board of Sweden sent him to Jönköping to examine a group of Swedish immigrants from the Ukraine, many of whom had trachoma and tear deficiency. Following their cases, Henrik Sjögren became interested in surfocular dryness.[5,7,8,10]

In 1930, Henrik Sjögren observed a middle-aged woman with lachrymal, salivary, and sweat hyposecretion and "rheumatismus chronicus." He introduced the neologism *keratoconjunctivitis sicca (KCS)* to describe her ocular manifestations, which were assessed with rose bengal and methylene blue. This patient's case, together with four other cases, was included in his first paper in *Hygiea*, the proceedings of the Swedish Medical Association.[18]

In May 1933, in his application for a PhD degree, he presented a doctoral dissertation, "Zur Kenntnis der Keratoconjunctivitis Sicca Keratitis filiformis bei hypofunction der Tranendriisen," in which he described in detail the clinical and pathological features of 19 females with KCS, of whom most were postmenopausal and 13 had arthritis. Henrik Sjögren concluded that this was a generalized systemic disease, not just an ocular disorder, and that it may represent a new nosologic entity. Sjögren stressed that KCS had no resemblance to xerophthalmia caused by vitamin A deficiency, emphasizing that KCS was mainly the result of water deficiency, whereas hypovitaminosis A resulted largely in a deficiency of mucin. In general, Sjögren did not consider his discoveries to represent a new disease but he aimed at confirming the previous experience on keratitis filamentosa, focusing for the first time on the systemic nature of this entity.[4]

Sjögren's presentation of his thesis was unsuccessful, and he was disqualified from a "teaching" grade, stopping his academic career.

Sjögren's 150-page doctoral thesis was in German, and it was not until 1940 that an English translation was published by an Australian ophthalmologist, J.B. Hamilton. This latter (1933) was the basis for the creation of the term *Sjögren's syndrome*.[19]

In 1936, Stephan von Gròsz, an assistant at the University of Budapest, proposed combining the various clinical pictures with the characteristics described by Sjögren and to name the entity *Sjögren's syndrome*. The Concilium Ophthalmologicum Internationale of Cairo in 1937 and the publications of Hamilton obtained much more attention than the original German version, greatly enhancing the international recognition of the term and making Henrik Sjögren well recognized internationally.[5] In 1951, Sjögren described 80 cases of the syndrome, the second largest population of patients at that time. By 1960, he had published 28 new papers related to KCS.[5]

## 1.3 The History of Sjögren's Syndrome: The Concept of Sjögren's Syndrome as an Autoimmune Disease

The currently accepted definition of SS as an autoimmune disease was first proposed in the 1950s and spread rapidly in the 1960s and 1970s. The studies by Jones (1958), aimed at identifying circulating autoantibodies responsible for an autoimmune attack in patients with SS, were the basis for a new line of research.[20] Between 1958 and 1960, Bunim and his team at the National Institutes of Health (Bethesda, MD, United States) collected 40 cases of SS that were isolated or associated with other systemic autoimmune diseases, and detected in these patients a positivity for rheumatoid arthritis, hypergammaglobulinemia, complement-fixing antibodies, antinuclear antibodies, and thyroglobulin antibodies.[21] In 1963, Bloch et al. stated that "the occurrence of a variety of autoantibodies strongly suggested that an abnormal immunologic mechanism was either primary or secondary involved in SS."[22] In 1965, Bloch et al. presented a study of 62 patients with SS isolated or associated with other connective tissue diseases including rheumatoid arthritis, systemic sclerosis, and polymyositis.[23]

The observation that a variety of autoantibodies occurred in SS strongly supported the idea that autoimmune mechanisms were involved in the disease pathogenesis. From this perspective, an important acquisition was provided by Alspaugh, who identified anti-SSA (anti-Ro) and anti-SSB (anti-La) autoantibodies as being present in SS patients.[24] Moreover, in 1968, histologic grading assessing the infiltration of labial glands was published.[25]

During the 1970s and 1980s, clinical and serologic research continued under the leadership of Norman Talal, Norman Cummings, Thomas Chused, and Haralampos Moutsopoulos, who together with their coworkers extensively investigated the clinical manifestations of the disease and the underlying immunologic mechanisms, describing SS as a chronic autoimmune disease characterized by T and B lymphocyte infiltration of exocrine glands, leading to xerostomia and xerophthalmia.[26] In particular, Moutsopoulos et al. suggested that the epithelium may play a pivotal role in orchestrating the immune response in the histopathologic lesions of SS, and proposed the term *autoimmune epitheliitis* as an etiologic term.[10,27] In 1978, Moutsopoulos and coworkers also reported for the first time that patients with SS have up to 44 times increased risk of developing lymphoma compared with the general population.[28] In 1980 the same group formally coined the terms *primary SS* and *secondary SS* to identify respectively patients with "disease limited to the exocrine gland or with additional extraglandular disease," or "the disease occurring as a component of another connective tissue disease, such as rheumatoid arthritis or systemic lupus erythematosus."[10,29]

## 1.4 The History of Sjögren's Syndrome: Subsequent Milestones

The subsequent history of SS moved though different complementary directions. Great efforts were put into developing universally accepted classification criteria for the disease. A number of sets of criteria have been proposed over time; however, because of the complexity of the disease and its different phenotypes, it has been quite challenging to elaborate a unique set of classification criteria able to identify patients with homogenous clinical and serologic manifestations[30,31] (Table 1.1). In 1993 the preliminary European classification criteria for SS were proposed and they were largely employed for the subsequent 10 years, both in clinical practice and in observational and interventional studies (Fig. 1.1).[32] These criteria were subsequently reexamined in 2002 and their revised version, the American–European Consensus Group (AECG) criteria set, has rapidly become the standard reference for SS.[33]

Nowadays, the AECG criteria are the most commonly used tool for classification of patients with primary SS and secondary SS, both in clinical trials and

**TABLE 1.1** Milestones in the Development of Classification Criteria

| Year | Classification Criteria |
| --- | --- |
| 1975 (Subsequently revised in 1984) | San Francisco criteria |
| 1986 | Copenhagen, Japanese, Greek, and San Diego criteria |
| 1993 | Preliminary EU classification criteria |
| 2002 | AECG criteria |
| 2012 | ACR criteria |

*ACR*, American College of Rheumatology; *AECG*, American–European Consensus Group; *EU*, European.

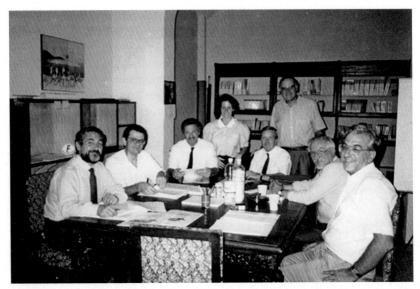

**FIGURE 1.1** Editorial office of *Clinical and Experimental Rheumatology*, Pisa (Italy). 1990: International meeting for the application for the preliminary classification criteria (1993).

in epidemiologic studies; moreover, given their high sensitivity and specificity, they have been largely employed in clinical practice for the diagnosis of the disease. However, although the criteria are widely adopted by the scientific community, it has nonetheless become a common belief that some aspects of these criteria still deserve to be properly readdressed. Recently the American College of Rheumatology (ACR)/Sjögren's International Collaborative Clinical Alliance endorsed new classification criteria for SS.[34] In 2013 an ACR-European classification criteria working group was founded in order to elaborate new classification criteria derived from the existing ones. This new set of criteria is expected to be published in the near future.

International efforts have also been made for the development of a consensus for a systemic disease activity index and a patient index for primary SS. These efforts resulted in two novel instruments: the European League Against Rheumatism (EULAR) SS disease activity index and the EULAR SS Patient Reported Index published respectively in 2010[35] and in 2011,[36] which are useful tools in patients' clinical assessment and for clinical trials. These clinical achievements have been paralleled over time by the huge amount of novel insights into the disease pathogenesis. Although the precise etiology and pathogenesis of SS remain elusive, the role of innate immune mechanisms in the early phases of the disease, as well as the importance of the subsequent activation of the adaptive immune system and the role of T and B cells in the disease progression, have been at least partially clarified.[37] In turn, these new acquisitions have opened and will continue to open new avenues for the early diagnosis of the disease and its treatment.[38] The "-omics" era has offered the opportunity to search for new and specific biomarkers in SS that may also represent attractive options for SS treatment.[39] It is not by chance that the first randomized clinical trials have been performed in patients with primary SS using biologic agents such as rituximab,[40] belimumab,[41] and abatacept,[42] changing our approach to the treatment of the disease. Hopefully, taking full advantage from a wealth of past experience, we will be ready in the near future to write new chapters in the history of SS.

## REFERENCES

1. Tzioufas AG, Voulgarelis M. Update on Sjögren's syndrome autoimmune epitheliitis: from classification to increased neoplasias. *Best Pract Res Clin Rheumatol* 2007;**21**:989–1010.
2. Ramos-Casals M, Brito-Zeron P, Font J. The overlap of Sjögren's syndrome with other systemic autoimmune diseases. *Semin Arthritis Rheum* 2007;**36**:246–55.
3. Baldini C, Mosca M, Della Rossa A, Pepe P, Notarstefano C, Ferro F, et al. Overlap of ACA-positive systemic sclerosis and Sjögren's syndrome: a distinct clinical entity with mild organ involvement but at high risk of lymphoma. *Clin Exp Rheumatol* 2013;**31**:272–80.
4. Sjögren H. Zur filiformis bei Hypofunktion der Tranendrusen. *Acta Ophthalmol* 1933;**2**:1–151.
5. Murube J. The first definition of Sjögren's syndrome. *Ocul Surf* 2010;**8**:101–10.
6. Ghafoor M. Sjögren's before Sjögren: did Henrik Sjögren (1899–1986) really discover Sjögren's disease? *J Maxillofac Oral Surg* 2012;**11**:373–4.
7. Parke AL, Buchanan WW. Sjögren's syndrome: history, clinical and pathological features. *Inflammopharmacology* 1998;**6**:271–87.
8. Talal N. Historical overview of Sjögren's syndrome. *Clin Exp Rheumatol* 1994;**12**:S3–4.
9. Leber T. Praparate zu dem Vortag uber Entstehung der Netzhautablosung und über verschei-edene Hornhautaffektionen. *Klin Monatsblatter Augenheilkd* 1882;**14**:165–6.
10. Moutsopoulos HM, Chused TM, Mann DL, Klippel JH, Fauci AS, Frank MM, et al. Sjögren's syndrome (sicca syndrome): current issues. *Ann Intern Med* 1980;**92**:212–26.
11. Osler W. *The principles and practice of medicine.* New York: D Appleton and Co.; 1892. p. 328.
12. Hadden WB. On "dry mouth", or suppression of the salivary and buccal secretions. *Trans Clin Soc Lond* 1888;**21**:176–9.
13. Von Mikulicz-Radecki J. Uebereine eigenartige symmetrische Erkrankung des Thranen: und Mundspeicheldrusen. In: *Beitrage zur Chirurgie. Festschrift gewidmet Theodore Billroth, Stuttgart.* 1892. p. 610–30.
14. Schaffer AJ, Jacobsen AW. Mikulicz's syndrome: a report of ten cases. *Am J Dis Child* 1927;**34**:327–46.
15. Morgan WS, Castleman B. A clinicopathologic study of Mikulicz's disease. *Am J Pathol* 1953;**29**:471–503.
16. Gougerot H. Insuffisance progressive et atrophie des glandes salivaires et muqueuses de la bouche, des conjonctives. Secheresse de la bouche, des conjonctives, etc. *Bull Med Paris* 1926;**40**:360–8.
17. Houwer AWM. IV. Diseases of cornea: keratitis filamentosa and chronic arthritis. *Trans Ophthalmol Soc UK* 1927;**47**:88–96.
18. Sjögren H. Keratoconjunctivitis sicca. *Hygiea* 1930;**92**:829.
19. Hamilton JB. Keratitis sicca, including Sjögren's syndrome. *Trans Ophthalmol Soc Aust* 1940;**2**:63.

20. Jones BR. Lacrimal and salivary precipitating antibodies in Sjögren's syndrome. *Lancet* 1958;**2**:773–6.

21. Bunim JJ. A broader spectrum of Sjögren's syndrome and its pathogenetic implications. *Ann Rheum Dis* 1961;**20**:1–10.

22. Bloch KJ, Wohl MJ, Ship II, Oglesby BB, Bunim JJ. Sjögren's syndrome. Part 1. Serologic reactions in patients with Sjögren's syndrome with and without rheumatoid arthritis. *Arthritis Rheum* 1960;**3**:287–97.

23. Bloch KJ, Buchanan WW, Wohl MJ, Bunim JJ. Sjögren's syndrome: a clinical, pathological, and serological study of sixty-two cases. *Med Baltim (1965)* 1992;**71**:386–401. discussion 401–3.

24. Alspaugh MA, Tan EM. Antibodies to cellular antigens in Sjögren's syndrome. *J Clin Invest* 1975;**55**:1067–73.

25. Chisholm DM, Mason DK. Labial salivary gland biopsy in Sjögren's disease. *J Clin Pathol* 1968;**21**:656–60.

26. Murube J. The second definition of Sjögren's syndrome as an autoimmune disorder. *Ocul Surf* 2010;**8**:163–72.

27. Moutsopoulos HM. Sjögren's syndrome: autoimmune epitheliitis. *Clin Immunol Immunopathol* 1994;**72**:162–5.

28. Kassan SS, Thomas TL, Moutsopoulos HM, Hoover R, Kimberly RP, Budman DR, et al. Increased risk of lymphoma in sicca syndrome. *Ann Intern Med* 1978;**89**:888–92.

29. Moutsopoulos HM, Fauci AS. Immunoregulation in Sjögren's syndrome: influence of serum factors on T-cell subpopulations. *J Clin Invest* 1980;**65**:519–28.

30. Baldini C, Talarico R, Tzioufas AG, Bombardieri S. Classification criteria for Sjögren's syndrome: a critical review. *J Autoimmun* 2012;**39**:9–14.

31. Goules AV, Tzioufas AG, Moutsopoulos HM. Classification criteria of Sjögren's syndrome. *J Autoimmun* 2014;**48–49**:42–5.

32. Vitali C, Bombardieri S, Moutsopoulos HM, Balestrieri G, Bencivelli W, Bernstein RM, et al. Preliminary criteria for the classification of Sjögren's syndrome: results of a prospective concerted action supported by the European Community. *Arthritis Rheum* 1993;**36**:340–7.

33. Vitali C, Bombardieri S, Jonsson R, Moutsopoulos HM, Alexander EL, Carsons SE, et al. Classification criteria for Sjögren's syndrome: a revised version of the European criteria proposed by the American-European Consensus Group. *Ann Rheum Dis* 2002;**61**:554–8.

34. Shiboski SC, Shiboski CH, Criswell L, Baer A, Challacombe S, Lanfranchi H, et al. American College of Rheumatology classification criteria for Sjögren's syndrome: a data-driven, expert consensus approach in the Sjögren's International Collaborative Clinical Alliance cohort. *Arthritis Care Res* 2012;**64**:475–87.

35. Seror R, Ravaud P, Bowman SJ, Baron G, Tzioufas A, Theander E, et al. EULAR Sjögren's syndrome disease activity index: development of a consensus systemic disease activity index for primary Sjögren's syndrome. *Ann Rheum Dis* 2010;**69**:1103–9.

36. Seror R, Ravaud P, Mariette X, Bootsma H, Theander E, Hansen A, et al. EULAR Sjögren's Syndrome Patient Reported Index (ESSPRI): development of a consensus patient index for primary Sjögren's syndrome. *Ann Rheum Dis* 2011;**70**:968–72.

37. Luciano N, Valentini V, Calabrò A, Elefante E, Vitale A, Baldini C, et al. One year in review 2015: Sjögren's syndrome. *Clin Exp Rheumatol* 2015;**33**:259–71.

38. Tzioufas AG, Kapsogeorgou EK, Moutsopoulos HM. Pathogenesis of Sjögren's syndrome: what we know and what we should learn. *J Autoimmun* 2012;**39**:4–8.

39. Baldini C, Gallo A, Perez P, Mosca M, Alevizos I, Bombardieri S. Saliva as an ideal milieu for emerging diagnostic approaches in primary Sjögren's syndrome. *Clin Exp Rheumatol* 2012;**30**:785–90.

40. Devauchelle-Pensec V, Mariette X, Jousse-Joulin S, Berthelot JM, Perdriger A, Puéchal X, et al. Treatment of primary Sjögren syndrome with rituximab: a randomized trial. *Ann Intern Med* 2014;**160**:233–42.

41. Mariette X, Seror R, Quartuccio L, Baron G, Salvin S, Fabris M, et al. Efficacy and safety of belimumab in primary Sjögren's syndrome: results of the BELISS open-label phase II study. *Ann Rheum Dis* 2015;**74**:526–31.

42. Meiners PM, Vissink A, Kroese FG, Spijkervet FK, Smitt-Kamminga NS, Abdulahad WH, et al. Abatacept treatment reduces disease activity in early primary Sjögren's syndrome (open-label proof of concept ASAP study). *Ann Rheum Dis* 2014;**73**:1393–6.

Chapter 2

# Clinical Features

E. Bartoloni, A. Alunno, R. Gerli
*University of Perugia, Perugia, Italy*

## 1. INTRODUCTION

The clear identification of primary Sjögren's syndrome (pSS) as a systemic disease occurred only in the 1980s and 1990s. Indeed, in the early 1970s, the only characterized systemic manifestations were bronchitis sicca, interstitial nephritis, and the risk of developing lymphoma in the same patients.[1] Later on, some nonspecific manifestations, including Raynaud phenomenon and arthralgias, were described, and in the early 1980s, clinical and immunopathological features of vasculitis associated with pSS were recognized as characteristic disease manifestations.[2,3] Finally, several systemic manifestations, including arthritis, different patterns of esophageal dysfunction, and liver and muscular inflammatory involvement, were recognized, thus confirming the wide spectrum of disease clinical appearance.[4–6]

## 2. THE MANY FACETS OF THE DISEASE

pSS is a protean systemic disease and the clinical picture can vary considerably from relatively mild sicca symptoms, arthralgias, and fatigue to severe systemic symptoms. As a consequence, the heterogeneity of signs and symptoms often leads to a delay in diagnosis and the estimated disease incidence and prevalence vary significantly depending on the classification criteria applied, the study design, and the ethnicity.[7–13] Interestingly, clinical appearance may vary according to several variables, including age at onset, sex, immunological profile, and clinical subsets. A significant influence of age on serological abnormalities and clinical expression of pSS has been demonstrated (Table 2.1). Younger pSS onset is associated with greater immunological expression and lower prevalence of sicca symptoms in comparison with patients who are older at the onset of disease. Patients aged younger than 35–40 years, in comparison with older ones, display a higher prevalence of circulating anti-Ro/SSA, anti-La/SSB antibodies, rheumatoid factor (RF), and immunological markers associated with a more active disease, including pancytopenia, low complement levels, and hypergammaglobulinemia.[14–18] On the other hand, pSS patients older than 65 years appear

Sjögren's Syndrome. http://dx.doi.org/10.1016/B978-0-12-803604-4.00002-2

## 12 Sjögren's Syndrome

**TABLE 2.1 Clinical and Serological Features in pSS According to Patient Age at Disease Onset**

| References | No. of Pts | pSS Classification Criteria | % of Pts With Age ≤35–40yrs | % of Pts With Age ≥65–70yrs | Pts With Age ≤35–40 Versus >40yrs | Pts With Age ≥65–70 Versus <65yrs |
|---|---|---|---|---|---|---|
| Ramos-Casals[14] | 144 | ECCG | 9% | | ↑Lymphadenopathy ↑RF, ↑anti-Ro/SSA | |
| Haga[15] | 67 | ECCG | 24% | 36% | ↑RF, anti-Ro/SSA, anti-La/SSB, hypergammaglobulinemia | |
| Tishler[19] | 85 | San Diego criteria | | 20% | | ↓RF ↓Anti-Ro/SSA |
| Garcia-Garrasco[16] | 400 | ECCG | 15% | 11% | ↑Lymphadenopathy ↑anti-Ro/SSA | |
| Ramos-Casals[17] | 1010 | ECCG | 14% | 15% | ↓Xerostomia ↓Altered ocular tests ↑Anti-Ro/SSA ↓Low C3–C4 | ↓Arthralgia ↑Lung involvement ↑Anemia ↓Anti-Ro/SSA |
| Botsios[21] | 336 | AECG | 39% | 6% | No difference | No difference |
| Malladi[20] | 886 | AECG | | 17% | | ↓RF, hypergammaglobulinemia, leukopenia, anti-Ro/ SSA, anti-La/SSB ↑Reduced UWS flow rate |
| Zhao[18] | 483 | AECG | 5% | | ↑Pancytopenia ↑Low C3 | |

*AECG*, American-European Consensus Group; *ECCG*, European Classification Criteria Group; *Pts*, patients; *RF*, rheumatoid factor; *UWS*, unstimulated whole salivary; *yrs*, years; ↑, higher frequency; ↓, lower frequency.

less likely to have RF, hypergammaglobulinemia, leukopenia, and anti-Ro/SSA or anti-La/SSB antibodies, but more likely to have a decreased unstimulated whole salivary flow rate and lung involvement.[17,19,20] Ethnicity and demographic factors may influence age-related variability in disease manifestations and the lower autoimmune characterization of the disease in older subjects may reflect senescence of the immune system.[21,22]

Gender may also influence disease immunological and clinical expression. Indeed, about 3% to 11% of pSS patients are men (Table 2.2). A lesser autoimmune expression, either clinical, histological, sialographic or immunological, has been described in males. In particular, pSS in males is characterized by a lower rate of altered ocular tests and lower prevalence of some immunological features, including RF, anti-La/SSB and anti-Ro/SSA.[16–18,23] Similarly, the prevalence of some specific extraglandular manifestations, such as Raynaud phenomenon, autoimmune thyroiditis, arthritis, cutaneous vasculitis and renal involvement, appears to be slightly lower in men.[16,17,24]

Although some immunological markers, in particular anti-Ro/SSA, anti-La/SSB, RF and cryoglobulins, have an undeniably important diagnostic and prognostic role, a seronegative form of pSS, first described in 1996, has been reported in up to one-third of patients.[25] The analysis of this "immuno-negative" subset showed a lower incidence of extraglandular features, mainly Raynaud phenomenon and cutaneous vasculitis, in these patients.[26] On the other hand, positivity for antinuclear antibodies, anti-Ro/SSA, anti-La/SSB, RF, or cryoglobulins is associated with a more active immunological profile with higher risk of hematological and systemic involvement. Indeed, the presence of more systemic autoantibodies may be considered a reflection of B cell hyperreactivity and a clear direct relationship has been demonstrated between the number of autoantibodies and extraglandular manifestations.[26] The subset of patients with pSS and anti-Ro/SSA and/or La/SSB probably represents the most clinically and immunologically "active" presentation of the disease, characterized by severe systemic complications, polyclonal B cell activation profile, and higher need for corticosteroids and immunosuppressive drugs.[16,26] In particular, anti-Ro/SSA positivity has been shown to be the strongest contributor for systemic extraglandular manifestations, including parotid swelling, lymphadenopathy, cutaneous vasculitis, and neurologic involvement in different SS cohorts.[17,27–29] Key phenotypic SS features are more prevalent and disease activity is higher in anti-Ro/SSA positive subjects with respect to those who are anti-La/SSB positive alone or negative for both.[30] RF and cryoglobulins are commonly observed in seropositive patients and contribute to higher risk of extraglandular and immunological features, including articular involvement and cutaneous vasculitis.[16] Of interest, pSS patients displaying at least two serological markers of severe disease, including low levels of C3/C4, RF positivity, hypergammaglobulinemia, and cryoglobulins, are at a higher risk of developing both disease-related systemic manifestations, requiring immunosuppressive therapy, and non-Hodgkin lymphoma in comparison

**TABLE 2.2** Extraglandular Manifestations in pSS Cohorts (Values are Expressed in Percentage Unless Specified)

| References | Pertovaara[35] | Garcia-Garrasco[16] | Alamanos[7] | Ramos-Casals[17] | Borg[27] | Martel[26] | Malladi[20] | Baldini[31] | Abrol[38] | Li[33] | Zhao[18] | Kvarnström[36] | Sandhya[32] |
|---|---|---|---|---|---|---|---|---|---|---|---|---|---|
| No. of patients | 110 | 400 | 422 | 1010 | 65 | 445 | 886 | 1115 | 152 | 315 | 483 | 199 | 332 |
| Country | Finland | Spain | Greece | Spain | NL | France | USA | Italy | UK | China | China | Sweden | India |
| Classification criteria | ECCG | ECCG | AECG | ECCG | AECG | AECG | AECG | ECCG AECG | AECG | AECG | AECG | AECG | AECG ACR |
| Female | 97 | 93 | 95 | 93 | 89 | 90 | 95 | 96 | 91 | 96 | 94 | 93 | 95 |
| Age (yrs) at diagnosis, mean (SD) | 62 (13) | 53 (1) | 55 (12) | 53 (1) | 51 (14) | 54 (1) | – | 52 (14) | 5 (13) | 47 (14) | 4 (11) | 55 (14) | 44 (11) |
| Xerostomia | 88 | 98 | – | 96 | 97 | 86 | 93 | 93 | – | 50 | 77 | – | 94 |
| Xerophthalmia | 72 | 93 | – | 96 | 89 | 86 | 87 | 94 | – | 31 | 60 | – | 89 |
| Parotid enlargement | 46 | 18 | 26 | 27 | 9 | 23 | – | 31 | 14 | – | 20 | – | 8 |
| Arthralgias | 75 | 37 | 39 | 48 | – | 50 | – | 61 | – | 25 | – | 67 | 83 |
| Arthritis | 22 | – | – | 15 | 1 | – | 8 | 11 | 20 | – | 18 | 14 | – |
| Raynaud phenomenon | 50 | 16 | 35 | 18 | – | 42 | 14 | 21 | 31 | 10 | – | 20 | – |
| Lung involvement | 33 | 9 | 3 | 11 | 6 | 12 | – | 5 | 7 | 21 | 30 | 1 | 12 |

| | | | | | | | | | | | | | |
|---|---|---|---|---|---|---|---|---|---|---|---|---|---|
| CNS involvement | 11 | 1 | – | 2 | 3 | – | – | – | – | 9 | – | – | – |
| PNS involvement | 21 | 7 | – | 11 | 15 | 16 | – | 5 | 5 | 16 | – | 5 | 10 |
| Skin involvement | 20 | 12 | 5 | 9 | 5 | 16 | 1 | 9 | 9 | – | 9 | 4 | 11 |
| Renal involvement | – | 6 | – | 5 | 6 | 8 | 1 | 2 | 7 | 19 | 7 | 0.5 | 14 |
| Myositis | 0 | 1 | – | – | – | 17 | – | 1 | 2 | – | – | – | 7 |
| Lymphoma | – | 2 | – | – | 0 | 4 | 1 | 4 | 10 | – | – | 0 | – |
| ANA | 67 | 74 | 94 | 85 | 77 | 78 | 64 | 84 | 76 | 98 | 90 | 52 | 66 |
| Anti-Ro/SSA | – | 40 | 50 | 52 | 74 | 48 | 76 | 68 | 56 | 93 | 77 | 52 | 64 |
| Anti-La/SSB | – | 26 | 40 | 34 | 52 | 31 | 49 | 37 | 35 | 49 | 48 | 30 | 38 |
| Rheumatoid factor | 46 | 38 | 32 | 48 | 68 | 41 | 60 | 52 | 55 | – | 65 | – | 60 |
| Cryoglobulins | – | 9 | 28 | 10 | – | 15 | | 5 | – | – | – | – | 0 |
| Low C3 | – | 3 | – | 9 | – | 16 | 16 | – | – | – | 40 | – | – |
| Low C4 | – | 8 | – | 9 | – | 18 | 11 | – | – | – | 7 | – | – |

*ACR*, American College Rheumatology; *AECG*, American-European Consensus Group; *CNS*, central nervous system; *ECCG*, European Classification Criteria Group; *NL*, Netherlands; *PNS*, peripheral nervous system; *UK*, United Kingdom.

to patients with one or no serological marker. These findings confirm that an active serological profile suggestive of B cell chronic activation is associated with a higher risk of systemic complications.[31]

Ethnicity and genetic background may also influence disease expression. As depicted in Table 2.2, Indian and Chinese patients are younger at diagnosis by a decade as compared with European cohorts.[18,32,33] Moreover, a smaller percentage of Chinese patients presented sicca symptoms with respect to the other cohorts of different ancestry. This could imply a difference in genetic and environmental factors contributing to the variability of disease appearance.[34] The relevance of both innate and adaptive immune responses in the pathogenesis of the disease may also be reflected by the substantial variability of extraglandular manifestation prevalence in the different cohorts (see Table 2.2). For example, Raynaud phenomenon has been described in 50% of a Finland cohort and only 10% of Chinese patients.[33,35] Similarly, arthritis was detected in 48% of Hungarian patients, in 14% of Swedish patients, and only 1% of cases in the Netherlands.[27,36,37] The influence of different genetic, lifestyle, and geographical factors in association with differences in the recruitment criteria employed and in methods for assessing the single extraglandular involvement may account for this variability. Moreover, development of systemic manifestations may affect disease prognosis and patients with extraglandular involvement have a twofold to threefold higher mortality risk in comparison to the glandular group.[37] Finally, it is relevant to consider that about half of pSS patients may develop an associated autoimmune disease, mainly autoimmune thyroid disease, and that up to 40% of patients are at risk of developing more than one concomitant autoimmune disease.[38] This risk seems particularly increased in female patients and in subjects with circulating anti-Ro/SSA and/or anti-La/SSB antibodies.[38]

## 3. GLANDULAR MANIFESTATIONS

The lymphocytic infiltration of lacrimal and salivary glands results in dry eye and dry mouth, the hallmarks of pSS. Aqueous-deficient dry eye represents the main mechanism associated with reduced tear production in pSS, leading to a typical condition of keratoconjunctivitis sicca. An evaporative dry eye, in which the evaporation of tear film is abnormally high, has been reported in SS as adjunctive mechanism.[39] Recurrent sensation of gritty eyes; daily, persistent dry eyes; frequent need for tear substitutes; intolerance of contact lenses in association with redness, photophobia, and burning; and fluctuating blurry vision exacerbated by prolonged visual effort or a low-humidity environment represent the most common symptoms. Almost all pSS patients have a history of dry eyes for an average of 10 years before presentation and about 10% of all subjects with clinically significant dry eye have a subsequent diagnosis of pSS.[40,41] Moreover, about a quarter of SS patients may experience extraglandular ocular involvement, including corneal scarring, ulcer or perforation, conjunctivitis, or conjunctival chemosis, uveitis, scleritis, optic neuropathy, or orbital inflammation.[40] Patients with vision-threatening extraglandular ocular findings are four times more likely to have systemic disease manifestations, in particular peripheral neuropathy, vasculitis, and interstitial nephritis.[40] Of interest, men with pSS have a sevenfold higher risk of developing vision-threatening extraglandular ocular complications, in particular corneal melt or perforation, with respect to women.[42]

Evaluation of tear stability, by tear film breakup time, tear secretion and composition, and ocular surface represent valuable tools that can be employed in the assessment of dry eye. In particular, determination of tear secretion rate by Schirmer test differentiates aqueous-deficient dry eye from evaporative dry eye.[39] Recently, experimental in vitro and in vivo studies identified specific molecules that have been proposed as useful biomarkers of ocular surface damage. In this setting, downregulation of *PAX6,* a key regulator of corneal lineage integrity, and activation of nucleotide oligomerization domain (NOD)-like receptor family pyrin domain containing 3 (NLRP3) inflammasome, a protein involved in modulation of inflammation and immune response in conjunctival cytology specimens of pSS patients correlated with the extent of corneal damage and level of local inflammation.[43,44]

The decrease in salivary flow in pSS patients causes xerostomia and indirect signs of mucosal dryness, including dry and cracked lips, oral mucosal sores, and tongue depapillation. Dry mouth makes talking difficult, impedes tasting and chewing properly, and causes dysphagia and dysgeusia, thus impairing quality of life of these patients. The impairment of saliva protein content, in particular of secretory immunoglobulin (Ig) A, reduces the antibacterial defense system against caries with consequent recurrent oral bacterial and fungal infections (in particular *Candida albicans*), periodontal inflammation, traumatic oral lesions with angular cheilitis, high incidence of caries, and earlier tooth loss.[45–47] Moreover, patients may complain of a sensation of oral burning or glossodynia, generally resulting from secondary fungal infection or SS-associated peripheral neuropathy.[47] Swelling of salivary glands can also occur alongside with dry mouth. About 25% to 66% of pSS patients have enlarged parotid or submandibular glands and persistent salivary gland swelling has been associated with a higher risk of developing lymphoproliferative disorder.[47]

As previously mentioned, pSS alters the protein profile and composition of saliva. Surface-enhanced laser mass spectrometry and two-dimensional gel electrophoresis have been employed in screening and profiling the proteins characterizing the saliva of these patients. An increase in the amounts of lactoferrin, $\beta_2$-microglobulin (B2M), lysozyme C, and cystatin, related to the inflammatory activity in the salivary gland, and a decrease in salivary amylase and carbonic anhydrase have been demonstrated in patients with pSS.[45] Indeed, recent progress in proteomics and genomics has shown that the proteomic and genomic profile may be more sensitive and specific in diagnosing SS. In particular, three protein biomarkers (cathepsin D, a-enolase and B2M) and three mRNA biomarkers (myeloid cell nuclear differentiation antigen, guanylate-binding protein 2, and the low-affinity IIIb receptor for the Fc fragment of IgG) were all significantly increased in patients with pSS compared with both patients with systemic lupus erythematosus and healthy controls. The combination of cathepsin D, a-enolase, and B2M yielded a very high value in distinguishing pSS from healthy subjects, thus confirming the important role of salivary flow proteomic as early diagnostic and prognostic tool in pSS patients.[48]

All exocrine glands, other than salivary and lacrimal ones, may be affected. About 70% of pSS women report reduced vaginal secretion with consequent dyspareunia and sexual dysfunction with a subsequent significant impairment on quality of life.[49,50] Moreover, dry skin (xeroderma) and dry hair are commonly reported symptoms.[51] Voice disorders and hoarseness related to dryness or thick mucus coating the vocal cords are relatively common in pSS and are more common as disease severity worsens.[52] Finally, about 50% of pSS patients complain of a constant dry cough related to reduced or absent mucociliary clearance (xerotrachea).[53] Patients with xerotrachea usually have difficulties in clearing thickened secretions and are thus predisposed to atelectasis, bronchiectasis, recurrent bronchitis, and bronchopneumonia.

## 4. SYSTEMIC INVOLVEMENT

The complex T and B cell network characterizing disease pathogenesis and the importance of the dysregulation of innate and adaptive immune system involved in disease initiation and perpetuation mirror the wide spectrum of systemic disease manifestations. Indeed, in association with nonspecific symptoms and glandular manifestation, the disease clinical picture encompasses a wide spectrum of extraglandular features (Fig. 2.1). Systemic manifestations are traditionally categorized in two main subsets, including a periepithelial one, which reflects the lymphocytic infiltration around epithelial tissues in parenchymal organs, and a set of manifestations related to the deposition of immune complexes in small vessels of different tissues as result of B cell hyperactivity.[54]

## 5. NONSPECIFIC MANIFESTATIONS

About 70% of patients complain of nonspecific signs and symptoms, including fatigue, myalgias, low-grade fever, Raynaud phenomenon, and a widespread musculoskeletal pain that often reflects a concomitant fibromyalgic syndrome. Fibromyalgia has been reported in about 20% of pSS patients. No differences have been depicted in SS-related activity and damage and in the number of tender points between patients with pSS and concomitant fibromyalgia and patients with primary fibromyalgia. This finding suggests that fibromyalgia can contribute to fatigue and pain in pSS but does not completely account for it.[55,56]

Arthritis and arthralgias represent some of the most common extraglandular manifestations in pSS patients (see Table 2.2). Articular manifestations are reported as the presenting manifestation in 50% of patients and in about 17%

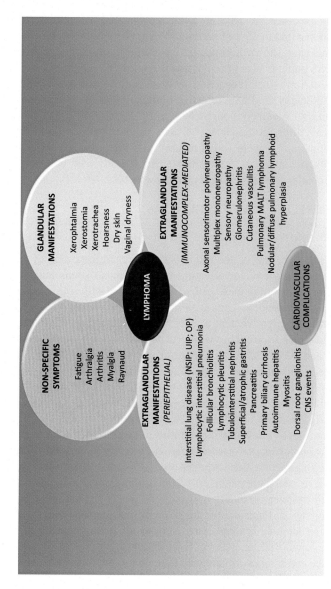

**FIGURE 2.1**  The wide spectrum of constitutional symptoms and glandular and extraglandular manifestations in primary Sjögren's syndrome. *MALT*, Mucosa-associated lymphoid tissue; *NSIP*, nonspecific interstitial pneumonia; *OP*, organizing pneumonia; *UIP*, usual interstitial pneumonia.

**NON-SPECIFIC SYMPTOMS**

Fatigue
Arthralgia
Arthritis
Myalgia
Raynaud

**GLANDULAR MANIFESTATIONS**

Xerophtalmia
Xerostomia
Xerotrachea
Hoarsness
Dry skin
Vaginal dryness

**LYMPHOMA**

**EXTRAGLANDULAR MANIFESTATIONS**
*(PERIEPITHELIAL)*

Interstitial lung disease (NSIP; UIP; OP)
Lymphocytic interstitial pneumonia
Follicular bronchiolitis
Lymphocytic pleuritis
Tubulointerstitial nephritis
Superficial/atrophic gastritis
Pancreatitis
Primary biliary cirrhosis
Autoimmune hepatitis
Myositis
Dorsal root ganglionitis
CNS events

**EXTRAGLANDULAR MANIFESTATIONS**
*(IMMUNOCOMPLEX-MEDIATED)*

Axonal sensorimotor polyneuropathy
Multiplex mononeuropathy
Sensory neuropathy
Glomerulonephritis
Cutaneous vasculitis
Pulmonary MALT lymphoma
Nodular/diffuse pulmonary lymphoid hyperplasia

**CARDIOVASCULAR COMPLICATIONS**

of cases, joint symptoms occur before sicca symptoms.[57] Arthralgias involving equally small and large joints are the most common reported symptoms, in association with episodes of intermittent, symmetrical, nonerosive polyarthritis, mainly affecting the small joints, or recurrent monoarthritis or oligoarthritis in 4% to 20% of cases.[57,58] Mild or moderate synovial hypertrophy has been detected by ultrasound in 15% of patients.[59] Synovial biopsies have rarely been performed and have shown nonspecific infiltration with mononuclear cells.[58] Of interest, pSS patients with articular manifestations have a higher risk of systemic manifestations, including renal involvement, cutaneous vasculitis, and peripheral neuropathy, and a more active immunological profile.[57] An inflammatory articular involvement consistent with rheumatoid arthritis can develop months or years after SS diagnosis. Of note, patients with concomitant rheumatoid arthritis and SS were found to have less salivary gland enlargement, vasculitis, leukopenia, and positive antinuclear antibody titer, but more severe radiographic changes compared with patients with pSS.[58,60]

## 6. PERIEPITHELIAL MANIFESTATIONS

### 6.1 Lung

Lung involvement is one of the major systemic manifestations of pSS and represents an important factor affecting patient clinical status and outcome. Indeed, lung involvement in these patients is associated with a reduced physical functioning with consequent significant impairment of patient quality of life.[61] Although pulmonary involvement usually has a stable and mild course in pSS, it is associated with a fourfold higher mortality risk after 10 years of disease and a reduced 5- and 10-year survival rate, resulting in one of the highest risk factors for mortality, in particular in the Chinese population.[61–63] The prevalence of pulmonary involvement in pSS is highly variable, ranging from 9% to 75%, according to the different methods employed for its detection, patient selection, ethnicity, environmental, or genetic factors; definition of lung involvement; and underdiagnosis as a result of nonsignificant symptoms.[64] Older age at disease diagnosis and/or longer disease duration represent factors associated with higher risk of lung involvement, whereas the association with a specific immunologic profile is more uncertain.[17,61,65] Initial and typical symptoms include dry cough and dyspnea on exertion, occasionally accompanied by chest pain. Abnormal findings at auscultation are often absent, but inspiratory bibasilar crackles may be depicted in some cases. Nonspecific radiographic changes may commonly be found in these patients. Such findings, however, have poor clinical significance and rarely correlate with pulmonary function testing (PFT) pattern, reduction in degree of diffusing capacity of the lungs for carbon monoxide (DLCO), or patient-reported symptoms.[64] Generally up to 85% of patients with lung involvement have abnormal findings at high-resolution computed tomography (HRCT), including reticular pattern, cysts, air trapping, ground-glass attenuation, bronchiectasis, small nodules, emphysema, enlarged mediastinal lymph nodes, and honeycombing. The relative frequency of these findings is highly variable from study to study and often airway disease and interstitial changes may coexist in the same subject.[64,66]

Nonspecific interstitial pneumonia (NSIP) represents the most common form of interstitial lung involvement in pSS, both at imaging and histological analysis, followed by organizing pneumonia and usual interstitial pneumonia (UIP). A lymphocytic infiltration with diffuse thickening of alveolar septa represents typical histological features in NSIP. Occasionally, foci of intraluminal polypoid organization, lymphoid follicles, and, in patients with more advanced disease or with UIP pattern, patchy areas of collagenous fibrosis with or without honeycombing may be observed.[64,66]

In 1966, Carrington and Liebow described the first case of lymphocytic interstitial pneumonia (LIP), a form of parenchyma involvement characterized by diffuse interstitial infiltration of lymphocytes and plasma cells to the alveolar septa and small airways.[67] Patients experience respiratory symptoms including cough and slowly progressive dyspnea, sometimes associated with pleuritic chest pain. PFTs typically reveal a restrictive pattern with reduced DLCO. Bilateral reticular or reticulonodular opacities, more prominent in the lower lung zones and diffuse ground-glass opacity and consolidation with occasional thin-walled cysts represent the more common findings at chest radiography and CT, respectively. The disease has a progressive course in one-third of patients despite corticosteroid and immunosuppressive therapy. Of interest, LIP must be distinguished from follicular bronchiolitis (FB), a rare type of cellular bronchiolitis characterized by hyperplastic lymphoid follicles with reactive germinal centers distributed along the bronchovascular bundles without significant extension into parenchyma. HRCT findings of FB include areas of nodular centrilobular or ground-glass attenuation, thickening of interlobular septa and bronchovascular bundles, and, occasionally, air cysts.[66] With respect to LIP, the course of FB is generally fairly benign, with 75% to 100% of treated patients presenting improvement of symptoms and/or PFTs or chest radiograph after therapy introduction.

Finally, multiple thin-walled air cysts mainly affecting the lower lobes and bronchiectasis have been reported in 10% and 23% to 50% of pSS patients, respectively.[64,66] Cystic lung disease may be detected in association with other pulmonary complications of pSS, including amyloidosis, malignant lymphoma, and LIP. At PFT, the number of small cysts on HRCT appears to correlate with the severity of obstructive findings and the severity of interstitial inflammation appears to correlate with restrictive findings. Cysts, such as fibrosis, are an irreversible manifestation of pulmonary SS, and early diagnosis and treatment, especially in cases associated with LIP, may successfully halt the process. Similarly, cylindrical bronchiectasis may have clinical relevance, because it is associated with a higher incidence of respiratory tract infections and pneumonia.

Lymphocytic pleuritis with or without effusion and/or pleural thickening has rarely been described in pSS. Pleural fluid of these patients is usually characterized by a predominant lymphocytic component and high levels of immune complexes, RF, anti-Ro/SSA, and anti-La/SSB antibodies.[64]

## 6.2 Kidney

An epithelial disease characterized by mononuclear lymphocytic tubulointerstitial infiltration of renal parenchyma, resulting in tubulointerstitial nephritis (TIN), represents the most common form of kidney involvement in pSS, as first described in the 1960s.[68] Interstitial kidney disease may produce complete or, more often, incomplete distal tubular acidosis characterized by persistent alkaline urinary pH and hyposthenuria, hyperchloremic hypokalemic metabolic acidosis with anion gap, and nephrolithiasis/nephrocalcinosis along with recurrent renal colics. Rarely, interstitial kidney disease may affect the proximal renal tubules, which is clinically expressed as Fanconi syndrome (type II renal tubular acidosis).[69,70] It is noteworthy that patients with TIN have a higher risk of developing long-term chronic renal failure.[71] In addition, patients with pSS and renal involvement, in particular with glomerulonephritis (GN), have significantly reduced survival for increased incidence of lymphoma.[71]

## 6.3 Gastrointestinal Tract

Prevalence of gastrointestinal involvement in pSS is highly variable according to the method used for its detection and symptoms largely differ according to the tract involved. Dysphagia, the main symptoms reported by 30% to 80% of patients, does not correlate with esophageal dysmotility, suggesting reduced salivary flow, more than an organic mechanism, as the leading cause of this disorder.[72] A chronic superficial gastritis, characterized by an inflammatory CD4+ cell infiltration affecting the superficial layer or the deeper part of gastric mucosa, and/or a chronic atrophic gastritis, characterized by a variable degree of gland atrophy, have been detected in up to 80% of pSS patients. Consistent with these findings, hypopepsinogenemia has been demonstrated in 69% of patients and elevated serum gastrin in half of these.[73] However, a clear correlation between histological findings and symptoms (dyspepsia) has not been demonstrated.[74] Although up to 23% of pSS patients complain of intestinal symptoms, including abdominal discomfort, constipation, nausea and diarrhea, there is no evidence of intestinal involvement.[74] It is important to consider, however, that prevalence of celiac disease diagnosed by small bowel biopsy is higher in pSS patients with respect to other connective tissue diseases, thus suggesting the importance of screening for celiac disease in pSS patients with suggestive abdominal symptoms.[75]

Pancreatic exocrine insufficiency demonstrated by an impaired response to secretin and resulting from an autoimmune pancreatitis has been documented.[74] Although clinically silent, abnormal exocrine pancreas function occurred from 18% to 37% of patients and morphologic changes of the pancreas or pancreatitis-like changes by magnetic resonance (MR) cholangiopancreatography may be detected in these patients.[76] Finally, primary biliary cirrhosis (PBC), a chronic cholestatic liver disease characterized by an inflammatory infiltrate leading to destruction of bile duct epithelial cells, is the most common cause of liver disease in pSS, followed by autoimmune hepatitis and nonalcoholic fatty liver disease.[77] Fatigue and pruritus are classically described as the most common symptoms in PBC at onset and both can also characterize up to 50% of pSS. The coexistence of PBC and pSS appears to have a prognostic value, being PBC cases with SS characterized by more advanced disease. On the other hand, 2% of pSS patients with PBC manifest some degree of subclinical liver disease and 5% have asymptomatic increased liver enzymes with positive serum antimitochondrial antibodies in 2% to 7% of patients.[74,77]

## 6.4 Muscle

Although subclinical histopathological evidence of muscle perimysial or endomysial inflammatory cell infiltrate has been reported in a wide range (5% to 73%) of patients with pSS, only a minority displays clinical evidence of inflammatory muscle disease.[78] Invalidating muscular weakness, usually involving the upper and lower limbs, and severe myalgias with increased serum level of creatine–phosphokinase and/or abnormal electromyography represent the most common findings in pSS patients with concomitant inflammatory myopathy.[79] Dysphagia, dropped head, or symptoms related to a possible muscular involvement of respiratory system are very rare. Muscular and sicca symptoms usually occur together at onset. Serological findings generally depict positivity for anti-Ro/SSA even though the demonstration of positivity for anti-Jo1 in some patients may suggest that inflammatory myopathy can occur in pSS as an overlapping syndrome.[79]

## 6.5 Nervous System

Although an immunocomplex-mediated pathogenic mechanism has been mainly associated with neurologic involvement in pSS, a dorsal root ganglionitis with degeneration of dorsal root ganglion neurons and mononuclear T cell infiltration without vasculitis have been associated with the sensory ataxic form of SS-associated neuropathy.[80] In this form, neurological manifestations typically precede disease diagnosis and are characterized by acute or subacute gait instability caused by impaired proprioception progressing to severe loss of muscle strength as a result of muscle atrophy.[81] Moreover, an inflammatory T cell infiltration may also be observed within vessel walls. This can lead to endothelial cell destruction, vessel lumen occlusion, and ischemia. Such findings may correlate with some subsets of peripheral neurological involvement, including mononeuropathy and multiple mononeuropathy, as well as with specific patterns of CNS involvement, including stroke-like episodes, optic neuritis, seizures, encephalitis, and spinal cord involvement characterized by acute transverse myelitis or progressive myelopathy.[82] In fact, the CNS is less affected than the peripheral nervous system (PNS) and the variable prevalence reported is likely as a result of selection bias. CNS involvement is most commonly focal (brain, spinal cord, and optic nerve), but symptoms occurring in pSS may mimic relapsing–remitting multiple sclerosis. On MR imaging, white matter changes compatible with multiple sclerosis may be detected in about 40% of patients.[82]

## 7. IMMUNE COMPLEX–MEDIATED MANIFESTATIONS

### 7.1 Nervous System

Axonal sensorimotor polyneuropathy and mononeuropathy multiplex are the most common types of PNS involvement in pSS. However, a variety of forms of neuropathy have been described in these patients, including sensory ataxic neuropathy, trigeminal neuropathy, radiculoneuropathy, painful sensory neuropathy without sensory ataxia, autonomic neuropathy with anhidrosis, and multiple cranial neuropathy.[80] Vasa nervorum injury from immune complexes and from antiendothelial cell antibodies are considered the principal immunological mechanisms associated with PNS involvement.[83] Symptoms are highly variable and differ according to the type of PNS involvement. Patients complain of burning pain in the extremities, numbness, dysesthesia, distal chronic or subacute onset of symmetric sensory deficit in a "glove–stocking" distribution and paresthesias in the feet. The lower limbs are initially affected and deficits may spread proximally over years as the neuropathy worsens. In more severe cases, distal upper limbs may also be affected and muscle weakness may be associated. Deep tendon reflexes may be diminished or absent in the affected limbs. Constitutional symptoms may be present, as well as systemic manifestations of palpable purpura, indicative of generalized vasculitis.[81] Indeed, extraglandular disease is more common and more severe in these patients and polyneuropathy is often associated with palpable purpura, vasculitis, low C4, and cryoglobulinemia. Rarely, autonomic nervous symptoms such as vertigo, facial flushes, palpitation, hypohidrosis or hyperhidrosis, and diarrhea or constipation may be referred. Electrodiagnostic tests are helpful in identifying the predominant pathophysiology of PNS involvement (demyelinating or axonal) and the anatomical distribution. Male sex and higher incidence of vasculitis have been identified as risk factors significantly associated with PNS involvement.[84] Axonal sensorimotor polyneuropathy is usually characterized by a good evolution. Sensory neuropathy represents the most disabling form with a poor response to treatment and, notably, precedes pSS diagnosis in a large proportion of patients. Mononeuropathy multiplex is strictly linked with a high systemic activity profile characterized by cryoglobulinemic vasculitis, cytopenia, and salivary gland swelling.[84] Of note, peripheral neuropathy is associated with a poor prognosis. Indeed, patients with mononeuropathy multiplex and axonal polyneuropathy are characterized by a reduced survival in comparison with patients without such involvement.[84]

## 7.2 Cutaneous Vasculitis

Cutaneous vasculitis associated with cryoglobulinemia, hypergammaglobulin-emic vasculitis (HGV), urticarial vasculitis, and purpura without cryoglobulins are the most common findings in pSS with cutaneous involvement.[85] Generally, patients with cutaneous vasculitis, generally classified as leukocytoclastic vasculitis or lymphocytic vasculitis, have more severe disease and more diffuse extraglandular involvement than those without this manifestation.[86] About half of such patients have a single episode, mainly involving the lower extremities, whereas the other half of these patients are characterized by recurrent episodes requiring corticosteroids and immunosuppressive therapy.[85] In particular, HGV represents a typical vasculitis in pSS related to benign B cell proliferation and characterized by lower extremity recurrent purpura, polyclonal hypergamma-globulinemia, and Ig deposition along the blood vessel walls. In pSS, HGV must be differentiated from cryoglobulinemia, a cutaneous vasculitis charac-terized by higher rates of systemic manifestations, including PNS and renal involvement, complement activation, leukopenia, serum monoclonal compo-nent, and, of more relevance, by a higher risk of lymphoma.[87]

Recently, cases of antineutrophil cytoplasmic antibody (ANCA)–associated vas-culitis (AAV) with systemic involvement in patients with pSS have been reported.[88] These are most commonly *p*-ANCA–associated vasculitis with antimyeloperoxi-dase specificity. All pSS patients with AAV experience at least one systemic mani-festation characteristic of pSS, suggesting that AAV onset could be correlated with pSS extraglandular manifestations. Moreover, these data suggest that AAV occurs in pSS patients with an important B cell activation, which could explain both most common systemic manifestations and the development of ANCA.[88]

## 7.3 Lung

The microscopic demonstration of plexiform lesions with depositions of IgG and complement in samples of pulmonary artery of pSS patients with associ-ated pulmonary arterial hypertension (PAH) suggests the involvement of B cell activation and immune complex–mediated mechanism. In the setting of pSS, moreover, PAH may be the result of pulmonary veno-occlusive disease, valvular heart disease, or interstitial lung disease. Primary PAH in pSS is rare and most patients exhibit advanced functional class and evidence of right heart failure resulting from a delay of diagnosis. Typically, pSS precedes the diagnosis of PAH and patients are more likely to have Raynaud phenomenon, cutaneous vasculitis, interstitial lung disease, and a more active serologic profile. More-over, hypocomplementemia and cryoglobulinemia have been demonstrated to be strong predictors of PAH.[64]

Pulmonary mucosa-associated lymphoid tissue (MALT) lymphoma is a tumor derived from bronchus-associated lymphoid tissue characterized by a predominance of small B cells. Clinically, primary pulmonary lymphoma presents cough, dyspnea, weight loss, and fatigue. Radiographically, it appears as solitary or multifocal nodules, bilateral alveolar infiltrates, or interstitial findings randomly distributed.[66] At CT, MALT lymphoma may appear as a solitary nodule or multiple nodules or masses, with areas of air-space consolidation or ground-glass attenuation. Of note, CT appearance of MALT pulmonary lymphoma is similar to some benign lymphoproliferative disorders, including nodular lymphoid hyperplasia and diffuse lymphoid hyperplasia, characterized by infiltration of mature polyclonal lymphocytes and plasma cells and presenting as solitary nodule or mass or parenchymal consolidation with air bronchograms or even as multiple nodules. Patients are usually asymptomatic or may refer dry cough and dyspnea. Rarely, benign lymphoproliferative disorders can progress to frank lymphoma.[89]

## 7.4 Kidney

The most common immune-mediated glomerular disease in pSS is the mesangioproliferative GN (MPGN) followed by mesangial GN. The MPGN is caused by the glomerular deposition of immune complexes with C3 and IgM, often in association with cryoglobulins, causing kidney small-vessel vasculitis. The clinical picture may be variable according to histological lesions, ranging from asymptomatic urinary abnormalities such as microscopic hematuria, proteinuria, and urinary casts, to hypertension, reduced excretory function, and, finally, nephrotic syndrome.[90] GN usually develops later than TIN during the course of the disease and is more commonly associated with low complement levels.[71] As stated, GN displays a less favorable prognosis in comparison with TIN and is associated with lymphoma development as a part of extraepithelial manifestations mediated by cryoprecipitable immune complexes possibly caused by cryoglobulinemia, which is considered to be an independent risk factor for mortality and morbidity in pSS.

## 8. CARDIOVASCULAR MANIFESTATIONS

In recent years, research has focused on the effects and mechanisms underlying cardiovascular (CV) involvement in pSS. Indeed, growing evidence suggests that CV involvement in pSS occurs much more often than initially thought. Similarly to other systemic autoimmune connective diseases, pSS may be considered an independent predictor of subclinical atherosclerosis, mainly through endothelial injury and dysfunction. Indeed, case-control studies have demonstrated signs of endothelial dysfunction, expressed as altered flow- or nitrate-mediated vasodilation or increased pulse-wave velocity or coronary flow impairment, and precocious arterial wall damage in pSS patients without previous CV disorders.[91–95] Disease duration, disease-related damage, and several clinical and immunological features, including joint involvement, parotid swelling, Raynaud phenomenon, leukopenia, anti-Ro/SSA and anti-La/SSB antibodies, seem to be associated with subclinical atherosclerotic damage in these patients. Moreover, chronic endothelial fragmentation characterized by an increased release of endothelial microparticles in association with a defective vascular endothelium restoration related to progressive exhaustion of endothelial progenitor cells has been demonstrated as adjunctive mechanisms leading to endothelial dysfunction in these patients.[96] On the other hand, although pSS women are characterized by a significantly higher prevalence of hypertension and hypercholesterolemia with respect to control subjects, the independent role of traditional CV risk factors with respect to disease-specific immunological features in the induction and perpetuation of precocious atherosclerosis should be further investigated.[97–99] It is of note that an increased prevalence of major CV events, including myocardial infarction and cerebrovascular events, has been demonstrated in pSS women in comparison to the general population.[99] Older age and longer disease duration contribute to this increased risk. Moreover, CV events appear to be more common in patients with more severe disease, including those with lung and central nervous system involvement, and patients in greater need of glucocorticoids and immunosuppressive therapy. The evidence that the disease may have a role in promoting CV events is also strengthened by the demonstration that patients with leukopenia, a marker of more severe disease, have a sixfold higher risk of developing angina compared with those with a normal number of circulating white cells.[99]

Findings derived from echocardiographic studies have shown that cardiac complications are common in pSS. Pericardial involvement may manifest in forms of either echogenic pericardium and clinically silent pericardial effusion or as overt pericarditis.[100] Other commonly reported echocardiographic abnormalities include thickening of mainly mitral, aortic and tricuspid valves, as well as aortic, mitral, and tricuspid regurgitation.[100] Finally, disorders of the heart rhythm, mainly conduction disorders and tachyarrhythmias, have been reported in the setting of pSS, in particular in patients carrying anti-Ro/SSA antibodies.[101,102]

## 9. CONCLUSIONS

Despite its relatively recent discovery, pSS has been extensively investigated and characterized. Indeed, it represents a complex disease in which multiple genetic, environmental, hormonal, autoimmune, and inflammatory factors interact, thereby contributing to the wide spectrum of disease manifestations. Initially considered the most indolent and benign disease in the entire world of connective tissue disorders, it is now evident that the disease may exert a significant impact on long-term patient outcome and that patients experience more clinical complications over time than previously described. Indeed, some specific disease systemic manifestations and high disease activity not only have been associated with significant reduced survival in these patients but also exert a relevant impact on patient quality of life. Moreover, the recent demonstration of increased risk of CV events in young women with pSS as compared with the general population and the evidence that pSS patients are at higher risk of developing malignancy during the course of the disease is of value. As a consequence, important areas for future research should include the identification of disease phenotypes associated with worst prognosis and the creation of universal recommendations for the proper management and follow-up care of these classes of patients.

## REFERENCES

1. Talal N. Sjögren's syndrome, lymphoproliferation, and renal tubular acidosis. *Ann Intern Med* 1971;**74**:633–4.
2. Pavlidis NA, Karsh J, Moutsopoulos HM. The clinical picture of primary Sjögren's syndrome: a retrospective study. *J Rheumatol* 1982;**9**:685e90.
3. Tsokos M, Lazarou SA, Moutsopoulos HM. Vasculitis in primary Sjögren's syndrome: histologic classification and clinical presentation. *Am J Clin Pathol* 1987;**88**:26e31.
4. Tsampoulas CG, Skopouli FN, Sartoris DJ, Kaplan P, Kursunoglu S, Pineda C. Hand radiographic changes in patients with primary and secondary Sjögren's syndrome. *Scand J Rheumatol* 1986;**15**:333e9.
5. Skopouli FN, Barbatis C, Moutsopoulos HM. Liver involvement in primary Sjögren's syndrome. *Br J Rheumatol* 1994;**33**:745e8.
6. Leroy JP, Drosos AA, Yiannopoulos DI, Youinou P, Moutsopoulos HM. Intravenous pulse cyclophosphamide therapy in myositis and Sjögren's syndrome. *Arthritis Rheum* 1990;**33**:1579–81.
7. Alamanos Y, Tsifetaki N, Voulgari PV, Venetsanopoulou AI, Siozos C, Drosos AA. Epidemiology of primary Sjögren's syndrome in north-west Greece, 1982–2003. *Rheumatology* 2006;**45**:187–91.
8. Thomas E, Hay EM, Hajeer A, Silman AJ. Sjögren's syndrome: a community-based study of prevalence and impact. *Br J Rheumatol* 1998;**37**:1069–76.
9. Tomsic M, Logar D, Grmek M, Perkovic T, Kveder T. Prevalence of Sjögren's syndrome in Slovenia. *Rheumatology* 1999;**38**:164–70.
10. Dafni UG, Tzioufas AG, Staikos P, Skopouli FN, Moutsopoulos HM. Prevalence of Sjögren's syndrome in a closed rural community. *Ann Rheum Dis* 1997;**56**:521–5.
11. Zhang NZ, Shi CS, Yao QP. Prevalence of primary Sjögren's syndrome in China. *J Rheumatol* 1995;**22**:659–61.
12. Pillemer SR, Matteson EL, Jacobsson LT. Incidence of physician-diagnosed primary Sjögren syndrome in residents of Olmsted County, Minnesota. *Mayo Clin Proc* 2001;**76**:593–9.
13. Patel R, Shahane A. The epidemiology of Sjögren's syndrome. *Clin Epidemiol* 2014;**6**:247–55.
14. Ramos-Casals M, Cervera R, Font J, García-Carrasco M, Espinosa G, Reino S, et al. Young onset of primary Sjögren's syndrome: clinical and immunological characteristics. *Lupus* 1998;**7**:202–6.
15. Haga HJ, Jonsson R. The influence of age on disease manifestations and serological characteristics in primary Sjögren's syndrome. *Scand J Rheumatol* 1999;**28**:227–32.

16. Garcìa-Carrasco M, Ramos-Casals M, Rosas J, Pallarès L, Calvo-Alen J, Cervera R, et al. Primary Sjögren syndrome: clinical and immunologic disease patterns in a cohort of 400 patients. *Medicine* 2002;**81**:270–80.

17. Ramos-Casals M, Solans R, Rosas J, Camps MT, Gil A, del Pino-Montes J, et al. Primary Sjögren syndrome in Spain: clinical and immunologic expression in 1010 patients. *Medicine* 2008;**87**:210–9.

18. Zhao Y, Li Y, Wang L, Li XF, Huang CB, Wang CG, et al. Primary Sjögren syndrome in Han Chinese: clinical and immunological characteristics of 483 patients. *Medicine* 2015;**94**:e667.

19. Tishler M, Yaron I, Shirazi I, Yaron M. Clinical and immunological characteristics of elderly onset Sjögren's syndrome: a comparison with younger onset disease. *J Rheumatol* 2001;**28**:795–7.

20. Malladi A, Sack KE, Shiboski S, Shiboski C, Baer AN, Banushree R, et al. Primary Sjögren's syndrome as a systemic disease: a study of participants enrolled in an international Sjögren's syndrome registry. *Arthritis Care Res* 2012;**64**:911–8.

21. Botsios C, Furlan A, Ostuni P, Sfriso P, Andretta M, Ometto F, et al. Elderly onset of primary Sjögren's syndrome: clinical manifestations, serological features and oral/ocular diagnostic tests. Comparison with adult and young onset of the disease in a cohort of 336 Italian patients. *Jt Bone Spine* 2011;**78**:171–4.

22. Gubbels Bupp MR. Sex, the aging immune system, and chronic disease. *Cell Immunol* 2015;**294**:102–10.

23. Molina R, Provost TT, Arnett FC, Bias WB, Hochberg MC, Wilson RW, et al. Primary Sjögren's syndrome in men. *Am J Med* 1986;**80**:23–31.

24. Drosos AA, Tsiakou EK, Tsifetaki N, Politi EN, Siamopoulo-Mavridou A. Subgroups of primary Sjögren's syndrome: Sjögren's syndrome in male and paediatric Greek patients. *Ann Rheum Dis* 1997;**56**:333–5.

25. Nishikai M, Akiya K, Tojo T, Onoda N, Tani M, Shimizu K. Seronegative Sjögren's syndrome manifested as a subset of chronic fatigue syndrome. *Br J Rheumatol* 1996;**35**:471–4.

26. Martel C, Gondran G, Launay D, Lalloué F, Palat S, Lambert M, et al. Active immunological profile is associated with systemic Sjögren's Syndrome. *J Clin Immunol* 2011;**31**:840–7.

27. Borg E, Risselada AP, Kelder JP. Relation of systemic autoantibodies to the number of extraglandular manifestations in primary Sjögren's syndrome: a retrospective analysis of 65 patients in the Netherlands. *Semin Arthritis Rheum* 2011;**40**:547–51.

28. Alexander EL, Arnett FC, Provost TT, Stevens MB. Sjögren's syndrome: association of anti-Ro(SS-A) antibodies with vasculitis, hematologic abnormalities and serologic hyperreactivity. *Ann Intern Med* 1983;**98**:155–9.

29. Moutsopoulos HM, Zerva LV. Anti-Ro (SS-A)/La (SS-B) antibodies and Sjögren's syndrome. *Clin Rheumatol* 1990;**9**(Suppl. 1):123–30.

30. Baer A, McAdams DeMarco M, Shiboski S, Lam MY, Challacombe S, Daniels TE, et al. The SSB-positive/SSA-negative antibody profile is not associated with key phenotypic features of Sjögren's syndrome. *Ann Rheum Dis* 2015;**74**:1557–61.

31. Baldini C, Pepe P, Quartuccio L, Priori R, Bartoloni E, Alunno A, et al. Primary Sjögren's syndrome as a multi-organ disease: impact of the serological profile on the clinical presentation of the disease in a large cohort of Italian patients. *Rheumatology* 2014;**53**:839–44.

32. Sandhya P, Jeyaseelan L, Scofield RH, Danda D. Clinical characteristics and outcome of primary Sjögren's syndrome: a large Asian Indian cohort. *Open Rheumatol J* 2015;**9**:36–45.

33. Li X, Xu B, Ma Y, Li X, Cheng Q, Wang X, et al. Clinical and laboratory profiles of primary Sjögren's syndrome in a Chinese population: a retrospective analysis of 315 patients. *Intern J Rheum Dis* 2015;**18**:439–46.

34. Miceli-Richard C, Criswell LA. Genetic, genomic and epigenetic studies as tools for elucidating disease pathogenesis in primary Sjögren's syndrome. *Expert Rev Clin Immunol* 2014;**10**:437–44.

35. Pertovaara M, Pukkala E, Laippala P, Miettinen A, Pasternack A. A longitudinal cohort study of Finnish patients with primary Sjögren's syndrome: clinical, immunological, and epidemiological aspects. *Ann Rheum Dis* 2001;**60**:467–72.

36. Kvarnström M, Ottosson V, Nordmark B, Wahren-Herlenius M. Incident cases of primary Sjögren's syndrome during a 5-year period in Stockholm County: a descriptive study of the patients and their characteristics. *Scand J Rheumatol* 2015;**44**:135–42.

37. Horvath I, Szanto A, Papp G, Zeher M. Clinical course, prognosis, and cause of death in primary Sjögren's syndrome. *J Immunol Res* 2014;**2014**:647507.

38. Abrol E, González-Pulido AC, Juan B, Praena-Fernández M, Isenberg D. A retrospective study of long-term outcomes in 152 patients with primary Sjögren's syndrome: 25-year experience. *Clin Med* 2014;**14**:157–64.

39. Foulks G, Forstot S, Donshik P, Forstot P, Goldstein M, Lemp M, et al. Clinical guidelines for management of dry eye associated with Sjögren disease. *Ocul Surf* 2015;**13**(118):132.

40. Akpek E, Mathews P, Hahn S, Hessen M, Kim J, Grader-Beck T, et al. Ocular and systemic morbidity in a longitudinal cohort of Sjögren's syndrome. *Ophthalmology* 2015;**122**:56–61.

41. Liew M, Zhang M, Kim E, Akpek E. Prevalence and predictors of Sjögren's syndrome in a prospective cohort of patients with aqueous-deficient dry eye. *B J Ophthalmol* 2012;**96**:1498–503.

42. Mathews PM, Hahn S, Hessen M, Kim J, Grader-Beck T, Birnbaum J, et al. Ocular complications of primary Sjögren's syndrome in men. *Am J Ophthalmol* 2015. http://dx.doi.org/10.1016/j.ajo.2015.06.004. [Epub ahead of print].

43. McNamara N, Gallup M, Porco T. Establishing *PAX6* as a biomarker to detect early loss of ocular phenotype in human patients with Sjögren's syndrome. *Invest Ophthalmol Vis Sci* 2014;**55**:7079–84.

44. Niu L, Zhang S, Wu J, Chen L, Wang Y. Upregulation of NLRP3 inflammasome in the tears and ocular surface of dry eye patients. *PLoS One* 2015;**10**:e0126277.

45. Mathews SA, Kurien BT, Scofield RH. Oral manifestations of Sjögren's syndrome. *J Dent Res* 2008;**87**:308–18.

46. Olate S, Muñoz D, Neumann S, Pozzer L, Cavalieri-Pereira L, de Moraes M. A descriptive study of the oral status in subjects with Sjögren's syndrome. *Int J Clin Exp Med* 2014;**7**:1140–4.

47. Napeñas J, Rouleau T. Oral complications of Sjögren's syndrome. *Oral Maxillofac Surg Clin N Am* 2014;**26**:55–62.

48. Jensen S, Vissink A. Salivary gland dysfunction and xerostomia in Sjögren's syndrome. *Oral Maxillofac Surg Clin N Am* 2014;**26**:35–53.

49. Maddali Bongi S, Del Rosso A, Orlandi M, Matucci-Cerinic M. Gynaecological symptoms and sexual disability in women with primary Sjögren's syndrome and sicca syndrome. *Clin Exp Rheumatol* 2013;**31**:683–90.

50. van Nimwegen J, Arends S, van Zuiden G, Vissink A, Kroese F, Bootsma H. The impact of primary Sjögren's syndrome on female sexual function. *Rheumatology* 2015;**54**:1286–93.

51. Kittridge A, Routhouska SB, Korman NJ. Dermatologic manifestations of Sjögren's syndrome. *J Cutan Med Surg* 2011;**15**:8–14.

52. Pierce J, Tanner K, Merrill R, Miller K, Ambati B, Kendall K, et al. Voice disorders in Sjögren's syndrome: prevalence and related risk factors. *Laryngoscope* 2015;**125**:1385–92.

53. Mathieu A, Cauli A, Pala R, Satta L, Nurchis P, Loi GL. Tracheo-bronchial mucociliary clearance in patients with primary and secondary Sjögren's syndrome. *Scand J Rheumatol* 1995;**24**:300–4.

54. Moutsopoulos HM. Sjögren's syndrome: a forty-year scientific journey. *J Autoimmun* 2014;**51**:1–9.

55. Ostuni P, Botsios C, Sfriso P, Punzi L, Chieco-Bianchi F, Semerano L, et al. Fibromyalgia in Italian patients with primary Sjogren's syndrome. *Jt Bone Spine* 2002;**69**:51–7.

56. Priori R, Iannuccelli C, Alessandri C, Modesti M, Antonazzo B, Di Lollo AC, et al. Fatigue in Sjogren's syndrome: relationship with fibromyalgia, clinical and biologic features. *Clin Exp Rheumatol* 2010;**28**:S82–6.

57. Fauchais A, Ouattara B, Gondran G, Lalloué F, Petit D, Ly K, et al. Articular manifestations in primary Sjögren's syndrome: clinical significance and prognosis of 188 patients. *Rheumatology* 2010;**49**:1164–72.

58. Pease CT, Shattles W, Barrett NK, Maini RN. The arthropathy of Sjögren's syndrome. *Br J Rheumatol* 1993;**32**:609–13.

59. Fujimura T, Fujimoto T, Hara R, Shimmyo N, Kobata Y, Kido A, et al. Subclinical articular involvement in primary Sjögren's syndrome assessed by ultrasonography and its negative association with anti-centromere antibody. *Mod Rheumatol* 2015;**25**(6). [Epub ahead of print].

60. Khan O, Carsons S. Occurrence of rheumatoid arthritis requiring oral and/or biologic disease-modifying antirheumatic drug therapy following a diagnosis of primary Sjögren's syndrome. *J Clin Rheumatol* 2012;**18**:356–8.

61. Palm O, Garen T, Berge Enger T, Liaaen Jensen J, Lund M, Mogens Aaløkken T, et al. Clinical pulmonary involvement in primary Sjögren's syndrome: prevalence, quality of life and mortality—a retrospective study based on registry data. *Rheumatology* 2013;**52**:173–9.

62. Lin DF, Yan SM, Zhao Y, Zhang W, Li MT, Zeng XF, et al. Clinical and prognostic characteristics of 573 cases of primary Sjögren's syndrome. *Chin Med J* 2010;**123**:3252–7.

63. Chen M, Chou HP, Lai CC, Chen YD, Chen MH, Lin HY. Lung involvement in primary Sjögren's syndrome: correlation between high-resolution computed tomography score and mortality. *J Chin Med Ass* 2014;**77**:75–82.

64. Kreider M, Highland K. Pulmonary involvement in Sjögren syndrome. *Semin Respir Crit Care Med* 2014;**35**:255–64.

65. Yazisiz V, Arslan G, Ozbudak IH, Turker S, Erbasan F, Avci AB, et al. Lung involvement in patients with primary Sjögren's syndrome: what are the predictors? *Rheumatol Int* 2010;**30**:1317–24.

66. Egashira R, Kondo T, Hirai T, Kamochi N, Yakushiji M, Yamasaki F, et al. CT Findings of thoracic manifestations of primary Sjögren syndrome: radiologic–pathologic correlation. *RadioGraphics* 2013;**33**:1933–49.

67. Liebow AA, Carrington CB. Lymphocytic interstitial pneumonia. *Am J Pathol* 1966;**48**:36a.

68. Tu WH, Shearn MA, Lee JC, Hopper J. Interstitial nephritis in Sjögren's syndrome. *Ann Intern Med* 1968;**69**:1163–70.

69. Both T, Hoorn EJ, Zietse R, van Laar A, Dalm V, Brkic Z, et al. Prevalence of distal renal tubular acidosis in primary Sjögren's syndrome. *Rheumatology* 2015;**54**:933–9.

70. Ram R, Swarnalatha G, Dakshinamurty G. Renal tubular acidosis in Sjögren's syndrome: a case series. *Am J Nephrol* 2014;**40**:123–30.

71. Goules A, Tatouli I, Moutsopoulos HM, Tzioufas A. Clinically significant renal involvement in primary Sjögren's syndrome: clinical presentation and outcome. *Arthritis Rheum* 2013;**65**:2945–63.

72. Mandl T, Ekberg O, Wollmer P, Manthorpe R, Jacobsson LT. Dysphagia and dysmotility of the pharynx and oesophagus in patients with primary Sjögren's syndrome. *Scand J Rheumatol* 2007;**36**:394–401.

73. Maury CP, Tornoth T, Teppo AM. Atrophic gastritis in Sjögren's syndrome: morphologic, biochemical, and immunologic findings. *Arthritis Rheum* 1985;**28**:388–94.

74. Ebert EC. Gastrointestinal and hepatic manifestations of Sjögren's syndrome. *J Clin Gastro-enterol* 2012;**46**:25–30.

75. Roblin X, Helluwaert F, Bonaz B. Celiac disease must be evaluated in patients with Sjögren's syndrome. *Arch Intern Med* 2004;**164**:2387.

76. Afzelius P, Fallentin EM, Larsen S, Møller S, Schiødt M. Pancreatic function and morphology in Sjögren's syndrome. *Scand J Gastroenterol* 2010;**45**:752–8.

77. Sun Y, Zhang W, Li B, Zou Z, Selmi C, Gershwin E. The coexistence of Sjögren's syndrome and primary biliary cirrhosis: a comprehensive review. *Clin Rev Allergy Immunol* 2015;**48**:301–15.

78. Lindvall B, Bengtsson A, Ernerudh J, Eriksson P. Subclinical myositis is common in primary Sjögren's syndrome and is not related to muscle pain. *J Rheumatol* 2002;**29**:717–25.

79. Colafrancesco S, Priori R, Gattamelata A, Picarelli G, Minniti A, Brancatisano F, et al. Myositis in primary Sjögren's syndrome: data from a multicenter cohort. *Clin Exp Rheumatol* 2015;**33**(4). [Epub ahead of print].

80. Mori K, Iijima M, Koike H, Hattori N, Tanaka F, Watanabe H, et al. The wide spectrum of clinical manifestations in Sjögren's syndrome–associated neuropathy. *Brain* 2005;**128**:2518–34.

81. Pavlakis P, Alexopoulos H, Kosmidis M, Mamali I, Moutsopoulos HM, Tzioufas AG, et al. Peripheral neuropathies in Sjögren's syndrome: a critical update on clinical features and pathogenetic mechanisms. *J Autoimmun* 2012;**39**:27–33.

82. Delalande S, de Seze J, Fauchais AL, Hachulla E, Stojkovic T, Ferriby D, et al. Neurologic manifestations in primary Sjögren syndrome: a study of 82 patients. *Medicine* 2004;**83**:280–91.

83. Chai J, Logigianb E. Neurological manifestations of primary Sjogren's syndrome. *Curr Opin Neurol* 2010;**23**:509–13.

84. Brito-Zerón P, Akasbi M, Bosch X, Bové A, Pérez-De-Lis M, Diaz-Lagares C, et al. Classification and characterisation of peripheral neuropathies in 102 patients with primary Sjögren's syndrome. *Clin Exp Rheumatol* 2013;**31**:103–10.

85. Scofield RH. Vasculitis in Sjögren's syndrome. *Curr Rheumatol Rep* 2011;**13**:482–8.

86. Ienopoli S, Carsons S. Extraglandular manifestations of primary Sjögren's syndrome. *Oral Maxillofac Surg Clin N Am* 2014;**26**:91–9.

87. Quartuccio L, Isola M, Baldini C, Priori R, Bartoloni E, Carubbi F, et al. Clinical and biological differences between cryoglobulinaemic and hypergammaglobulinaemic purpura in primary Sjögren's syndrome: results of a large multicentre study. *Scand J Rheumatol* 2015;**44**:36–41.

88. Guellec D, Cornec-Le Gall E, Groh M, Hachulla E, Karras A, Charles P, et al. ANCA-associated vasculitis in patients with primary Sjögren's syndrome: detailed analysis of 7 new cases and systematic literature review. *Autoimmun Rev* 2015;**14**:742–50.

89. Song MK, Seol YM, Park YE, Kim YS, Lee MK, Lee CH, et al. Pulmonary nodular lymphoid hyperplasia associated with Sjögren's syndrome. *Korean J Intern Med* 2007;**22**:192–6.

90. Evans R, Zdebik A, Ciurtin C, Walsh S. Renal involvement in primary Sjögren's syndrome. *Rheumatology* 2015;**54**(9). [Epub ahead of print].

91. Gerli R, Vaudo G, Bartoloni E, Schillaci G, Alunno A, Luccioli F, et al. Functional impairment of the arterial wall in primary Sjögren's syndrome: combined action of immunologic and inflammatory factors. *Arthritis Care Res* 2010;**62**:712–8.

92. Vaudo G, Bartoloni E, Shoenfeld Y, Schillaci G, Wu R, Del Papa N, et al. Precocious intima media thickening in patients with primary Sjögren's syndrome. *Arthritis Rheum* 2005;**52**:3890–7.

93. Pirildar T, Tikiz C, Ozkaya S, Tarhan S, Utük O, Tikiz H, et al. Endothelial dysfunction in patients with primary Sjögren's syndrome. *Rheumatol Int* 2005;**25**:536–9.

94. Atzeni F, Sarzi-Puttini P, Signorello MC, Gianturco L, Stella D, Boccassini L, et al. New parameters for identifying subclinical atherosclerosis in patients with primary Sjögren's syndrome: a pilot study. *Clin Exp Rheumatol* 2014;**32**:361–8.

95. Sabio J, Sanchez-Berna I, Martinez-Bordonado J, Vargas-Hitos J, Navarrete-Navarrete N, Exposito Ruiz M, et al. Prevalence of and factors associated with increased arterial stiffness in patients with primary Sjögren's syndrome. *Arthritis Care Res* 2015;**67**:554–62.

96. Bartoloni E, Alunno A, Bistoni O, Caterbi S, Luccioli F, Santoboni G, et al. Characterization of circulating endothelial microparticles and endothelial progenitor cells in primary Sjögren's syndrome: new markers of chronic endothelial damage? *Rheumatology* 2015;**54**:536–44.

97. Pèrez-De-Lis M, Akasbi M, Sisò A, Diez-Cascon P, Brito-Zerón P, Diaz-Lagares C, et al. Cardiovascular risk factors in primary Sjögren's syndrome: a case-control study in 624 patients. *Lupus* 2010;**19**:941–8.

98. Gerli R, Bartoloni E, Vaudo G, Marchesi S, Vitali C, Shoenfeld Y. Traditional cardiovascular risk factors in primary Sjögren's syndrome: role of dyslipidaemia. *Rheumatology* 2006;**45**:1580–1.

99. Bartoloni E, Baldini C, Schillaci G, Quartuccio L, Priori R, Carubbi F, et al. Cardiovascular disease risk burden in primary Sjögren's syndrome: results of a population-based multicentre cohort study. *J Intern Med* 2015;**278**:185–92.

100. Vassiliou VA, Moyssakis I, Boki KA, Moutsopoulos HM. Is the heart affected in primary Sjögren's syndrome? An echocardiographic study. *Clin Exp Rheumatol* 2008;**26**:109–12.

101. Lazzerini P, Capecchi P, Guideri F, Acampa M, Galeazzi M, Laghi Pasini F. Connective tissue diseases and cardiac rhythm disorders: an overview. *Autoimmun Rev* 2006;**5**:306–13.

102. Lazzerini P, Capecchi P, Guideri F, Bellisai F, Selvi E, Acampa M, et al. Comparison of frequency of complex ventricular arrhythmias in patients with positive versus negative anti-Ro/SSA and connective tissue disease. *Am J Cardiol* 2007;**100**:1029–34.

Chapter 3

# Management of Sjögren's Syndrome

C.P. Mavragani, M.N. Manoussakis

*National and Kapodistrian University of Athens, Athens, Greece*

## 1. INTRODUCTION

Sjögren's syndrome (SS) is a chronic autoimmune exocrinopathy affecting predominantly middle-aged women and displaying lymphocytic infiltration and secretory dysfunction of the exocrine glands (primarily the salivary and lacrimal glands, resulting in oral and ocular dryness). Depending on the absence or presence of other connective tissue disorders, SS can be classified into primary SS and SS associated with other systemic autoimmune disorders, respectively.[1] Though classically designated as a local disease, systemic manifestations are not uncommon, affecting more than one-third of patients. Systemic features in the context of SS can be classified into nonspecific, periepithelial (caused by the presence of lymphocytic infiltrations around tubular epithelia), and those arising from immune complex deposition (such as peripheral neuropathy, purpura, cryoglobulinemic vasculitis, and glomerulonephritis). The latter have been consistently revealed as major adverse predictors of lymphoma development, the most serious SS-related complication.[2] The symptoms of SS are chronic and sometimes so devastating that quality of life can be significantly compromised. SS management is primarily aimed at alleviating sicca complaints using both local measures and stimulators of salivary secretion, with the role of synthetic disease-modifying antirheumatic drugs (DMARDs) being rather inconclusive. Recent progress in our understanding of SS pathogenesis, together with the availability of several biological agents already licensed for other chronic inflammatory and autoimmune disorders, has stimulated new efforts toward SS treatment.

## 2. MANAGEMENT OF GLANDULAR COMPLICATIONS

### 2.1 Dry Mouth and Salivary Gland Component

Secretory compromise in patients with SS results in heightened rates of dental caries, friability of the mucosal membranes, and fungal infections, especially

Sjögren's Syndrome. http://dx.doi.org/10.1016/B978-0-12-803604-4.00003-4

candidiasis. Prevention and treatment of oral infections and the use of salivary substitutes together with stimulation of salivary flow remain the main lines of management (Table 3.1).[3]

To prevent dental caries, routine dental care and preventive dental treatment is mandatory. Administration of topical fluoride contributes to the effective mineralization of the hydroxyapatite component of the enamel, rendering it less susceptible to decay development. Stimulation of salivary flow through administration of formulations such as sugar-free lozenges, chewing gum, xylitol mannitol, and the US Food and Drug Administration (FDA)–approved oral muscarinic agonist agents pilocarpine and cevimeline is of major importance in improving oral dryness in approximately two-thirds of patients.[4–6] Excessive sweating, present in half of the patients, represents the major adverse effect, with nausea, diarrhea, and palpitations being quite

**TABLE 3.1 Treatment of SS-Related Glandular Manifestations**

| Manifestations | | Treatment |
| --- | --- | --- |
| Oral involvement | Oral dryness | Salivary substitutes<br>Muscarinic agonists (pilocarpine, cevimeline)[5,6,22]<br>Biological agents (RTX in patients with residual salivary function and abatacept in patients with secondary SS)[9,10,12,13] |
| | Dental caries | Local antimicrobials (chlorhexidine) |
| | Oral candidiasis | Fluconazole or itraconazole |
| Ocular involvement | Ocular dryness | Artificial tears[17]<br>Lubricant solutions<br>Calcineurin inhibitors (cyclosporine, tacrolimus drops)[19,21]<br>Rebamipide[20]<br>Muscarinic agonists (pilocarpine, cevimeline)[22,23]<br>Autologous serum drops[24]<br>Scleral contact lenses[25]<br>Biologic agents (RTX)[10] |
| Other glandular manifestations | Upper respiratory involvement | Humidification<br>Bromhexine<br>Prevention of infections (immunization, antibiotic treatment) |
| | Vaginal dryness | Vaginal lubricants |

*RTX*, Rituximab; *SS*, Sjögren's syndrome.

common. Patients who tolerate $M_2$ agonists well should be encouraged to increase the daily dose for an extended period of several weeks before quitting because of ineffectiveness. In a recent report, cevimeline showed a better profile compared with pilocarpine in terms of safety profile, because primary SS patients were more likely to continue cevimeline than pilocarpine long term.[7]

The use of local antimicrobials such as chlorhexidine in a form of varnish, gel, or rinses may be considered in SS patients with severe dry mouth and a high rate of dental caries. Nonfluoride demineralizing agents may be also considered as an adjunct therapy in xerostomic SS patients (unpublished personal observation).

The enlargement of parotid and/or other major salivary glands is asymptomatic and self-limiting in the majority of cases. For tender salivary gland enlargement, local application of moist heat and nonsteroidal antiinflammatory drugs may be beneficial. However, persistent enlargement should be meticulously evaluated to exclude bacterial superinfection and most importantly non-Hodgkin lymphoma (NHL) development.

Oral candidiasis must be treated, because it worsens sicca symptoms. It usually responds to local treatments such as clotrimazole troches and nystatin suspension. Systemic antifungal medications including fluconazole or itraconazole should be implemented in cases of extended oropharyngeal infections.

Conventional therapy with DMARDs has not proven efficacious in the management of sicca complaints.[3] A recent randomized study on hydroxychloroquine (HCQ) administration had confirmed previous observations, showing no improvement in oral dryness features.[8] The administration of the monoclonal antibody against CD20 rituximab has been reported to improve oral dryness, unstimulated salivary flow, and reduction in salivary gland infiltrates.[9,10] These findings, however, were not confirmed in a recent randomized trial.[11] In an interim analysis of an open-label abatacept trial in patients with rheumatoid arthritis (RA) and secondary SS, increases in saliva production by Saxon's test were observed together with control of arthritis-related complaints.[12] Similarly, increases in salivary production (after adjustment for disease duration) together with the reduction of lymphocytic infiltrates in the salivary gland tissues were also observed in a pilot study of abatacept in 11 primary SS patients.[13] Nevertheless, no differences in salivary gland function were noted in a subsequent open-label study including 15 early and active primary SS patients.[14] Blockade of the B-cell activating factor (BAFF or Blys) did not seem to improve measures of oral dryness, both subjective and objective.[15]

## 2.2 Dry Eyes

Ocular dryness is one of the most devastating features related to SS. Successful management can be achieved by patient education on avoiding aggravating environmental stimuli, such as very dry or windy environments and smoking, as well as by reducing tasks associated with reduced blinking, such as reading or using monitor screens for extended periods. Systemic medications known to reduce tear secretion, such as systemic antihistamines and tranquilizers with anticholinergic effects, should be avoided. Meibomian gland dysfunction should be carefully detected and appropriately managed with eyelid margin hygiene, topical antibiotic, or systemic doxycycline therapy when required. Adhering to a diet enriched in supplemental Ω-3 essential fatty acids may reduce the severity of ocular dryness, although further confirmatory data are required for SS.[16] In addition to preventive measures, tear replacement with topically applied artificial tears or lubricant solutions, antiinflammatory measures (eg, topical corticosteroids or cyclosporine), or oral secretagogues can be considered. When frequent use of artificial tears is required, preservative-free preparations are preferred because of the potential irritation effects of preservatives on the ocular surface. Amino acid–enriched preparations have also been shown to have beneficial effects.[17] Compared to tear substitutes, lubricating ointments and methylcellulose inserts have longer duration but can cause a transient blurring of vision. With regard to local antiinflammatory treatment, short-term local administration of steroid, as well as cyclosporine drops (0.05%), have been convincingly shown to provide symptomatic relief, improving both subjective and objective ocular signs in a randomized controlled trial.[18] According to recently published data, the local application of the macrolide tacrolimus (0.03% eye drops) may lead to the improvement of objective signs as early as 14 days after treatment initiation.[19] Of interest, beneficial effects in both subjective and objective signs of oral dryness were demonstrated in 30 patients with SS, with corneal fluorescein staining scores greater than 3, and conjunctival lissamine green staining scores greater than 3, treated four times daily for 4 weeks with 2% mucin secretagogue rebamipide ocular suspension, a derivative of quinolone-class antibiotics.[20] Additionally, administration of a single drop of cyclosporine led to improvement in eye redness, breakup time, and Schirmer test scores.[21] Patients with residual glandular function may benefit from the oral administration of the muscarinic $M_3$ receptor agonists pilocarpine[22] and cevimeline,[23] although the overall effects are considered less pronounced compared with alleviation of oral symptoms. Improvement of dryness scores was also observed following rituximab treatment.

Plugging of the lacrimal puncta can be offered as soon as local inflammation related to ocular dryness is controlled. For refractory cases, the use of topical autologous drops or partial closure of the interpalpebral fissure to reduce surface exposure can be alternative options.[24] Finally, scleral contact lenses may be needed to control severe ocular surface damage.[25]

## 2.3 Other Glandular Manifestations

Exocrine glands of the upper airways, gastrointestinal tract, and skin involvement can be also affected in the setting of SS, though less commonly. Desiccation of the upper respiratory tract mucosa can result into dry, crusted secretions in the nose, epistaxis, hoarseness, and bronchial hyperresponsiveness manifested as persistent dry cough and shortness of breath. A home humidifier to moisten the air and/or bromhexine at a dosage of 48 mg/day may be effective measures for alleviation of symptoms related to airways dryness, although data from controlled studies are lacking. Supportive measures such as immunization with pneumococcal polysaccharide, antibiotic treatment for sinusitis, and periodical removal of dry, crusted secretions using normal saline local infusions should be recommended. Exocrine pancreatic impairment dysfunction resulting from lymphocytic invasion of the pancreas tissue can also occur. Finally, vaginal lubricants may be used to treat vaginal dryness and dyspareunia.

## 3. MANAGEMENT OF SYSTEMIC COMPLICATIONS

### 3.1 Nonspecific Manifestations

#### 3.1.1 Fatigue

Fatigue is a major problem in SS, affecting a considerable proportion of patients, ranging from approximately 38% to 88%.[26–29] It is presented as lack of vitality contributing to the impaired quality of life documented in patients with primary SS.[30] According to recent findings from our group,[31] depression, neuroticism, and fibromyalgia were revealed as independent contributors to primary SS-related fatigue, with markers of B-cell activation being unrelated to fatigue scores in these patients. In this context, active collaboration with mental health professionals, early recognition, and appropriate treatment of both anxiety disorders and fibromyalgia seem appropriate. Aerobic exercise (Nordic walking) was previously shown to have a beneficial effect on depression, physical capacity, and fatigue in a controlled trial.[32] Caution should be taken when selective serotonin reuptake inhibitors (SSRI) or tricyclic antidepressants are prescribed, given their potential to exacerbate sicca complaints. Benzodiazepines such as clonazepam or low dosages of tricyclic antidepressants like amitriptyline 15–20 mg/day, or anticonvulsants such as pregabalin might be helpful to alleviate neuropathic or fibromyalgic pain (Table 3.2). SSRI agents or noradrenergic and specific serotonergic antidepressants (mirtazapine), which do not cause significant dryness, can be prescribed in depressive patients. Finally, the contribution of patient-based associations in the management of the disease should be emphasized through patient/family education, coping strategies reinforcement, and increased public awareness of the disease burden.

Beneficial effects on fatigue have been shown after treatment with certain biologicals, as yet via an unspecified mechanism. In an early randomized controlled study, administration of two infusions of rituximab of 1 gram each led to significant improvement of fatigue visual analog scale (VAS) scores at 6 months compared with placebo, as well as in the social functioning score of the Short Form (SF)-36 and a trend toward significance of the mental health domain score

**TABLE 3.2** Treatment of SS-Related Extraglandular (Systemic) Manifestations

| Manifestations | | Treatment |
|---|---|---|
| Nonspecific | Fatigue | Aerobic exercise<br>Tricyclic antidepressants or benzodiazepines<br>Biological agents (RTX, belimumab, anakinra, abatacept)[9,11,14,15,33,34] |
| | Arthralgias/arthritis | DMARDs (HCQ, MTX)[35]<br>Corticosteroids<br>Biological agents (RTX, abatacept)[37,41,12] |
| | Raynaud phenomenon | Avoidance of exposure to cold |
| Periepithelial | Renal tubular dysfunction/acidosis | Oral potassium and sodium bicarbonate |
| | Primary biliary cirrhosis<br>Autoimmune hepatitis | Ursodeoxycholic acid<br>Corticosteroids, azathioprine |
| | Lung–bronchial involvement/interstitial disease | β-Agonists, corticosteroids, cyclophosphamide, azathioprine |
| Immune-complex mediated | Palpable purpura, peripheral neuropathy, cryoglobulinemia, hypocomplementemia | Biological agents (RTX, belimumab)[11,33,37,41–44] |
| | Lymphoma | RTX alone or with CHOP[5,46] |

*CHOP*, Cyclophosphamide, doxorubicin, vincristine, prednisone; *DMARDs*, disease-modifying antirheumatic drugs; *HCQ*, hydroxychloroquine; *MTX*, methotrexate; *RTX*, rituximab; *SS*, Sjögren's syndrome.

of the SF-36.[33] In a recent randomized controlled trial, an improvement of at least 30 mm in VAS fatigue score was more common with rituximab at weeks 6 and 16, and improvement in fatigue from baseline to week 24 was greater with rituximab.[11] Improvement on the patient-reported outcomes was also shown in the study reported by St Clair at 26th week after a single dose of rituximab; however, the effect was modest.[9] In a recent bicentric prospective 1-year open-label trial study aiming at blocking BAFF, an improvement of fatigue scores was also observed.[15] Because several efforts have so far failed to correlate fatigue with markers of B-cell hyperactivity, the beneficial effect of B-cell blockade remains to be further clarified.

In addition, a recent post-hoc analysis of a double-blind, placebo-controlled clinical trial using the interleukin (IL)-1 receptor antagonist (IL-1ra, anakinra) showed a 50% reduction in fatigue in patients taking the active drug compared with those receiving placebo.[34] Fatigue and health-related quality of life were also reported to significantly improve after abatacept treatment.[14]

### 3.1.2 Arthralgias/Arthritis

Administration of HCQ in cases of joint involvement is the first line treatment, with methotrexate[35] and combination therapy being used when HCQ is required to control arthritic complaints. Short-term use of low-dose oral corticosteroids (<10 mg/day of prednisone or equivalent) can be also implemented in refractory cases. Of note, in a recent report, administration of leflunomide 20 mg/day for 3 months (after a loading dose) in addition to methotrexate in RA with associated SS resulted in deterioration of keratoconjunctivitis sicca in some patients and reduction of Schirmer test scores and therefore caution is mandatory.[36]

Among biological agents, administration of rituximab has been shown to improve joint symptoms and thus is reserved for resistant forms of inflammatory arthritis.[37] In a recent open label trial with belimumab, a monoclonal antibody against BAFF, no improvement in pain scores was detected.[15] In another study the use of abatacept in RA patients with secondary SS led to improvement of both joint and sicca-related clinical features.[12] Studies on antitumor necrosis factor agents (both infliximab and etanercept) failed to demonstrate clinical efficacy in SS patients. Augmentation of interferon/BAFF axis seems to account for the reduced efficacy.[38–40]

### 3.1.3 Raynaud Phenomenon

For Raynaud phenomenon, avoidance of exposure to cold, emotional stress, and smoking should be recommended.

## 3.2 Periepithelial Disease

### 3.2.1 Renal Involvement

Tubular renal dysfunction with or without acidosis and Fanconi syndrome are usual manifestations of interstitial nephritis, with nephrocalcinosis being an undesired complication. Hypokalemic hyperchloremic acidosis is the most severe manifestation, as a result of tubular dysfunction and can be managed with oral potassium and sodium bicarbonate. The administration of sodium bicarbonate should begin with 1 g three times daily, but up to 12 g daily administration may be required. In the presence of gastrointestinal disturbances, a sodium citrate solution may be alternatively given.

### 3.2.2 Liver Involvement

Liver involvement in primary SS patients occurs in approximately 5% of patients and is manifested by increased levels of liver enzymes, the occurrence of anti-mitochondrial antibodies and/or histopathological lesions of stage I primary biliary cirrhosis. Evidence of autoimmune hepatitis may be also encountered. In cases of persistent and progressive liver enzyme elevation, prednisone and azathioprine 1 mg/kg may be required.

### 3.2.3 Lung Involvement

Increasing evidence suggests that bronchial/bronchiolar disease is the predominant pattern of lung involvement in patients with primary SS compared with interstitial lung disease. Small airway involvement may be demonstrated by both functional pulmonary tests and chest computed tomography. In such cases, the use of β-agonists and corticosteroids may provide limited benefit. Although it seems to occur early in disease course, the natural history of lung disease seems to be indolent and nonprogressive in the majority of these patients. Lymphoid interstitial pneumonitis should be treated with corticosteroids (0.5–1.0 mg/kg). In addition, cyclophosphamide, cyclosporine, or azathioprine can be considered under selected circumstances.

## 4. IMMUNE COMPLEX–MEDIATED DISEASE

A vast majority of systemic manifestations in SS arise from the deposition of immune complexes as a result of B-cell hyperactivity, which constitutes a cardinal SS feature. These include palpable purpura (vasculitis), peripheral neuropathy, and glomerulonephritis, as well as the occurrence of laboratory test abnormalities such as cryoglobulinemia and hypocomplementemia, all of which have been shown to connote NHL development. In this context, B-cell depletion and/or inhibition of B signals for B-cell differentiation, and survival appears to provide a reasonable therapeutic approach with beneficial results.[11,33,37,41–45] In a report from a French registry, administration of rituximab in 78 primary SS patients with mainly systemic manifestations observed for a median period around 3 years led to a decrease of the European Sjögren's Syndrome Disease Activity Index score, as well as in a remarkable improvement in purpura, peripheral neuropathy, and cryoglobulinemic vasculitis[37] therefore it should be mainly reserved for threatening systemic manifestations.

Although peripheral neurological involvement occurs commonly in SS patients, CNS involvement is a rare event. Given the lack of controlled studies, management of SS-related CNS disease is mainly based on expert opinion and anecdotal reports. Thus in the presence of stable, self-limiting disease, no intervention is required. In contrast, when signs of activity or progression are evident (eg, abnormalities in magnetic resonance imaging or in the cerebrospinal fluid), aggressive treatment, initially with intravenous pulses of methylprednisolone (1.0 g/day for 3 consecutive days) and monthly intravenous pulses of cyclophosphamide is warranted (at a dosage of 700–1000 mg/m$^2$ body surface). Intravenous γ-globulin may be useful in the treatment of SS-associated sensorimotor neuropathies or nonataxic sensory neuropathy without any necrotizing vasculitis.

The treatment of malignant lymphoma in SS patients, based on histological type and extent, is more extensively discussed in the specific chapter of this book. Patients with localized low-grade lymphoma affecting exocrine glands should be closely monitored (wait and watch policy). In patients with disseminated lymphoma, the chemotherapy regimen should be adapted to the histological grade. The implication of ongoing B-cell activation in the SS pathophysiology suggests targeted anti-B-cell therapies as a major therapeutic strategy.[5,46] Thus there is an increasingly appreciated therapeutic role for rituximab and possibly for belimumab in SS-related lymphomas, alone in low-grade lymphomas, or in combination with cyclophosphamide, doxorubicin, vincristine, and prednisone in diffuse large B-cell lymphomas. Data from randomized controlled trials are required before definite recommendations can be offered.

## REFERENCES

1. Manoussakis MN, Georgopoulou C, Zintzaras E, Spyropoulou M, Stavropoulou A, Skopouli FN, et al. Sjögren's syndrome associated with systemic lupus erythematosus: clinical and laboratory profiles and comparison with primary Sjögren's syndrome. *Arthritis Rheum* 2004;**50**:882–91.
2. Mavragani CP, Moutsopoulos HM. Sjögren syndrome. *CMAJ* 2014;**186**:E579–86.
3. Mavragani CP, Moutsopoulos HM. Conventional therapy of Sjögren's syndrome. *Clin Rev Allergy Immunol* 2007;**32**:284–91.
4. Vivino FB, Al-Hashimi I, Khan Z, Le Vewue FG, Salisbury PL, Tran-Johnson TK, et al. Pilocarpine tablets for the treatment of dry mouth and dry eye symptoms in patients with Sjögren's syndrome. *Arch Intern Med* 1999;**159**:174–81.
5. Mavragani CP, Moutsopoulos NM, Moutsopoulos HM. The management of Sjögren's syndrome. *Nat Clin Pract Rheumatol* 2006;**2**:252–61.
6. Ramos-Casals M, Tzioufas AG, Stone JH, Siso A, Bosch X. Treatment of primary Sjögren syndrome: a systematic review. *JAMA* 2010;**304**:452–60.
7. Noaiseh G, Baker JF, Vivino FB. Comparison of the discontinuation rates and side-effect profiles of pilocarpine and cevimeline for xerostomia in primary Sjögren's syndrome. *Clin Exp Rheumatol* 2014;**32**:575–7.
8. Gottenberg JE, Ravaud P, Puechal X, Le Guern V, Sibilia J, Goeb V, et al. Effects of hydroxychloroquine on symptomatic improvement in primary Sjögren syndrome: the Joquer randomized clinical trial. *JAMA* 2014;**312**:249–58.
9. St Clair EW, Levesque MC, Luning Prak ET, Vivino FB, Alappatt CJ, Spychala ME, et al. Rituximab therapy for primary Sjögren's syndrome: an open-label clinical trial and mechanistic analysis. *Arthritis Rheum* 2013;**65**:1097–106.
10. Carubbi F, Cipriani P, Marrelli A, Benedetto P, Ruscitti P, Berardicurti O, et al. Efficacy and safety of rituximab treatment in early primary Sjögren's syndrome: a prospective, multi-center, follow-up study. *Arthritis Res Ther* 2013;**15**:R172.
11. Devauchelle-Pensec V, Mariette X, Jousse-Joulin S, Berthelot JM, Perdriger A, Puechal X, et al. Treatment of primary Sjögren syndrome with rituximab: a randomized trial. *Ann Intern Med* 2014;**160**:233–42.
12. Tsuboi H, Matsumoto I, Hagiwara S, Hirota T, Takahashi H, Ebe H, et al. Efficacy and safety of abatacept for patients with Sjögren's syndrome associated with rheumatoid arthritis: rheumatoid arthritis with orencia trial toward Sjögren's syndrome endocrinopathy (ROSE) trial-an open-label, one-year, prospective study, interim analysis of 32 patients for 24 weeks. *Mod Rheumatol* 2014;**25**:187–93.

13. Adler S, Korner M, Forger F, Huscher D, Caversaccio MD, Villiger PM. Evaluation of histologic, serologic, and clinical changes in response to abatacept treatment of primary Sjögren's syndrome: a pilot study. *Arthritis Care Res (Hoboken)* 2013;**65**:1862–8.

14. Meiners PM, Vissink A, Kroese FG, Spijkervet FK, Smitt-Kamminga NS, Abdulahad WH, et al. Abatacept treatment reduces disease activity in early primary Sjögren's syndrome (open-label proof of concept ASAP study). *Ann Rheum Dis* 2014;**73**:1393–6.

15. Mariette X, Seror R, Quartuccio L, Baron G, Salvin S, Fabris M, et al. Efficacy and safety of belimumab in primary Sjogren's syndrome: results of the BELISS open-label phase II study. *Ann Rheum Dis* 2015;**74**:526–31.

16. Kokke KH, Morris JA, Lawrenson JG. Oral omega-6 essential fatty acid treatment in contact lens associated dry eye. *Cont Lens Anterior Eye* 2008;**31**:141–6. quiz 70.

17. Aragona P, Rania L, Roszkowska AM, Spinella R, Postorino E, Puzzolo D, et al. Effects of amino acids enriched tears substitutes on the cornea of patients with dysfunctional tear syndrome. *Acta Ophthalmol* 2013;**91**:e437–44.

18. Stevenson D, Tauber J, Reis BL. Efficacy and safety of cyclosporin A ophthalmic emulsion in the treatment of moderate-to-severe dry eye disease: a dose-ranging, randomized trial. The cyclosporin a phase-2 study group. *Ophthalmology* 2000;**107**:967–74.

19. Moscovici BK, Holzchuh R, Chiacchio BB, Santo RM, Shimazaki J, Hida RY. Clinical treatment of dry eye using 0.03% tacrolimus eye drops. *Cornea* 2012;**31**:945–9.

20. Arimoto A, Kitagawa K, Mita N, Takahashi Y, Shibuya E, Sasaki H. Effect of rebamipide ophthalmic suspension on signs and symptoms of keratoconjunctivitis sicca in Sjögren syndrome patients with or without punctal occlusions. *Cornea* 2015;**33**:806–11.

21. Deveci H, Kobak S. The efficacy of topical 0.05% cyclosporine A in patients with dry eye disease associated with Sjögren's syndrome. *Int Ophthalmol* 2014;**34**:1043–8.

22. Vivino FB, Al-Hashimi I, Khan Z, LeVeque FG, Salisbury 3rd PL, Tran-Johnson TK, et al. Pilocarpine tablets for the treatment of dry mouth and dry eye symptoms in patients with Sjögren syndrome: a randomized, placebo-controlled, fixed-dose, multicenter trial. P92-01 study group. *Arch Intern Med* 1999;**159**:174–81.

23. Petrone D, Condemi JJ, Fife R, Gluck O, Cohen S, Dalgin P. A double-blind, randomized, placebo-controlled study of cevimeline in Sjögren's syndrome patients with xerostomia and keratoconjunctivitis sicca. *Arthritis Rheum* 2002;**46**:748–54.

24. Hwang J, Chung SH, Jeon S, Kwok SK, Park SH, Kim MS. Comparison of clinical efficacies of autologous serum eye drops in patients with primary and secondary Sjögren syndrome. *Cornea* 2014;**33**:663–7.

25. Foulks GN, Forstot SL, Donshik PC, Forstot JZ, Goldstein MH, Lemp MA, et al. Clinical guidelines for management of dry eye associated with Sjögren disease. *Ocul Surf* 2015;**13**:118–32.

26. Theander L, Strombeck B, Mandl T, Theander E. Sleepiness or fatigue? Can we detect treatable causes of tiredness in primary Sjögren's syndrome? *Rheumatology (Oxford)* 2010;**49**:1177–83.

27. Haldorsen K, Bjelland I, Bolstad AI, Jonsson R, Brun JG. A five-year prospective study of fatigue in primary Sjögren's syndrome. *Arthritis Res Ther* 2011;**13**:R167.

28. Segal B, Thomas W, Rogers T, Leon JM, Hughes P, Patel D, et al. Prevalence, severity, and predictors of fatigue in subjects with primary Sjögren's syndrome. *Arthritis Rheum* 2008;**59**:1780–7.

29. Iannuccelli C, Spinelli FR, Guzzo MP, Priori R, Conti F, Ceccarelli F, et al. Fatigue and widespread pain in systemic lupus erythematosus and Sjögren's syndrome: symptoms of the inflammatory disease or associated fibromyalgia? *Clin Exp Rheumatol* 2012;**30**:117–21.

30. Champey J, Corruble E, Gottenberg JE, Buhl C, Meyer T, Caudmont C, et al. Quality of life and psychological status in patients with primary Sjögren's syndrome and sicca symptoms without autoimmune features. *Arthritis Rheum* 2006;**55**:451–7.

31. Karageorgas T, Fragioudaki S, Nezos A, Karaiskos D, Moutsopoulos HM, Mavragani CP. Fatigue in primary Sjögren's syndrome: clinical, laboratory, psychometric and biological associations. *Arthritis Care Res (Hoboken)* 2015;**68**(1):123–31.

32. Strombeck BE, Theander E, Jacobsson LT. Effects of exercise on aerobic capacity and fatigue in women with primary Sjögren's syndrome. *Rheumatology (Oxford)* 2007;**46**:567–71.

33. Dass S, Bowman SJ, Vital EM, Ikeda K, Pease CT, Hamburger J, et al. Reduction of fatigue in Sjögren syndrome with rituximab: results of a randomised, double-blind, placebo-controlled pilot study. *Ann Rheum Dis* 2008;**67**:1541–4.

34. Norheim KB, Harboe E, Goransson LG, Omdal R. Interleukin-1 inhibition and fatigue in primary Sjögren's syndrome: a double blind, randomised clinical trial. *PLoS One* 2012;**7**:e30123.

35. Skopouli FN, Jagiello P, Tsifetaki N, Moutsopoulos HM. Methotrexate in primary Sjögren's syndrome. *Clin Exp Rheumatol* 1996;**14**:555–8.

36. Shahin AA, El-Agha S, El-Azkalany GS. The effect of leflunomide on the eye dryness in secondary Sjögren's syndrome associated with rheumatoid arthritis and in rheumatoid arthritis patients. *Clin Rheumatol* 2014;**33**:925–30.

37. Gottenberg JE, Cinquetti G, Larroche C, Combe B, Hachulla E, Meyer O, et al. Efficacy of rituximab in systemic manifestations of primary Sjögren's syndrome: results in 78 patients of the autoimmune and rituximab registry. *Ann Rheum Dis* 2012;**72**(6):1026–31.

38. Zandbelt MM, de Wilde PCM, van Damme PA, Hoyng CB, van der Putte LBA, van den Hoogen FHJ. Etanercept in the treatment of patients with primary Sjögren's syndrome: a pilot study. *J Rheumatology* 2004;**31**:96–101.

39. Mavragani CP, Niewold TB, Moutsopoulos NM, Pillemer SR, Wahl SM, Crow MK. Augmented interferon-alpha pathway activation in patients with Sjögren's syndrome treated with etanercept. *Arthritis Rheum* 2007;**56**:3995–4004.

40. Mariette X, Ravaud P, Steinfeld S, Baron G, Goetz J, Hachulla E, et al. Inefficacy of infliximab in primary Sjögren's syndrome: results of the randomized, controlled Trial of Remicade in Primary Sjögren's Syndrome (TRIPSS). *Arthritis Rheum* 2004;**50**:1270–6.

41. Seror R, Sordet C, Guillevin L, Hachulla E, Masson C, Ittah M, et al. Tolerance and efficacy of rituximab and changes in serum B cell biomarkers in patients with systemic complications of primary Sjögren's syndrome. *Ann Rheum Dis* 2007;**66**:351–7.

42. Meiners PM, Arends S, Brouwer E, Spijkervet FK, Vissink A, Bootsma H. Responsiveness of disease activity indices ESSPRI and ESSDAI in patients with primary Sjögren's syndrome treated with rituximab. *Ann Rheum Dis* 2012;**71**:1297–302.

43. Mekinian A, Ravaud P, Hatron PY, Larroche C, Leone J, Gombert B, et al. Efficacy of rituximab in primary Sjögren's syndrome with peripheral nervous system involvement: results from the air registry. *Ann Rheum Dis* 2012;**71**:84–7.

44. Meijer JM, Meiners PM, Vissink A, Spijkervet FK, Abdulahad W, Kamminga N, et al. Effectiveness of rituximab treatment in primary Sjögren's syndrome: a randomized, double-blind, placebo-controlled trial. *Arthritis Rheum* 2010;**62**:960–8.

45. Meiners PM, Arends S, Meijer JM, Moerman RV, Spijkervet FK, Vissink A, et al. Efficacy of retreatment with rituximab in patients with primary Sjögren's syndrome. *Clin Exp Rheumatol* 2015;**33**:443–4.

46. Voulgarelis M, Ziakas PD, Papageorgiou A, Baimpa E, Tzioufas AG, Moutsopoulos HM. Prognosis and outcome of non-Hodgkin lymphoma in primary Sjögren syndrome. *Medicine (Baltimore)* 2012;**91**:1–9.

# Chapter 4

# Classification Criteria for Sjögren's Syndrome

C. Vitali
*Casa di Cura of Lecco, Lecco, Italy; Istituto S. Stefano, Como, Italy*

N. Del Papa
*Istituto G. Pini, Milan, Italy*

## 1. GENERAL CONCEPTS ON CLASSIFICATION CRITERIA

Sjögren's syndrome (SS) is a systemic autoimmune disease (SAD) that primarily affects the exocrine glands, predominantly the salivary and lachrymal glands, and leads to their functional impairment with consequent persistent dryness of the eye and mouth. The pathological hallmark of the disorder is a focal lympho-monocytic infiltration of the target tissue.[1,2]

In addition to the disease-specific exocrine manifestations, SS is also characterized in most patients by the production of a variety of autoantibodies and by a systemic and multiorgan involvement, where constitutional symptoms, joint, skin, lung, renal, and neurological manifestations may be present.[3] This justifies the inclusion of SS in the SAD family.

Similarly to what happens in all of the SADs, SS does not present itself with a single distinguishing feature that can allow a correct diagnosis. Hence only a certain number of specific clinical and laboratory features can lead to and confirm a correct diagnosis.

Theoretically, classification criteria and diagnostic criteria can be considered alike. This is particularly true when the sensitivity and specificity of the criteria are equal up to nearly 100%. However, the main purpose of the classification criteria is to distinguish patients with the disease from patients without and from normal subjects, thus to define homogeneous disease groups for clinical and epidemiological studies. Ideally, classification criteria should possess a high-level sensitivity in order to be able to identify the particular disease they are created for, and an equally high specificity, so as to avoid the inclusion of patients with other similar diseases. If they are not valid, participants without the disease may be included in the disease group, and participants with clear-cut disease may be excluded. Conversely, valid classification criteria facilitate the selection of cohorts of patients with a given disease to be enrolled in clinical trials and epidemiologic studies, thus allowing comparison of results across studies.[4,5]

## 2. THE HISTORICAL SETS OF CLASSIFICATION CRITERIA PROPOSED BEFORE THE 1990s

Leading experts in the field proposed a number of classification criteria sets for SS before the 1990s. Most of these criteria sets were presented and discussed during the first International Symposium on SS, held in Copenhagen in 1986.[6] These historical criteria sets include the San Francisco criteria (proposed in 1975 and subsequently revised in 1984[7,8]) and the Copenhagen,[9] Japanese,[10] Greek,[11] and San Diego criteria.[12] The Japanese criteria have been subsequently updated and the latest version was proposed in 1999.[13]

Nearly all of them were chiefly addressed to precisely define the involvement of the lachrymal and salivary glands; that is, the evidence of tear and saliva flow reduction, as well as the presence of superficial lesions of the conjunctival epithelial surface and abnormalities in salivary gland imaging.

An important discrepancy among the different criteria sets concerned the subjective symptoms of either dry eye or dry mouth. Some criteria sets gave prominence to them for diagnostic assessment, whereas others focused on more specific and reproducible objective findings (Table 4.1). Moreover, other important differences concerned the tests included in the criteria sets, the cut-offs chosen for each test, and the number of tests needed for the diagnostic definition of either ocular or salivary involvement. The differences among the proposed criteria sets are shown in Table 4.1.[7–13] For instance, only the Japanese criteria took into account sialography as a criterion for salivary gland assessment in SS.[9–13] Conversely, the Copenhagen criteria included salivary gland scintigraphy, an expensive method for a functional evaluation of all the major salivary glands.[9]

All the criteria sets included minor salivary gland biopsy, but only the Greek and the San Diego criteria sets considered it to be mandatory to classify a patient as having SS.[11,12] In the Japanese criteria set, the tear gland biopsy could replace the minor salivary gland biopsy.[10–13]

As to the modalities for performing the biopsy, all of the criteria sets adopted the guidelines proposed by Daniels et al. in 1975,[7] where a focal sialoadenitis was defined by the presence of focal infiltrates and a focus score (FS) as a cluster of at least 50 mononuclear cells. To diagnose primary SS, an average FS per $4\,mm^2$ was required, based on the evaluation of at least four glands.[7,8] However, the FS considered as indicative for a diagnosis of SS was not the same in all of the criteria sets (see Table 4.1).

Subsequent studies confirmed that the focal sialoadenitis, quantified by the FS, was closely associated with parotid flow rate, evidence of keratoconjunctivitis sicca (KCS), and the presence of autoantibodies.[13–15] Significantly, the presence of autoantibodies (anti-nuclear antibodies [ANAs], anti-Ro/SSA, anti-La/SSB, and immunoglobulin (Ig) M–rheumatoid factor [RF]) as an additional

**TABLE 4.1** Comparison Among the Different Items, Considered According to the Historical Criteria for SS Proposed Before the 1990s

| | Copenhagen[9] | Japan[10,13,a] | Greek[11] | San Diego[12] | San Francisco[7,8,a] |
|---|---|---|---|---|---|
| Definition of probable/definite diagnosis of SS | – | + | + | + | + |
| Definition of primary vs secondary SS | + | – | + | – | – |
| Subjective dry eye | – | + | + | – | – |
| Subjective dry mouth | – | + | + | + | – |
| Patient reported past parotid gland swelling | – | + | + | – | – |
| Ocular Tests | | | | | |
| • Schirmer-I test | + (≤10 mm/5′) | + (≤10 mm/5′) | + (≤10 mm/5′) | + (≤9 mm/5′) | + (≤10 mm/5′) |
| • Break-up time | + (≤10 s) | – | – | – | + |
| • Rose bengal (van Bijsterveld score) | + (≥4) | + (≥2) | + (≥4) | + (≥4) | + (≥4) |
| • Fluorescein test | – | + | – | + | – |
| • KCS defined by the abnormality of 2 tests | + | + | – | + | + |
| Oral Parameters | | | | | |
| • Unstimulated whole saliva | + | – | – | + | – |
| • Stimulated parotid flow rate | – | – | + | + | – |

*Continued*

**TABLE 4.1 Comparison Among the Different Items, Considered According to the Historical Criteria for SS Proposed Before the 1990s—cont'd**

|  | Copenhagen[9] | Japan[10,13,a] | Greek[11] | San Diego[12] | San Francisco[7,8,a] |
|---|---|---|---|---|---|
| • Scintigraphy | + | − | − | − | − |
| • Sialography | − | + | − | − | − |
| Minor salivary gland biopsy (mandatory) | No | No | Yes | Yes | Yes |
| Focus score | >1 | >1 | >2 | >2 | >1 |
| Serological Findings |  |  |  |  |  |
| • ANA | − | − | − | + | − |
| • Anti-Ro/SSA | − | −/+[b] | − | + | − |
| • Anti-La/SSB | − | −/+[b] | − | + | − |
| • IgM-RF | − | − | − | + | − |

*ANA*, Antinuclear antibodies; *Ig*, immunoglobulin; *KCS*, keratoconjunctivitis sicca; *RF*, rheumatoid factor.
[a]Japanese criteria were revised in 1999[13].
[b]Introduced in the 1999 revised version of Japanese criteria.

diagnostic domain was introduced only in the San Diego criteria set. This pointed out the autoimmune origin of the disease.[12]

Finally, all of the criteria sets except that from Copenhagen adopted the terms of "probable" and "definite" SS, whereas only the Copenhagen and Greek criteria distinguished the "primary" form of SS from the "secondary" one.[9–11]

Although the proposed criteria sets were all hypothetically able to correctly classify patients with SS, their application was limited to single centers, and none of them was validated by multicenter studies in the following years. For many years, this has made it difficult to compare data from epidemiological, clinical, and serological studies carried out by different investigators who had adopted different classification criteria in the selection of patients.

## 3. FROM THE PRELIMINARY EUROPEAN CRITERIA TO THE AMERICAN–EUROPEAN CONSENSUS GROUP CRITERIA

In 1988, because none of the proposed criteria had gained wide enough acceptance within the scientific community, the Epidemiology Committee of the Commission of the European Communities decided to support a multicenter study aimed at reaching a consensus on classification criteria for SS.[16] The study was carried out from 1989 to 1993, when the preliminary European Classification Criteria for SS were finally published.[17] The Delphi method, based on the consensus of the experts and adopted in previously proposed criteria, was not employed to develop the European criteria. Instead, it was decided to use the methodology and statistics previously adopted by the American College of Rheumatology (ACR) in setting their criteria for rheumatoid arthritis[18] and systemic lupus.[19] Consequently the criteria were derived directly from cohorts of patients with primary SS, with SADs, associated or not with SS, and patients with sicca symptoms without SS. The expert clinician at the best of her/his clinical skill was responsible for the inclusion of each patient in the different groups. Therefore the expert clinical judgment represented the gold standard for the diagnosis. Multivariate analyses allowed the development of a criteria set composed of six items. Any four of these six items were required for the diagnosis. The six items were as follows: (1) ocular symptoms; (2) oral symptoms (both defined on the basis of validated questionnaires); (3) ocular signs (defined by positive Schirmer-I test and/or rose bengal score); (4) signs of salivary gland involvement (assessed by parotid sialography, scintigraphy, and unstimulated salivary flow); (5) focal sialoadenitis (observed in lip biopsy); and (6) presence of autoantibodies. Sensitivity and specificity, obtained by selecting patients with primary SS who met four out of six criteria items, were equal to 93.5% and 94%, respectively.[17] A list of exclusion criteria were also formulated following the recommendations of Fox et al.[12] This included the presence of preexisting lymphoma, acquired immunodeficiency syndrome, sarcoidosis, and graft-versus-host disease.[12]

A validation of the European criteria set was performed in a following survey carried out on a different population of patients and controls. The criteria were confirmed to have both high sensitivity and specificity (97.5% and 94.2%, respectively).[20] When previously proposed criteria[7–12] were used to classify patients with primary SS and controls enrolled in the European validation cohort, they all showed a very high specificity (range 97.9% to 100%), but a much lower sensitivity (range 22.9% to 72.2%). This shows how much the application of the new European criteria were able to improve classification accuracy, and may explain why the validated European classification criteria were widely accepted by the scientific community and largely used in following studies on SS.

It is worth pointing out that the distinction between probable and definite diagnosis was finally abolished in the formulation of the validated European criteria,[20] because it was clearly in contrast with the concept of classification criteria itself, which should be aimed at selecting true patients for clinical, epidemiological, and therapeutic studies.[4,5]

Despite widespread acceptance over the following years, the European classification criteria set was the object of an extensive discussion. The main criticism was that the criteria might lead to classifying a patient as having a true SS even in absence of autoantibodies or focal sialoadenitis, considered to be a clear-cut demonstration of autoimmune activation in this disorder. An additional critical point of the European criteria set was that because two out of the six items were represented by subjective complaints, patients with SS but without symptoms would find it hard to meet the criteria for classification.[21,22]

To overcome these criticisms and expand the acceptance of the European classification criteria, a European group (the European Study Group on Classification Criteria for SS), and a group of American experts decided to conduct an additional analysis of the European cohort database. Based on the analysis of the derived sensitivity/specificity receiver operating characteristic curve, the condition "positivity of 4 out of 6 items with the exclusion of the cases in which both serology and histopathology were negative" showed the same accuracy (92.7%) as that obtained by applying the unlimited combination of any four out of six items, with an increase of specificity (95.2%), and an acceptable loss of sensitivity (89.5%). Furthermore, the combination of any three of the four objective criteria items also showed a slightly lower accuracy (90.5%), with a specificity of 95.2% and a sensitivity of 84.2%. In summary, the American–European Consensus Group (AECG) maintained the previous European scheme of six items but introduced the concept that either minor salivary gland biopsy or serology (limited to the more specific presence of anti-Ro/SSA and anti-La/SSB antibodies) was mandatory in order to correctly classify a patient as having primary SS.[23] Other small changes to the methodology to be used in performing ocular tests were integrated into the European criteria set in order to make the item definition more precise.[23]

Finally, it was decided to include hepatitis C virus infection as an exclusion criterion, considering that sicca symptoms and focal sialoadenitis, often observed in patients with this chronic infection, are not easy to distinguish from those of SS.[24]

More details on AECG criteria and rules for classification are reported in Table 4.2.

**TABLE 4.2 AECG Classification Criteria for Sjögren's Syndrome[23]**

I. Ocular symptoms: a positive response to at least one of the following questions:
1. Have you had daily, persistent, troublesome dry eyes for more than 3 months?
2. Do you have a recurrent sensation of sand or gravel in the eyes?
3. Do you use tear substitutes more than 3 times a day?

II. Oral symptoms: a positive response to at least one of the following questions:
1. Have you had a daily feeling of dry mouth for more than 3 months?
2. Have you had swollen salivary glands, recurrently or persistently, as an adult?
3. Do you frequently drink liquids to aid in swallowing dry food?

III. Ocular signs, that is, objective evidence of ocular involvement defined as a positive result for at least one of the following two tests:
1. Schirmer-I test, performed without anesthesia (<5 mm in 5 minutes)
2. Rose bengal score, or other ocular dye score (>4 according to van Bijsterveld scoring system)

IV. Histopathology:
   In minor salivary glands, the presence of focal lymphocytic sialoadenitis in normal-appearing mucosa, evaluated by an expert histopathologist, with a focus score ≥1, defined as a number of lymphocytic foci (adjacent to normal-appearing mucous acini, and containing more than 50 lymphocytes) per 4 mm² of glandular tissue.

V. Salivary gland involvement: objective evidence of salivary gland involvement, defined by a positive result for at least one of the following diagnostic tests:
1. Unstimulated whole salivary flow (<1.5 mL in 15 minutes)
2. Parotid sialography showing the presence of diffuse sialectasias (punctate, cavitary, or destructive pattern), without evidence of obstruction in the major ducts
3. Salivary scintigraphy showing delayed uptake, reduced concentration, and/or delayed excretion of tracer

VI. Autoantibodies: presence in the serum of the following autoantibodies:
1. Antibodies to SSA(Ro) or SSB(La) antigens, or both

**Rules for Classification**

For primary SS:
   In patients without any potentially associated disease, primary SS may be defined as follows:
a. The presence of any 4 of the 6 items is indicative of primary SS, as long as either item IV (Histopathology) or VI (Serology) is positive
b. The presence of any 3 of the 4 objective criteria items (ie, items III, IV, V, VI)
c. The classification tree procedure represents a valid alternative method for classification, although it should be more properly used in clinical-epidemiological surveys

For secondary SS:
   In patients with a potentially associated disease, eg, another well-defined connective tissue disease, the presence of item I, or item II, plus any 2 from among items III, IV, and V may be considered as indicative of secondary SS.

Exclusion criteria:
   Past head and neck radiation treatment
   Hepatitis C infection
   Acquired immunodeficiency syndrome (AIDS)
   Preexisting lymphoma
   Sarcoidosis
   Graft-versus-host disease
   Use of anticholinergic drugs (over a period shorter than fourfold the half life of the drug)

Since its publication in 2002, the AECG criteria set has been largely adopted by the scientific community, and has certainly become the worldwide gold standard for the classification of patients with SS. This is consistent with the thousands of citations that the AECG criteria have received in scientific literature since their appearance.

Despite widespread acceptance and diffusion of the AECG criteria, some points related to the sensitivity/specificity balance of the criteria, and to the methodology adopted to derive them, remained still unsolved.

As to their performance in an epidemiological survey, the AECG criteria have been considered too stringent, so much so as to have possibly led to underestimating the total prevalence of the disease obtained in general population surveys.[25–36] This varies from 0.1% to 0.6%, when applying the AECG criteria,[25–27,30–32] and from 0.2% to 4.5%[25–29,36] if the preliminary European and Copenhagen criteria are used. This is an obvious consequence of the introduction of mandatory items in the AECG formulation, which certainly enhances specificity to the disadvantage of sensitivity.

In addition, according to the statistical methodology employed to derive the European and the AECG criteria,[17,20,23] patients had to be preliminarily classified as having, or not having, a specific disease simply on the basis of the physician's clinical judgment. At a later time, the best combination of items able to more accurately distinguish between case patients, previously judged as having the disease, and case controls, initially classified as not having the disease, was derived from multivariate correlation analysis.[17,20,23] This method may bias the selection of the criteria items due to a circularity process, because the preliminary classification of patient cases is certainly influenced in the physician's judgment by the positivity of specific tests, which, at the end of the process, are most likely to be in the list of items selected by means of statistical tools.

Furthermore, nonequivalent tests, which are considered to be equivalent in some domains, and the inclusion in the criteria set of such an invasive and obsolete test like sialography, and an expensive one like salivary scintigraphy, are other important issues still being debated. This may undoubtedly lead to the opinion that the need for some revision is desirable.

## 4. THE NEW PRELIMINARY ACR CLASSIFICATION CRITERIA FOR SJÖGREN'S SYNDROME

A new approach to classification criteria for SS has been proposed more recently and published as the ACR preliminary classification criteria for SS.[37] This new set of criteria was the result of the analysis of data from a large cohort of patients enrolled during a multicenter study, ie, the Sjögren's International Collaborative Clinical Alliance (SICCA). These criteria state that a patient can be classified as having SS if at least two of the following three criteria items are met: (1) a positive serum anti-Ro/SSA and/or anti-La/SSB, or, alternatively, positive RF plus ANA (titer >1:320); (2) KCS, defined by an ocular staining score ≥3; (3) focal lymphocytic sialoadenitis, defined by a FS ≥1 focus per 4 mm$^2$ in labial salivary gland biopsy.[37]

The authors pointed out how the high specificity demonstrated by this criteria set in selecting true patients with SS could be a determinant aspect when one considers the employment of the criteria to enroll patients for clinical trials where new therapies with potentially severe side effects are tested. The authors also underlined that their criteria specificity was strongly reinforced by the exclusion of the symptoms of dry mouth and dry eye from the criteria set, because subjective complaints are much less specific than objective tests.[37]

The method employed to derive the ACR preliminary criteria was different from the methodologies previously adopted for the same purpose.[5] The Delphi method was used to select and restrict the number of diagnostic tests and candidates for entry into the criteria set. At the end of this process, 10 variables were selected by expert consensus as the best predictors of SS. Furthermore, a specific type of cluster analysis, ie, a latent class analysis, was adopted to define the number of disease classes present in the analyzed cohort, on the basis of the presence, or absence, of the selected items.[38] This statistical procedure produced a model formed of two classes into which disease cases and control cases can be separated. The three items included in the final ACR classification set proved to be the most accurate ones in distinguishing patients from controls, and the combined presence of two out of three of these items achieved the best performance in terms of classification accuracy.[37]

Since their appearance, a number of criticisms have been raised regarding the methodology and the results obtained by the whole procedure. First of all, subjective complaints were excluded from the criteria set because of their low specificity. However, the AECG questionnaire for dry eye and dry mouth symptoms was used as an entry criterion for the enrollment into the SICCA cohort.[37]

Two disease classes seem to be too few when compared with the clinical spectrum of SS, which includes at least three disease classes, ie, patients with primary SS, patients with SS associated with other SADs, and patients with only sicca complaints without true SS. The SICCA cohort included only a few patients with SS associated with other SADs, and these patients were excluded from the analysis. Nevertheless the ACR preliminary criteria were proposed as a valid tool to classify even this kind of patients, who are well known for showing different patterns of presentation, according to the associated SADs.[39]

Another important point is represented by the inclusion in the ACR criteria of a positive ANA and RF, instead of anti-Ro/SSA and anti-La/SSB antibodies, as an alternative serologic item. This came as a result of a consensus decision of the SICCA experts that was taken even if this alternative item had not demonstrated a solid sensitivity or specificity.[37]

The SICCA group had adopted the Ocular Staining Score (OSS)[40] and proposed a cut-off value of at least three points for selecting patients with KCS related to SS. The OSS was proposed as an alternative test to the van Bijsterveld scoring system. Both tests are aimed at scoring epithelial lesions, which become evident by staining the corneal surface with fluorescein and the conjunctiva with lissamine green. The OSS score may vary from 0 to 12, whereas the range of the van Bijsterveld score is more restricted (from 0 to 9) and considers a score of four or more to be specific for SS-related KCS.[40] Hence it appears evident that the OSS cut-off value of three points is probably too low and less specific than a van Bijsterveld score of four when selecting potential patients with SS. Moreover, the Schirmer-I test, which is acknowledged to be more specific for SS than ocular dye tests,[37] was excluded from the ACR classification set. Consequently, the ACR criteria might impair the performance of the diagnostic approach to eye involvement.

## 5. COMPARISON OF THE NEW ACR CRITERIA WITH THE AECG CLASSIFICATION CRITERIA

The ACR criteria were tentatively validated by comparing their accuracy with that of the AECG classification criteria, which were considered to be the gold standard for the comparison.[37] This was decided because, as the authors pointed out, the AECG criteria had shown better accuracy than all of the criteria previously proposed.[7-13] The statistical comparison between the AECG criteria and the newly described criteria, performed on the whole SICCA cohort, demonstrated that there was a strong agreement between the two criteria sets ($k$ measure of agreement with the ACR criteria was 0.88).[37]

An additional comparison between the ACR and the AECG classification criteria sets was performed on a cohort of 646 patients at the Sjögren's Research Clinics, Oklahoma City, OK, USA. This comparison confirmed the strong agreement between the two classification criteria ($k$ measure of agreement was 0.81).[41] However, in both comparisons there were a certain number of discordant cases, ie, patient cases classified as having SS only by one of the two criteria sets. The number of discordant cases was small but not completely irrelevant (around 6% in the SICCA[37] cohort and 9% in the Oklahoma cohort[43]). The detailed analysis of these discordant cases gave the following results:

1. Some cases met the ACR criteria only thanks to the presence of the alternative serological item; therefore they were negative for anti-Ro/SSA and anti-La/SSB antibodies, and had positive RF and ANA results. Such cases amounted to a very small number (around 1% in both the whole SICCA and Oklahoma cohorts).
2. Most of the other patients who met only the ACR criteria did so because of the positivity of OSS (with negative van Bijsterveld score and Schirmer-I test); these cases represented 2.6% and 1.9% of the totality of the patients in the Oklahoma and SICCA cohorts, respectively.

3. The totality of patients who met only the AECG, but not the ACR criteria, met one of the mandatory criteria (presence of anti-Ro/SSA or anti-La/SSB antibodies, or an FS ≥1) and showed a positive result in one objective test for KCS, or a reduction of unstimulated salivary flow, in addition to both oral and ocular sicca symptoms. This population, consisting of patients with probable SS, was not so marginal, accounting for 5.4% of the whole Oklahoma cohort, while being less represented in the SICCA cohort (2.4%).[37,41]

An additional comparison between the two criteria sets was carried out in Brest, in a smaller cohort of patients suspected to have SS.[44] The main conclusions of this further study were that the AECG criteria were certainly more specific. This final result largely benefited from adding the Schirmer-I test and unstimulated saliva collection (not included in the ACR set of criteria). Conversely, the contribution of the alternative serological item (positive RF and positive ANA included in ACR criteria) resulted as irrelevant. As the authors stated, the ACR criteria seemed to be better suited for the selection of younger and early patients, even though some of the patients classified according to this criteria set had an uncertain diagnosis of SS when judged by an expert clinician.[42]

## 6. THE ACR-EULAR INITIATIVE

Two different criteria sets are presently available to classify patients with SS. This may cause further problems for the community of researchers and clinicians interested in this field. Cohorts of patients selected for clinical studies, through different methods, may not be equivalent in terms of disease features, and the results obtained in the clinical studies and therapeutic trials may not be entirely comparable. This is obviously a crucial issue, especially nowadays, when new therapies (namely biological agents), potentially effective in this (until now) orphan disorder, are at hand. Consequently, it is now a high priority for the SS scientific community to achieve international consensus on a single set of definitive classification criteria for SS.

To overcome this problem SICCA-ACR team and the European League Against Rheumatism (EULAR) Sjögren's Task Force decided to join the ACR-EULAR Sjögren's Syndrome Classification Criteria Working Group, with the objective of deriving a single set of classification criteria for SS from the existing highly concordant AECG and ACR criteria. After some preliminary meetings, all of the group participants agreed to adopt, for the development of the new ACR-EULAR classification criteria, the methodology used for the development and validation of the 2010 ACR-EULAR classification criteria for rheumatoid arthritis,[43] and the 2013 ACR-EULAR classification criteria for systemic sclerosis.[44] This methodology is based on multicriteria decision analysis (or conjoint analysis).[45] Both the ACR and EULAR organizations defined this statistical procedure as the anchor method to be used for developing classification criteria for rheumatic diseases.[46,47]

The different steps of this methodology can be summarized as follows:

1. Candidate items for the classification criteria are generated by using consensus methods (Delphi method) among experts.
2. Multicriteria decision analysis and multivariate logistic regression model are employed to reduce the number of candidate items and assign preliminary weight to each item. The derived classification system is then tested and adapted by using existing cohort data on SS cases and non-SS controls and compared against expert clinical judgment.
3. The classification criteria are finally tested in a validation cohort that is different from the derivation cohort used for the initial testing and adaptation of the criteria.

The ACR-EULAR working group, after having obtained the official patronage of both the ACR and EULAR organizations, is now actively working. The final result of this joint effort is going to be reached in a relatively short time.

## REFERENCES

1. Fox RJ. Sjögren's syndrome. *Lancet* 2005;**366**:321–31.
2. Brito-Zerón P, Ramos-Casals M, EULAR-SS task force group. Advances in the understanding and treatment of systemic complications in Sjögren's syndrome. *Curr Opin Rheumatol* 2014;**26**:520–7.
3. Kassan SS, Moutsopoulos HM. Clinical manifestations and early diagnosis of Sjögren syndrome. *Arch Intern Med* 2004;**164**:1275–84.
4. Fries JF, Hochberg MC, Medsger Jr TA, Hunder GG, Bombardier C. Criteria for rheumatic disease: different types and different functions. The American College of Rheumatology Diagnostic and Therapeutic Criteria Committee. *Arthritis Rheum* 1994;**37**:454–62.
5. Johnson SR, Goek ON, Singh-Grewal D, et al. Classification criteria in rheumatic diseases: a review of methodologic properties. *Arthritis Rheum* 2007;**57**:1119–33.
6. Fox RI, Saito I. Criteria for diagnosis of Sjögren's syndrome. *Rheum Dis North Am* 1994;**20**: 391–407.
7. Daniels TE, Silverman S, Michalski JP, Greenspan JS, Sylvester RA, Talal N. The oral component of Sjögren's syndrome. *Oral Surg Oral Med Oral Pathol* 1975;**39**:875–85.
8. Daniels TE. Labial salivary gland biopsy in Sjögren's syndrome: assessment as a diagnostic criterion in 362 suspected cases. *Arthritis Rheum* 1984;**27**:147–56.
9. Manthorpe R, Oxholm P, Prause JU, Schiodt M. The Copenhagen criteria for Sjögren's syndrome. *Scand J Rheumatol* 1986;(Suppl. 61):19–21.
10. Homma M, Tojo T, Akizuki M, Yamagata H. Criteria for Sjögren's syndrome in Japan. *Scand J Rheumatol* 1986;(Suppl. 61):26–7.
11. Skopouli FN, Drosos AA, Papaioannou T, Moutsopoulos HM. Preliminary diagnostic criteria for Sjögren's syndrome. *Scand J Rheumatol* 1986;(Suppl. 61):22–5.
12. Fox RI, Robinson CA, Curd JG, Kozin F, Howell FV. Sjögren's syndrome: proposed criteria for classification. *Arthritis Rheum* 1986;**29**:577–85.
13. Fujibayashi T, Sugai S, Myasaka N, Tojo T, Miyawaki S, Ichikawa Y, et al. Criteria for the diagnosis of Sjögren's syndrome [Japanese criteria III]. *Annu Rep Res Group Autoimm Dis* 1999:135–8.
14. Atkinson JC, Travis WD, Slocum L, Ebbs WL, Fox PC. Serum anti-SS-B/La and IgA rheumatoid factor are markers of salivary gland disease activity in primary Sjögren's syndrome. *Arthritis Rheum* 1992;**35**:1368–72.

15. Daniels TE, Witcher JP. Association of patterns of labial salivary gland inflammation with keratoconjunctivitis sicca: analysis of 618 patients with suspected Sjögren's syndrome. *Arthritis Rheum* 1994;**6**:869–77.

16. Workshop on diagnostic criteria for Sjögren's syndrome: I. Questionnaires for dry eye and dry mouth. II. Manual of methods and procedures. *Clin Exp Rheumatol* 1989;**7**:212–9.

17. Vitali C, Bombardieri S, Moutsopoulos HM, Balestrieri G, Bencivelli W, Bernstein RM, et al. Preliminary criteria for the classification of Sjögren's syndrome: results of a prospective concerted action supported by the European Community. *Arthritis Rheum* 1993;**36**:340–7.

18. Arnett FC, Edworthy SM, Bloch DA, McShane DJ, Fries JF, Cooper NS, et al. The 1987 Revised American Association criteria for classification of rheumatoid arthritis. *Arthritis Rheum* 1988;**31**:315–24.

19. Tan EM, Cohen AS, Fries JF, Masi AT, McShane DJ, Rothfield NF, et al. The 1982 revised criteria for the classification of systemic lupus erythematosus. *Arthritis Rheum* 1982;**25**:1271–7.

20. Vitali C, Bombardieri S, Moutsopoulos HM, Coll J, Gerli R, Hatron PY, et al. Assessment of the European classification criteria for Sjögren's syndrome in a series of clinically defined cases: results of a prospective multicentre study. The European Study Group on Diagnostic Criteria for Sjögren's Syndrome. *Ann Rheum Dis* 1996;**55**:116–21.

21. Fox RI, Saito I. Summary of the IVth International Sjögren's syndrome meeting. *Arthritis Rheum* 1994;**37**:771–2.

22. Fox RI. Fifth international symposium on Sjögren's syndrome. *Arthritis Rheum* 1996;**39**:195–6.

23. Vitali C, Bombardieri S, Jonsson R, Moutsopoulos HM, Alexander EL, Carson SE, et al. Classification criteria for Sjögren's syndrome: a revised version of the European criteria proposed by the American–European Consensus Group. *Ann Rheum Dis* 2002;**61**:554–8.

24. Ramos-Casals M, Garcia Carrasco M, Cervera R, Rosas J, Trejo O, Dela Red G, et al. Hepatitis C virus infection mimicking primary Sjögren's syndrome: a clinical and immunologic description of 35 cases. *Med Baltim* 2001;**80**:1–8.

25. Birlik M, Akar S, Gurler O, Sari I, Birlik B, Sarioglu S, et al. Prevalence of primary Sjögren's syndrome in Turkey: a population-based epidemiological study. *Int J Clin Pract* 2009;**63**:954–61.

26. Haugen AJ, Peen E, Hultén B, Johannessen AC, Brun JG, Halse AK, et al. Estimation of the prevalence of primary Sjögren's syndrome in two age-different community-based populations using two sets of classification criteria: the Hordaland Health Study. *Scand J Rheumatol* 2008;**37**:30–4.

27. Kabasakal Y, Kitapcioglu G, Turk T, Oder G, Durusoy R, Mete N, et al. The prevalence of Sjögren's syndrome in adult women. *Scand J Rheumatol* 2006;**35**:379–83.

28. Bjerrum KB. Keratoconjunctivitis sicca and primary Sjögren's syndrome in a Danish population aged 30–60 years. *Acta Opthalmol Scand* 1997;**75**:281–6.

29. Zhang NZ, Shi CS, Yao QP, Pan GX, Wang LL, Wen ZX, et al. Prevalence of primary Sjögren's syndrome in China. *J Rheumatol* 1995;**22**:659–61.

30. Alamanos Y, Tsifetaki N, Voulgari PV, Venetsanopoulos AI, Siozos C, Drosos AA. Epidemiology of primary Sjögren's syndrome in North-West of Greece, 1982–2003. *Rheumatol Oxf* 2006;**45**:187–91.

31. Trontzas PI, Adianakos AA. Sjögren's syndrome: a population-based study of prevalence in Greece: the ESORDIG study. *Ann Rheum Dis* 2005;**64**:1240–1.

32. Bowman SJ, Ibrahim GH, Holmes G, Hamburger J, Ainsworth JR. Estimating the prevalence among Caucasian women of primary Sjögren's syndrome in two general practices in Birmingham, UK. *Scand J Rheumatol* 2004;**33**:39–43.

33. Tomsic M, Logar D, Grmek M, Perkovic T, Kveder T. Prevalence of Sjögren's syndrome in Slovenia. *Rheumatology* 1999;**38**:164–70.

34. Thomas E, Hay EM, Hajeer A, Silman AJ. Sjögren's syndrome: a community-based study of prevalence and impact. *Br J Rheumatol* 1998;**37**:1069–76.

35. Dafni UG, Tzioufas AG, Staikos P, Skopouli FN, Moutsopoulos HM. Prevalence of Sjögren's syndrome in a closed rural community. *Ann Rheum Dis* 1997;**56**:521–5.

36. Jacobsson LT, Axell TE, Hansen BU, Henricsson VJ, Larsson A, Lieberkind K, et al. Dry eye and mouth: an epidemiological study in Swedish adults, with special reference to primary Sjögren's syndrome. *J Autoimm* 1989;**2**:521–7.

37. Shiboski SC, Shiboski CH, Criswell L, et al. American College of Rheumatology classification criteria for Sjögren's syndrome: a data-driven, expert consensus approach in the Sjögren's International Collaborative Clinical Alliance Cohort. *Arthritis Care Res* 2012;**64**:475–87.

38. Qu Y, Tan M, Kutner MH. Random effect models in latent class analysis for evaluating accuracy of diagnostic tests. *Biometrics* 1996;**52**:797–810.

39. Hernandez-Molina G, Avila-Casado C, Cárdenas-Velázquez F, Hernández-Hernández C, Calderillo ML, Marroquín V, et al. Similarities and differences between primary and secondary Sjögren's syndrome. *J Rheumatol* 2010;**37**:800–8.

40. Whitcher JP, Shiboski CH, Shiboski SC, Heidenreich AM, Kitagawa K, Zhang S, et al. Sjögren's International Collaborative Clinical Alliance Research Group. A simplified quantitative method for assessing keratoconjunctivitis sicca from the Sjögren's syndrome international registry. *Am J Ophthalmol* 2010;**149**:405–15.

41. Rasmussen A, Ice J, Li H, Grundahl K, Kelly JA, Radfar L, et al. Comparison of the American–European Consensus Group. Sjögren's syndrome classification criteria to newly proposed American College of Rheumatology criteria in a large, carefully characterized SICCA cohort. *Ann Rheum Dis* 2014;**73**:31–8.

42. Cornec D, Saraux A, Cochener B, Pers J-O, Jousse-Joulin S, Renaudineau Y, et al. Level of agreement between 2002 American–European consensus group and 2012 American College of Rheumatology classification criteria for Sjögren's syndrome and reasons for discrepancies. *Arthritis Res Ther*, 2014;**16**:R74.

43. Neogi T, Aletaha D, Silman AJ, Naden RL, Felson DT, Aggarwal R, et al. The 2010 American College of Rheumatology/European League against Rheumatism classification criteria for rheumatoid arthritis: phase 2 methodological report. *Arthritis Rheum* 2010;**62**:2582–91.

44. van den Hoogen F, Khanna D, Fransen J, Johnson SR, Baron M, Tyndall A, et al. 2013 classification criteria for systemic sclerosis: an American College of Rheumatology/European League against Rheumatism Collaborative Initiative. *Arthritis Rheum* 2013;**65**:2737–47.

45. Hansen P, Ombler F. A new method for scoring multi-attribute value models using pairwise rankings of alternatives. *J Multi-Crit Decis Anal* 2009;**15**:87–107.

46. Singh JA, Solomon DH, Dougados M, Felson D, Hawker G, Katz P, et al. Classification and response criteria subcommittee of the committee on quality measures, American College of Rheumatology: development of classification and response criteria for rheumatic diseases. *Arthritis Rheum* 2006;**55**:348–52.

47. Dougados M, Gossec L. Classification criteria for rheumatic diseases: why and how? *Arthritis Rheum* 2007;**57**:1112–5.

Chapter 5

# Imaging Procedures Useful for the Diagnosis of Sjögren's Syndrome: Abnormalities of the Major Salivary Glands

V. Devauchelle-Pensec

*La Cavale Blanche University Hospital, Brest, France; University of Western Brittany (UBO), Brest, France*

Primary Sjögren's syndrome (pSS) is an autoimmune disease affecting predominantly the salivary glands. Most of the classification criteria have considered involvement of salivary glands as a major sign of the disease.[1–3] This involvement can be assessed by imaging procedures such as sialography or scialoscintigraphy (considered in the classification criteria currently used), which were the most commonly used procedures until 1990.[4] More recently the development of magnetic resonance imaging (MRI) and ultrasonography (US)[5] offers the opportunity to visualize specific abnormalities of major salivary glands using noninvasive and nonionizing procedures. Because of its easy accessibility and ability to save time in comparison with MRI, US appears to be the major imaging procedure used to classify Sjögren's syndrome[6] that has demonstrated its capacity to improve the diagnostic value of American-European Consensus Group (AECG) and American College of Rheumatology (ACR) criteria.[7,8] MRI has value for complications such as duct obstruction, abscess, or lymphoma. Positron emission tomography/computed tomography (PET/CT) scan should be evaluated to detect nodal and extranodal location.

## 1. SIALOGRAPHY

### 1.1 Procedure

Sialography is based on the injection of a dye into the salivary duct orifice (Wharton or Stensen duct) in order to visualize the entire ductal pattern.[9] It can induce discomfort for the patient, but the use of delicate catheters and gentle techniques can make the procedure painless.[4] The sialograph is evaluated with panoramic, posteroanterior, or lateral views of the mandible. It has a great sensitivity to detect

Sjögren's Syndrome. http://dx.doi.org/10.1016/B978-0-12-803604-4.00005-8

stone blocking of the duct. The presence of acute salivary gland infection and sialolithiasis of the duct, as well as allergy to contrast material, are contraindications for sialography. This procedure was commonly used until 1980 in Sjögren's syndrome (SS). However, the development of sialoendoscopy for the treatment of salivary gland obstruction[10] revitalized this radiographic technique.

## 1.2  Validity for Sjögren's Syndrome

Sialography has been used for several years in SS and allows classification of patients with abnormal patterns, although sialographic changes in SS are not specific. The major excretory ducts can be normal but also atrophic with intraglandular diffuse collections that persist during the evacuation time of the procedure. Stages are described as normal with no contrast media collection or with punctuate, globular, cavitary, or destructive stages.[11,12] The punctuated sialograph with sialectasias is considered as typical of SS. At a later stage, the cysts are enlarged and the gland is atrophic with complete destruction of the glandular parenchyma. Results of sialography correlated well with the diagnosis of SS, the presence of autoantibodies, or salivary gland biopsy (SGB) but appear to be less specific than labial SGB.[13,14] Following these results,[15,16] parotid sialography was included in the consensual classification criteria in 2002 and is considered abnormal if it shows diffuse sialectasias. However, this procedure is uncomfortable and can sometimes increase the sicca symptoms. Less invasive procedures, such as US, are now recommended.[17]

## 2. SIALOSCINTIGRAPHY

### 2.1  Procedure

Sialoscintigraphy is based on a scan after the injection of radioactive isotopes into the bloodstream (Fig. 5.1).[18] Technetium-99m is the most commonly used isotope, and is injected intravenously with simultaneous multiframe dynamic

(A)                                    (B)

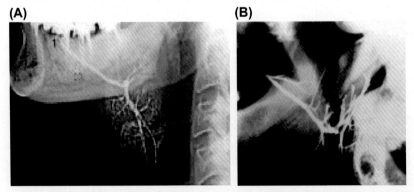

FIGURE 5.1   (A) Normal sialogram of the submandibular gland. (B) Typical lateral parotid sialogram in Sjögren (ie, four stages: punctate sialectasia; globular sialectasia; cavitary sialectasia; destructive sialectasia with complete loss of gland architecture).

acquisition performed for 20–40 min. The scintiscan is considered for each gland using qualitative or quantitative analysis and evaluates the uptake, concentration, and excretion of the radioisotope by the major salivary gland with a gamma camera. The maximum uptake, the ratio between the mean counts in the gland at 20 min and the background activity and outflow efficiency can be calculated. Lemon juice stimulation can be performed for SS. It reveals the functional activity of the gland more than anatomical structures.

## 2.2 Validity for Sjögren's Syndrome

The results of sialoscintigraphy, including delayed uptake, reduced concentration, and/or delayed excretion of tracer, are part of the 2002 classification criteria. The normal uptake of the radioisotopes in the salivary glands is diminished or patchy in SS, with a decrease in both excretion and uptake by the four glands.[19] Most studies demonstrated its diagnostic accuracy with a good correlation with patient's clinical symptoms of dryness, salivary flow rate, and sialography.[20] Milic et al.[21] evaluated its positive and negative predictive values (VVP and NPV), taking minor SGB as gold standard. She found VVP=74.3% and VPN=72.3%, and a good correlation with SGB or ultrasonography.[22] Sialoscintigraphy has not been so extensively evaluated in SS as sialography and some uncertainty persists concerning the most useful parameters for detection of impaired parenchymatous function of major salivary glands.[23–25]

## 3. ULTRASONOGRAPHY

### 3.1 Procedure

US of the major salivary glands has been used in SS since 1980,[5,26,27] but has been extensively developed in recent years. It concerns the parotid and submandibular glands that can be explored using superficial linear probes with a frequency varying from 5 to 15 MHz (Fig. 5.2). The pressure on the probe must be minimal to avoid any bias. The submandibular glands are scanned with the patient lying in the supine position with the neck hyperextended and the head slightly turned to the opposite side. The parotid glands are commonly scanned in both the longitudinal and transverse planes, and the submandibular glands in the longitudinal plane (Fig. 5.3). US is performed almost exclusively in B mode to visualize parenchymal abnormalities. Power or pulsed Doppler alone or combined to B mode can be used to obtain better sensitivity, and the resistive or pulsatility index reveals gland vascularizations.[28–30] However, these techniques required standardization. US is a noninvasive, nonionizing technique to study salivary glands that requires trained experts.

### 3.2 Validity for Sjögren's Syndrome

Echostructure abnormality of the salivary gland is not included in the recent classification criteria but is strongly associated with the diagnosis of the disease,

**(A)**  **(B)**

**(C)**

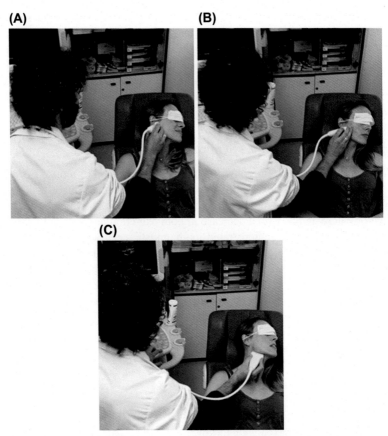

**FIGURE 5.2** Ultrasonography of the salivary glands. (A) Parotid. (B) Submandibular.

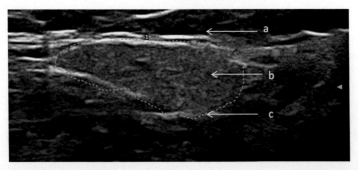

**FIGURE 5.3** Normal submandibular gland, longitudinal scan with the superficialis fascia (A), the homogeneous glandular parenchyma (B), and the border (C).

the salivary test, the presence of autoantibodies, the SGB, and the European League Against Rheumatism Sjögren's Syndrome Disease Activity index [30–33] and it has a good construct validity with a high sensitivity compared with other diagnosing methods.[34–36] More interestingly, it has demonstrated its capacity to

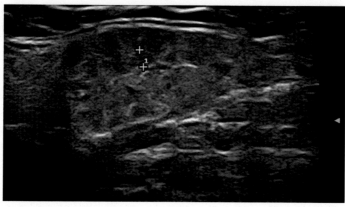

**FIGURE 5.4** Submandibular gland in Sjögren's disease with rare hyperechoic bands and multiple hypoechoic area.

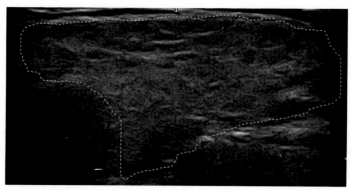

**FIGURE 5.5** Parotid gland in Sjögren's disease: longitudinal scan with hyperechoic bands and hypoechoic area.

improve the diagnostic value of AECG and ACR criteria[7,8] in newly diagnosed disease[8,33] as well as in established SS.

Several parenchymal abnormalities have been described with different scoring (echogenicity; homogeneity; presence of hypoechoic areas within the glands or hyperechoic bands (Figs. 5.4 and 5.5); clearness of the borders of the glands, presence of lymph nodes, and calcifications). The most relevant is probably the inhomogeneity of the parenchyma. The ability of US to detect lymphoma in SS has not yet been explored but large lymphomatous nodes can be suggestive or can guide biopsy.[5] However, MRI and biopsy are still the reference for this diagnosis. Some points have to be considered in order to improve its usefulness in SS. A general agreement on a US score is now required to have similar evaluation of SS, because its specificity must be measured, for example, in immunoglobulin (Ig) G4 disease[37] (in which recent studies demonstrated typical patterns) or in connective disease. In addition, the capacity of US to detect change (during the evolution of the disease or after treatment) has been poorly investigated,[38,39] although it could be a major element in evaluating treatment efficacy in SS[40] using the Sjögren's Syndrome Responder index.

## 4. MAGNETIC RESONANCE IMAGING

### 4.1 Procedure

MRI is also a noninvasive, nonionizing procedure that reveals characteristic changes of major salivary glands in SS.[41] It is more commonly performed on parotid glands for anatomical analysis, and sometimes coupled with sialography. Both axial and coronal T1 weighted and T2 scans are performed with a conventional spin echo structure and slice thickness of less than 5 mm. Intravenous injection of a contrast medium increases the detection of abnormalities but is not mandatory for the diagnosis of Sjögren (Fig. 5.6).

### 4.2 Validity for Sjögren's Syndrome

MRI is also a noninvasive procedure that reveals characteristic changes of major salivary glands in SS.[41] It has an excellent agreement with US in established pSS patients, whereas correlation was slightly decreased when compared with patients with sicca symptoms.[42–44] Parotid or submandibular glands involvement may give a "salt-and-pepper" appearance or a honeycomb appearance. Lacrimal glands may have possible change in size associated with fat deposition. Results of the MRI are associated with the presence of autoantibodies. A scoring system has been described[45] and modified[43] based on homogeneity of the parenchyma and on nodular structure. Takagi et al.[46] published a score based on three grades that considered parenchymal heterogeneity, fat infiltration, lymphocytic infiltrates and acinocanalar destruction. MRI has a good reliability and is considered as the reference imaging technique for the detection

**(A)**          **(B)**

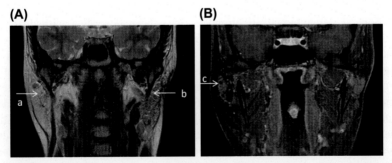

FIGURE 5.6   (A) MRI of salivary glands (coronal, T2, fast spin echo), and (B) After gadolinium injection. Right parotid gland with fat infiltrate and cyst (a). Left parotid gland with surgical sequelae and cysts (b). Moderate enhancement after gadolinium injection (c).

of intraparotideal tumors and for lymphoma, which always require histological confirmation. This technique in SS is interesting for diagnosis but because of inaccessibility, US is preferred.

## 5. ELASTOMETRY

### 5.1 Procedure

Based on the development of US, some techniques exist to objectively appreciate the real consistency of a structure. There are several types of elastographic examinations that were first developed for hepatitis, fibrosis, or tumors.[47] The "real-time" elastography provides semiquantitative results but can be operator-dependent (that is, the modality by which the region of interest is being pressed or the experience of the sonographer). Another elastographic procedure is the shear wave elastography, where the image is produced by successive pulses of different acoustic power ("pushing" waves). This technique has been used to discriminate between benign and malignant nodules. The acoustic radiation force impulse (ARFI) technique is based on a mechanical excitation of the tissue using short-duration acoustic pulses (<1 ms) that generate localized displacement within the selected region.

### 5.2 Validity for Sjögren's Syndrome

Elastometry can be applied to salivary glands[48,49] and more recently has been described in SS.[50] Knopf et al. evaluated shear wave velocities in 70 patients with SS as compared with healthy controls using a probe 9–14 MHz. They found a good reliability of the ARFI results for the parotid gland but modest results for submandibular glands. Healthy patients had mean shear wave velocities on parotid gland of 1870.02 m/s. In SS, velocities were significantly higher, with a mean of 2860.07 m/s for parotid glands. The cutoff for pathologic induration of the parotid gland in pSS was ≥2.4 m/s (AUC 0.84; 95% interval confidence: 0.78–0.90; $p < 0.0001$), with subsequent diagnostic sensitivity and specificity pSS of 77% and 56%, respectively.

However, these procedures need further validation in SS. Reliabilities and internal validity must be confirmed, but they could be interesting methods of evaluating the severity of the disease and treatment efficacy.

## 6. FDG PET/CT IMAGING

### 6.1 Procedure

Fluorodeoxyglucose positron emission tomography/computed tomography (FDG PET/CT) is widely used to evaluate therapeutic response in oncological diseases.[51] Tracer is intravenously infused in the patient and acquisition is performed after 60 min, coupled with CT or MRI. Several tracers exist with different avidities. Patients are scanned from the base of the skull to the mid-thigh

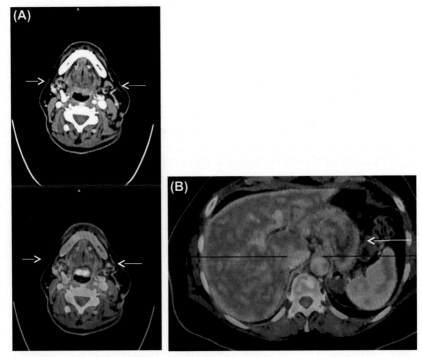

**FIGURE 5.7**  PET/CT scan with parotid glands and adenopathy in mucosa-associated lymphoid tissue (MALT) syndrome. (A) Submandibular adenopathies in MALT syndrome (axial plan); (B) gastric uptake in MALT syndrome.

in the arms-down position and the time for the PET and CT acquisition is approximately 1 h. Data is acquired in the three-dimensional mode and, for attenuation correction, is reconstructed using CT data and an algorithm, and analyzed using software by an experienced nuclear medicine physician. Regions of interest can be drawn. Semiquantitative FDG uptake is calculated and expressed as a standard uptake value.

## 6.2  Validity for SS

The few studies performed to validate usefulness of PET/CT for mucosa-associated lymphoid tissue (MALT) lymphoma suggested that delayed time-point imaging may improve sensitivity of FDG PET in MALT lymphoma[52] to detect nodal and extranodal localizations (Fig. 5.7). However, FDG avidity is different according to the location, because gastric MALT lymphoma is commonly more superficial with lower avidity.[53]

Data concerning the usefulness of PET in SS disease is limited[54] but should be evaluated for suspected lymphoproliferative disorder, an IgG4-related syndrome,[55] or multisystemic involvement with caution as a result of ionizing induced by this procedure.

## 7. CONCLUSION

Imaging procedures are very helpful to analyze objective parenchymal abnormalities of the salivary gland in SS and probably in the future to evaluate treatment efficacy. US is now one of the most important because of its accessibility and capacity to improve the sensitivity of the classification criteria. Trained experts are necessary to validate this tool as an outcome measure in SS.

## REFERENCES

1. Shiboski SC, Shiboski CH, Criswell L, Baer A, Challacombe S, Lanfranchi H, et al. American College of Rheumatology classification criteria for Sjögren's syndrome: a data-driven, expert consensus approach in the Sjögren's International Collaborative Clinical Alliance cohort. *Arthritis Care Res* 2012;**64**:475–7.

2. Tsuboi H, Hagiwara S, Asashima H, Umehara H, Kawakami A, Nakamura H, et al. Validation of different sets of criteria for the diagnosis of Sjögren's syndrome in Japanese patients. *Mod Rheumatol* 2013;**23**:219–25.

3. Vitali C, Bombardieri S, Jonsson R, Moutsopoulos HM, Alexander EL, Carsons SE, et al. Classification criteria for Sjögren's syndrome: a revised version of the European criteria proposed by the American-European Consensus Group. *Ann Rheum Dis* 2002;**61**:554–8.

4. Kalk WW, Vissink A, Spijkervet FK, Möller JM, Roodenburg JL. Morbidity from parotid sialography. *Oral Surg Oral Med Oral Pathol Oral Radiol Endod* 2001;**92**:572–5.

5. De Vita S, Lorenzon G, Rossi G, Sabella M, Fossaluzza V. Salivary gland echography in primary and secondary Sjögren's syndrome. *Clin Exp Rheumatol* 1992;**10**:351–6.

6. Vitali C, Carotti M, Salaffi F. Is it the time to adopt salivary gland ultrasonography as an alternative diagnostic tool for the classification of patients with Sjögren's syndrome? Comment on the article by Cornec et al. *Arthritis Rheum* 2013;**65**:1950.

7. Cornec D, Jousse-Joulin S, Marhadour T, Pers JO, Boisramé-Gastrin S, Renaudineau Y, et al. Salivary gland ultrasonography improves the diagnostic performance of the 2012 American College of Rheumatology classification criteria for Sjögren's syndrome. *Rheumatology* 2014;**53**:1604–7.

8. Cornec D, Jousse-Joulin S, Pers JO, Marhadour T, Cochener B, Boisramé-Gastrin S, et al. Contribution of salivary gland ultrasonography to the diagnosis of Sjögren's syndrome: toward new diagnostic criteria? *Arthritis Rheum* 2013;**65**:216–25.

9. Hasson O. Modern sialography for screening of salivary gland obstruction. *J Oral Maxillofac Surg* 2010;**68**:276–80.

10. Hasson O. Sialoendoscopy and sialography: strategies for assessment and treatment of salivary gland obstructions. *J Oral Maxillofac Surg* 2007;**65**:300–4.

11. Holt JF. Sialography. *Radiology* 1957;**68**:584–5.

12. Rubin P, Holt JF. Secretory sialography in diseases of the major salivary glands. *Am J Roentgenol Radium Ther Nucl Med* 1957;**77**:575–98.

13. Daniels TE, Benn DK. Is sialography effective in diagnosing the salivary component of Sjögren's syndrome? *Adv Dent Res* 1996;**10**:25–8.

14. Lindvall AM, Jonsson R. The salivary gland component of Sjögren's syndrome: an evaluation of diagnostic methods. *Oral Surg Oral Med Oral Pathol* 1986;**62**:32–42.

15. Vitali C, Monti P, Giuggioli C, Tavoni A, Neri R, Genovesi-Ebert F, et al. Parotid sialography and lip biopsy in the evaluation of oral component in Sjögren's syndrome. *Clin Exp Rheumatol* 1989;**7**:131–5.

16. Vitali C, Tavoni A, Simi U, Marchetti G, Vigorito P, d'Ascanio A, et al. Parotid sialography and minor salivary gland biopsy in the diagnosis of Sjögren's syndrome: a comparative study of 84 patients. *J Rheumatol* 1988;**15**:262–7.

17. Takagi Y, Kimura Y, Nakamura H, Sasaki M, Eguchi K, Nakamura T. Salivary gland ultrasonography: can it be an alternative to sialography as an imaging modality for Sjögren's syndrome? *Ann Rheum Dis* 2010;**69**:1321–4.

18. Van den Akker HP, Sokole EB, van der Schoot JB. Origin and location on the oral activity in sequential salivary gland scintigraphy with 99mTc-pertechnetate. *J Nucl Med* 1976;**17**:959–64.

19. Aung W, Yamada I, Umehara I, Ohbayashi N, Yoshino N, Shibuya H. Sjögren's syndrome: comparison of assessments with quantitative salivary gland scintigraphy and contrast sialography. *J Nucl Med* 2000;**41**:257–62.

20. Schall GL, Anderson LG, Wolf RO, Herdt JR, Tarpley Jr TM, Cummings NA, et al. Xerostomia in Sjögren's syndrome: evaluation by sequential salivary scintigraphy. *JAMA* 1971;**216**: 2109–16.

21. Milic VD, Petrovic RR, Boricic IV, Marinkovic-Eric J, Radunovic GL, Jeremic PD, et al. Diagnostic value of salivary gland ultrasonographic scoring system in primary Sjögren's syndrome: a comparison with scintigraphy and biopsy. *J Rheumatol* 2009;**36**:1495–500.

22. Milic V, Petrovic R, Boricic I, Radunovic G, Marinkovic-Eric J, Jeremic P, et al. Ultrasonography of major salivary glands could be an alternative tool to sialoscintigraphy in the American-European classification criteria for primary Sjögren's syndrome. *Rheumatol* 2012;**51**:1081–5.

23. Daniels TE, Powell MR, Sylvester RA, Talal N. An evaluation of salivary scintigraphy in Sjögren's syndrome. *Arthritis Rheum* 1979;**22**:809–14.

24. Hermann GA, Vivino FB, Shnier D, Krumm RP, Mayrin V, Shore JB. Variability of quantitative scintigraphic salivary indices in normal subjects. *J Nucl Med* 1998;**39**:1260–3.

25. Kalk WW, Vissink A, Spijkervet FK, Bootsma H, Kallenberg CG, Roodenburg JL. Parotid sialography for diagnosing Sjögren syndrome. *Oral Surg Oral Med Oral Pathol Oral Radiol Endod* July 2002;**91**(1):131–7.

26. de Clerck LS, Corthouts R, Francx L, Brussaard C, de Schepper A, Vercruysse HA, et al. Ultrasonography and computer tomography of the salivary glands in the evaluation of Sjögren's syndrome: comparison with parotid sialography. *J Rheumatol* 1988;**15**:1777–81.

27. Kawamura H, Taniguchi N, Itoh K, Kano S. Salivary gland echography in patients with Sjögren's syndrome. *Arthritis Rheum* 1990;**33**:505–10.

28. Jousse-Joulin S, Devauchelle-Pensec V, Morvan J, Guias B, Pennec Y, Pers JO, et al. Ultrasound assessment of salivary glands in patients with primary Sjögren's syndrome treated with rituximab: quantitative and Doppler waveform analysis. *Biologics* 2007;**1**:311–9.

29. Martinoli C, Derchi LE, Solbiati L, Rizzatto G, Silvestri E, Giannoni M. Color Doppler sonography of salivary glands. *AJR Am J Roentgenol* 1994;**163**:933–41.

30. Shimizu M, Okamura K, Yoshiura K, Ohyama Y, Nakamura S. Sonographic diagnosis of Sjögren syndrome: evaluation of parotid gland vascularity as a diagnostic tool. *Oral Surg Oral Med Oral Pathol Oral Radiol Endod* 2008;**106**:587–94.

31. Ariji Y, Ohki M, Eguchi K, Izumi M, Ariji E, Mizokami A, et al. Texture analysis of sonographic features of the parotid gland in Sjögren's syndrome. *AJR Am J Roentgenol* 1996;**166**:935–41.

32. Hocevar A, Ambrozic A, Rozman B, Kveder T, Tomsic M. Ultrasonographic changes of major salivary glands in primary Sjögren's syndrome: diagnostic value of a novel scoring system. *Rheumatol* 2005;**44**:768–72.

33. Baldini C, Luciano N, Tarantini G, Pascale R, Sernissi F, Mosca M, et al. Salivary gland ultrasonography: a highly specific tool for the early diagnosis of primary Sjögren's syndrome. *Arthritis Res Ther* 2015;**17**:146.

34. Hammenfors DS, Brun JG, Jonsson R, Jonsson MV. Diagnostic utility of major salivary gland ultrasonography in primary Sjögren's syndrome. *Clin Exp Rheumatol* 2015;**33**:56–62.
35. Theander E, Mandl T. Primary Sjögren's syndrome: diagnostic and prognostic value of salivary gland ultrasonography using a simplified scoring system. *Arthritis Care Res Hob* 2014;**66**:1102–7.
36. Jousse-Joulin S, Milic V, Jonsson MV, Plagou A, Theander E, Luciano N, et al. Is salivary gland ultrasonography a useful tool in Sjögren's syndrome? A systematic review. *Rheumatology (Oxford)* May 2016;**55**(5):789–800. http://dx.doi.org/10.1093/rheumatology/kev385. [Epub 2015 Dec 14].
37. Shimizu M, Okamura K, Kise Y, Takeshita Y, Furuhashi H, Weerawanich W, et al. Effectiveness of imaging modalities for screening IgG4-related dacryoadenitis and sialadenitis (Mikulicz's disease) and for differentiating it from Sjögren's syndrome (SS), with an emphasis on sonography. *Arthritis Res Ther* 2015;**17**:223.
38. Devauchelle-Pensec V, Gottenberg JE, Jousse-Joulin S, Berthelot JM, Perdriger A, Hachulla E, et al. Which and how many patients should be included in randomised controlled trials to demonstrate the efficacy of biologics in primary Sjögren's syndrome? *PLoS One* 2015;**10**:e0133907.
39. Jousse-Joulin S, Devauchelle-Pensec V, Cornec D, Marhadour T, Bressollette L, Gestin S, et al. Brief report: ultrasonographic assessment of salivary gland response to rituximab in primary Sjögren's syndrome. *Arthritis Rheumatol* 2015;**67**:1623–8.
40. Cornec D, Devauchelle-Pensec V, Mariette X, Jousse-Joulin S, Berthelot JM, Perdriger A. Development of the Sjögren's Syndrome Responder Index: a data-driven composite endpoint for assessing treatment efficacy. *Rheumatol* 2015;**54**:1699–708.
41. Traxler M, Hajek P, Solar P, Ulm C. Magnetic resonance in lesions of the parotid gland. *Int J Oral Maxillofac Surg* 1991;**20**:170–4.
42. El Miedany YM, Ahmed I, Mourad HG, Mehanna AN, Aty SA, Gamal HM, et al. Quantitative ultrasonography and magnetic resonance imaging of the parotid gland: can they replace the histopathologic studies in patients with Sjögren's syndrome? *Jt Bone Spine* 2004;**71**:29–38.
43. Makula E, Pokorny G, Kiss M, Vörös E, Kovács L, Kovács A, et al. The place of magnetic resonance and ultrasonographic examinations of the parotid gland in the diagnosis and follow-up of primary Sjögren's syndrome. *Rheumatol* 2000;**39**:97–104.
44. Niemelä RK, Takalo R, Pääkkö E, Suramo I, Päivänsalo M, Salo T, et al. Ultrasonography of salivary glands in primary Sjögren's syndrome: a comparison with magnetic resonance imaging and magnetic resonance sialography of parotid glands. *Rheumatol* 2004;**43**:875–9.
45. Späth M, Krüger K, Dresel S, Grevers G, Vogl T, Schattenkirchner M. Magnetic resonance imaging of the parotid gland in patients with Sjögren's syndrome. *J Rheumatol* 1991;**18**:1372–8.
46. Takagi Y, Sumi M, Sumi T, Ichikawa Y, Nakamura T. MR microscopy of the parotid glands in patients with Sjogren's syndrome: quantitative MR diagnostic criteria. *AJNR Am J Neuroradiol* 2005;**26**(5):1207–14.
47. Westerland O, Howlett D. Sonoelastography techniques in the evaluation and diagnosis of parotid neoplasms. *Eur Radiol* 2012;**22**:966–9.
48. Dumitriu D, Dudea SM, Botar-Jid C, Băciuț G. Ultrasonographic and sonoelastographic features of pleomorphic adenomas of the salivary glands. *Med Ultrason* 2010;**12**:175–83.
49. Badea AF, Tamas Szora A, Ciuleanu E, Chioreanu I, Băciuț G, Lupșor Platon M, et al. ARFI quantitative elastography of the submandibular glands: normal measurements and the diagnosis value of the method in radiation submaxillitis. *Med Ultrason* 2013;**15**:173–9.
50. Knopf A, Hofauer B, Thürmel K, Meier R, Stock K, Bas M, et al. Diagnostic utility of acoustic radiation force impulse (ARFI) imaging in primary Sjögren's syndrome. *Eur Radiol* 2015;**25**:3027–34.

51. Barrington SF, Mikhaeel NG, Kostakoglu L, Meignan M, Hutchings M, Müeller SP, et al. Role of imaging in the staging and response assessment of lymphoma: consensus of the International Conference on Malignant Lymphomas Imaging working group. *J Clin Oncol* 2014;**32**:3048–58.

52. Mayerhoefer ME, Giraudo C, Senn D, Hartenbach M, Weber M, Rausch I, et al. Does delayed-time-point imaging improve 18F-FDG-PET in patients with MALT lymphoma? Observations in a series of 13 patients. *Clin Nucl Med* 2015. [Epub ahead of print].

53. Carrillo-Cruz E, Marín-Oyaga VA, de la Cruz Vicente F, Borrego-Dorado I, Ruiz Mercado M, Acevedo Báñez I, et al. Role of 18F-FDG-PET/CT in the management of marginal zone B cell lymphoma. *Hematol Oncol* 2014. [Epub ahead of print].

54. Sharma P, Chatterjee P. 18F-FDG PET/CT in multisystem Sjögren syndrome. *Clin Nucl Med* 2015;**40**:e293–4.

55. Ebbo M, Grados A, Guedj E, Gobert D, Colavolpe C, Zaidan M, et al. Usefulness of 2-[$^{18}$F]-fluoro-2-deoxy-D-glucose-positron emission tomography/computed tomography for staging and evaluation of treatment response in IgG4-related disease: a retrospective multicenter study. *Arthritis Care Res* 2014;**66**:86–96.

Chapter 6

# Sjögren's Syndrome–Associated Lymphoma

S. Gandolfo, L. Quartuccio, S. De Vita
*Udine University Hospital, Udine, Italy*

## 1. INTRODUCTION

Sjögren's syndrome (SS) is an autoimmune systemic disease associated with B-cell lymphoproliferation and an increased risk of B-cell non-Hodgkin lymphoma (NHL) development compared with the general population.[1–4]

NHLs are a highly heterogeneous group of malignancies that originate in lymphatic hematopoietic tissue, classified into B-cell and T-cell lymphomas, which account for about 90% and 10% of lymphomas respectively. The distinct subtypes of NHL show significant differences in epidemiological and geographical distribution and in histological patterns, suggesting a potential interplaying role of many different factors, such as infectious triggers, individual genetic status, and environment influences, in the development of NHL. Despite this heterogeneity, new insights into NHL etiology have focused on possible underlying common mechanisms, considering immune modulation and chronic antigenic stimulation as the main shared basis of NHL pathophysiology.[5]

The association between autoimmune chronic inflammatory diseases and NHL has been demonstrated by several studies.[6–9] In autoimmune disorders, an antigen-driven chronic stimulation in the context of specific genetic background would play a central role in generating and perpetuating a clonal lymphocytic expansion through a multistep oncogenic process, leading to an overt malignant disease at the end. The sustained risk of lymphoma observed in chronic autoimmune conditions over time, especially in SS, and the time-dependent increase of malignant transformation risk, strongly support this hypothesis.

A recent pooled analysis,[6] of 8692 NHL cases and 9260 controls from 14 studies (1988–2007) within the International Lymphoma Epidemiology Consortium, evaluated the interaction between immune system genetic variants and autoimmune conditions in NHL risk. The authors confirmed that autoimmune conditions mediated by B-cell responses were associated with increased NHL risk, specifically diffuse large B-cell lymphoma (DLBCL) (odds ratio [OR] = 3.11, 95% confidence interval [CI]: 2.25, 4.30) and marginal zone B-cell

*Sjögren's Syndrome.* http://dx.doi.org/10.1016/B978-0-12-803604-4.00006-X

lymphoma (MZBCL) (OR=5.80, 95% CI: 3.82, 8.80), whereas those mediated by T-cell responses were associated with peripheral T-cell lymphoma (OR=2.14, 95% CI: 1.35, 3.38). Moreover, in the presence of the rs1800629 AG/AA genotype of tumor necrosis factor (TNF) gene, the risk of NHL in B cell-mediated autoimmune conditions increased (OR=3.27, 95% CI: 2.07, 5.16; P-interaction=0.03).

## 2. EPIDEMIOLOGY AND HISTOLOGICAL SUBTYPES OF LYMPHOMA IN SJÖGREN'S SYNDROME

The analysis of NHL risk in different large cohorts of patients with autoimmune disease shows the highest risk in SS and in cryoglobulinemic vasculitis (CV) compared with the other autoimmune diseases. In SS, 6.1- to 44.4-fold increased risk of NHL was observed and followed by much lower risk in systemic lupus erythematosus (SLE) and rheumatoid arthritis.[1,2,9–11] The lifetime risk of NHL in SS is about 5% in most studies. It has become clear that the occurrence of lymphoma is a somewhat later complication of SS, with a median time from diagnosis of 7.5 years in the multicenter study by Voulgarelis et al.[12] In this study the incidence of lymphoma in primary SS (pSS) was estimated to be 4.3%. No gender differences in lymphoma evolution have been reported in a recent meta-analysis.

SS has been linked to an increased risk of specific subtypes of NHL, ie, MZBCL, with the mucosa-associated lymphoid tissue (MALT) lymphoma being much more common than the nodal MZBCL, and the more aggressive DLBCL. The distribution of these subtypes is not homogeneous in different cohorts of SS patients but MALT NHL has been widely recognized as the most common subtype.[1,2,13]

In the pooled analysis of autoimmune conditions and the risk of NHL subtypes conducted within the InterLymph Consortium,[7] SS was associated with a ninefold increase in risk of DLBCL (OR 8.92; 95% CI, 3.83–20.7) and with a 30-fold increase in risk of MZBCL (OR 30.6; 95% CI, 12.3–74.6), with a 1000-fold increased risk when the parotid gland MALT lymphoma was considered in detail (OR=995; 95% CI, 216–4596).

In a Swedish registry-based study,[9] the predominance of the DLBCL subtype has been reported. Trigger stimuli of lymphomagenesis in different geographic regions were speculated. However, in a large multicenter European analysis of SS-associated NHL by Voulgarelis et al.,[14] there was no difference in the distribution of different subtypes and grades of SS lymphoma between the north and south of Europe.

Whereas the multistep evolution of lymphoproliferative lesions in SS patients toward an overt MALT lymphoma has been widely studied, the development of DLBCL in the context of SS still remains ill-defined. Of note, it has been recently demonstrated that DLBCL may arise from the same B-cell clone of a previous indolent low-grade lymphoma, especially from a preexisting

MALT lymphoma, with the addition of genetic alterations, finally resulting in a high-grade and more aggressive malignant process. Thus the development of DLBCL complicating the course of SS may occur as an evolution of an indolent NHL, especially of the MALT type.[15,16]

SS patients with NHL have an increased mortality compared with the general population. A large retrospective Greek study[12] evaluated the outcome of 53 B-cell NHL cases in a cohort of 584 patients with pSS diagnosis. The median age at NHL diagnosis was 54 years (range, 28–90 years) and the median period from diagnosis of SS to NHL was 11 years (range, 1–23 years). Age and sex were not significantly different compared with the SS population without lymphoma. Thirty-one NHLs (59%) were of the MALT type, 8 (15%) DLBCL, 8 (15%) nodal marginal zone lymphomas (NMZLs), and 6 (11%) other lymphomas. The overall survival for the entire NHL cohort was 0.96 (95% CI, 0.83–0.99) at 3 years and 0.92 (95% CI, 0.76–0.97) at 5 years. The actual overall survival at 3 years was 0.97 for patients with MALT lymphoma, 0.80 for those with NMZL, and 1.0 for those with DLBCL (with a marked improvement from 0.37 to 1.0 after the introduction of rituximab in the management of DLBCL).

In this study the age/sex-adjusted standardized mortality ratio (SMR) of the SS-NHL group compared with the general population in Greece was estimated at 3.25 (95% CI, 1.32–6.76), and the SMR of pSS without NHL was 1.08 (95% CI, 0.79–1.45), comparable to the general population. Notably, in another Greek study, Skopouli et al.[17] demonstrated that in SS the SMR increased to 2.07 (95% CI, 1.03–3.71) only in the presence of adverse predictors of NHL, such as purpura, mixed cryoglobulinemia and low C4 levels. When patients with adverse predictors were excluded from the analysis, the mortality rate of pSS was the same as the general population (SMR 1.02).

In a Swedish prospective cohort study,[18] excess mortality in pSS was found only for the subgroup of patients with a lymphoid malignancy (cause-specific SMR 7.89 [95% CI 2.89–17.18]), corresponding to 2.53 excess deaths per 1000 person-years at risk. Overall, no increased mortality has been found in SS patients without lymphoma, compared with the general population.

All this data demonstrate that malignant lymphomas have a very high impact on SS survival and mortality, supporting the efforts to identify the possible adverse predictors.

## 3. PREDICTORS OF LYMPHOMA IN SJÖGREN'S SYNDROME

The clinical manifestations during the course of SS that could predict an evolution to an NHL have been extensively studied since the 1970s.[10] The persistent enlargement of parotid glands and the presence of lymphadenopathy and/or splenomegaly were identified as the most important clinical signs.

The association between mixed monoclonal cryoglobulinemia (linked to a complement decrease) and the risk of lymphoma in SS was first documented by

Tzioufas et al.,[19] who also reported an increased risk related to the presence of specific monoclonal rheumatoid factor (mRF)–associated cross-reactive idiotypes (CRIs), such as 17,109 and G-6.

Skoupouli and coworkers[17] reported that the development of lymphoproliferative disorders in SS was associated with low levels of C4 complement (relative risk, 7.5; P=0.0016), the presence of mixed monoclonal cryoglobulins (relative risk, 7.9; P=0.0012), and purpura (relative risk, 3.9; P=0.037). Low levels of C4 were additionally indicated as the strongest predictor for mortality after adjusting for age (relative risk, 6.5; P=0.0041). Of interest, in this study the authors focused on the concept that the initial presentation of SS with these manifestations could determine the outcome and mortality of SS.

The need to stratify SS patients on the basis of their risk of developing lymphoproliferative disorders, including lymphoma, was assessed for the first time by Ioannidis et al.[20] At SS diagnosis, parotid enlargement (hazard ratio [HR] 5.21, 95% CI 1.76–15.4), palpable purpura (HR 4.16, 95% CI 1.65–10.5), and low C4 levels (HR 2.40, 95% CI 0.99–5.83) were independent predictors of lymphoproliferation in pSS. The authors then proposed a classification of pSS distinguishing two distinct categories according to the presence or absence of low C4 levels and/or palpable purpura, respectively: the type I high-risk pSS that accounts for about 20% of pSS at diagnosis and the more common (80%) type II low-risk pSS without a significant increase in risk of lymphoma evolution. Brito-Zeròn and coworkers[21] confirmed this data and identified besides palpable purpura and low C4, severe parotid involvement, demonstrated by scintigraphy, and serum cryoglobulinemia as two additional risk factors of lymphoma development in their study cohort analysis. A survival analysis performed in this study found that patients with at least two adverse factors at diagnosis (parotid involvement by scintigraphy, cryoglobulinemia, purpura, and low C4) had a significantly lower survival rate than patients without risk factors.

In a large retrospective Greek study investigating hematologic manifestations and predictors of lymphoma development in pSS by Baimpa and coworkers,[22] lymphocytopenia was the only independent variable predicting the development of any type of lymphoma other than MZBLC, especially the DLBCL type, whereas neutropenia, low C4 levels, cryoglobulinemia, lymphadenopathy, and splenomegaly were independent predictors for the development of MZBCL type.

Low lymphocyte cell count has also been reported as predictor of NHL in pSS in a cohort study on cancer incidence and lymphoma predictors in pSS by Theander et al.,[9] which identified the CD4+/CD8+ T-cell ratio≤0.8 (HR 10.92, 95% CI 2.80–41.83) as the strongest risk factor for developing lymphoma. Other predictors in this study were CD4+ T lymphocytopenia (HR 8.14, 95% CI 2.10–31.53), low C4 (HR 9.49, 95% CI 1.94–46.54), purpura/skin vasculitis (HR 4.64, 95% CI 1.13–16.45), and low complement factor C3 (HR 6.18, 95% CI 1.57–24.22).

Reduced complement levels are closely associated with the two worst adverse outcomes in SS: lymphoma development and death. Many authors[18,23,24] have reported that low levels of C3 and C4 were predictors of both lymphoma evolution risk and mortality in SS, mainly as the result of lymphoproliferative disease. Only in Ioannidis' study[20] were low C3 levels not significantly predictive for increased mortality, possibly because of a lower cut-off point of C3 used in the Greek study (0.50 g/L instead of 0.83 g/L).

Overall, based on these studies, it can be concluded that a heavy MALT involvement, mainly of the parotid glands (clinically leading to their persistent swelling), and cryoglobulinemia (often linked to complement consumption and with possible vasculitic features such as purpura) are the two main predictors of lymphoma in SS.

Two clinical entities of SS, ie, CV and the persistent enlargement of salivary glands (usually parotid swelling), can therefore be considered as prelymphomatous conditions. Focusing on this particular issue, a multicenter Italian study by Quartuccio et al.[25] investigated the association between laboratory biomarkers and lymphoma risk in pSS, differentiating patients with prelymphomatous conditions (CV and salivary glands (SGs)/parotid enlargement) as separate groups in order to better evaluate in specific different subsets the risk of lymphoma development. All the selected 601 pSS patients, fulfilling the American European Criteria for the classification of pSS,[26] were negative for hepatitis C virus (HCV) antibodies and were repeatedly tested for the presence of cryoglobulins. Patients were categorized into four groups: group 1/NHL, patients with lymphoma (including lymphoma patients with concomitant CV and/or SG swelling); group 2/CV, patients with CV and without lymphoma; group 3/SW (swelling), patients with SG swelling without lymphoma, with or without concomitant CV; and group 4/pSS controls, pSS patients without lymphoma and without CV or SG swelling. The study showed that four biomarkers, ie, cryoglobulinemia, low C4, anti-La/SSB antibodies, and leukopenia, were significantly associated to lymphoma in pSS. An interesting finding was that in the group of patients with persistent SG swelling without lymphoma, the presence of two of these four biomarkers identified a 9-fold higher risk of lymphoma, whereas the positivity of only one or no biomarker provided a negative predictive value for lymphoma of about 90% in the same subset.

Because SG swelling is a more common finding in SS (about 30%) compared with lymphoma (about 5%), this study better characterized for the first time the risk of NHL in SS patients with SG swelling, with an increased risk of lymphoma only in those patients with at least two negative predictors.

Additional new data has recently been provided comparing the clinical and laboratory features in pSS patients who are positive or negative for the anti-Ro/SSA and/or anti-La/SSB antibodies. Of note, anti-Ro/SSA–anti-La/SSB-negative pSS showed a lower risk of lymphoma evolution.[27] Moreover, a younger age at SS onset determined an increased risk for lymphoproliferation.[28]

## 4. LYMPHOMAGENESIS IN PRIMARY SJÖGREN'S SYNDROME

SS is characterized by both B- and T-cell lymphocytic infiltrates in inflamed SGs and a B-cell hyperactivity that leads to a significant expansion of B-cell clonal populations in different times, tissues, and stages, a process potentially evolving into a malignant B-cell monoclonal lymphoma.[29] Polyclonal autoantibodies such as anti-Ro/SSA, anti-La/SSB, and rheumatoid factor (RF) are produced in the inflamed MALT tissue.

MALT lymphoma arises from chronic inflamed tissues through a multistep process in which a local, chronic antigenic stimulation, together with a predisposing genetic background, allows the emergence of B-cell clonal expansion and the evolution to an overt malignant process.

### 4.1 The Classification of Sjögren's Syndrome–Related Lymphoproliferation

Lymphoproliferation in SS has been classified into two major categories: malignant and nonmalignant lymphoproliferation according to the current standard classification.[30] Nonmalignant lymphoproliferation in SS is further subdivided into fully benign lymphoproliferation (that is a feature of SS itself) and a nonmalignant lymphoproliferative form, which represents a more advanced stage toward B-cell malignancy. MALT sites, the lymph nodes, and rarely the bone marrow may be involved, and laboratory alterations such as hypergammaglobulinemia, positive M-component in biological fluids, and/or cryoglobulinemia (polyclonal, oligoclonal, or monoclonal) may be present.[31]

Fully benign lymphoproliferation consists of a fully benign infiltrate in MALT sites or a reactive lymphadenopathy, and it lacks an M-component in biological fluids.[31] In lymphoepithelial or myoepithelial sialadenitis (MESA) with fully benign lymphoid infiltrates, the lobular architecture of the gland is preserved. Lymphoepithelial lesions are prominent, monocytoid, and/or marginal zone B-cells (centrocyte-like) are restricted to the lymphoepithelial lesions, reactive follicles without expansion of the mantle; or marginal zones are prominent, and small lymphocytes and plasma cells (usually not in broad sheets) are present in the interfollicular regions. Moreover, this category includes gastric MALT lesions up to grade 2 according to Wotherspoon and Isaacson,[32] and fully benign lymphoid infiltrates in other sites,[33] as established by a reference hemopathologist.

Nonmalignant lymphoproliferative disorder includes cases with a "lymphoproliferative lesion" in MALT sites, cases with nodal atypical lymphoproliferative disorder, or cases with monoclonal cryoglobulinemia or an M-component persistently detected in biological fluids.[31] In MESA with lymphoproliferative lesion, the glands show a diffuse or multifocal process, islands of normal acini are often preserved, aggregates of centrocyte-like cells may be present within the diffuse lymphoid infiltrate, and nonconfluent centrocyte-like cell "halos" surround the lymphoepithelial lesions. Lymphoepithelial aggressiveness may be pronounced and areas of immunoglobulin (Ig) light-chain restriction may be present. Gastric MALT lesions of grades 3 and 4 according to Wotherspoon and Isaacson[32] and lymphoproliferative lesions without definite malignant features are considered SS-related nonmalignant lymphoproliferative disorders.[33]

MZBCL of MALT type is the most common subtype of SS-related lymphoma, generally indolent and with a good prognosis. Its histopathological picture consists of a dense lymphoid infiltrate diffusely involving the gland or forming a localized mass, with obliteration of acini. Lymphoid cells and plasma cells present monotypic Ig expression. Plasmocytic differentiation may occur. A large cell component may be detected. The prominence of reactive lymphoid follicles and lymphoepithelial lesions are shared features with MESA, whereas, in contrast with MESA, lymphoma shows centrocyte-like cells forming broad interconnecting strands between lymphoepithelial lesions as a key feature and broad "halos" around the epithelial cell (EC) nests.[31]

The other more common types of malignant lymphomas in SS are the more aggressive DLBCL and the nodal MZBCL.[22]

## 4.2 Genetic Alterations in Sjögren's Syndrome–Related Lymphoma

It has been observed that the most common genetic alteration of MALT lymphoma, t(11; 18)(q21; q21), was virtually absent in MALT lymphoma of the SGs. Similarly, other chromosomal abnormalities usually related to MALT lymphoma development, such as t(14; 18)(q32; q21), t(1; 14)(p22; q32), and t(3; 14)(p13; q32), have been found only in a few cases of MALT lymphomas.[34]

The acquisition of mutations in genes involved in cellular proliferation and the nuclear factor (NF)-κB pathway could favor lymphoma evolution. It has recently been demonstrated that the activation of NF-κB$_2$ pathway mediated by a specific mutation of B-cell activating factor receptor (BAFF-R) (His159Tyr) might contribute to SS lymphoproliferation.[28] A potential role of an alteration in the *TNFAIP3* gene that codifies for A20 protein (a factor also involved in NF-κB pathway) has been previously shown. Germinal mutations in *TNFAIP3* gene have been associated with autoimmune disease and somatic mutations with MALT lymphoma development. Specific variants of *TNFAIP3* are associated with pSS and functional polymorphisms of this gene are found in the subset of pSS patients with lymphoma.[35–37] This suggests the existence of a close genetic link between autoimmunity and lymphoproliferation in SS.

## 4.3 The Role of Infectious Triggers in Sjögren's Syndrome–Related Lymphoproliferation

Research into the role of antigenic stimulation for the acquisition of lymphoid tissue and the development of specific subtypes of MALT lymphoma identified in bacterial or viral trigger activity the first possible event.[38] The expanded B-cell clone, which often uses a combination of Ig genes encoding autoantibodies, may in turn become infectious trigger–independent, and the eradication of infection may no longer be sufficient to abolish clonal persistence and potential malignant evolution. Infectious triggers linked to B-cell lymphomagenesis have been identified in *Helicobacter pylori, Borrelia burgdorferi* and *Borrelia afzelii, Chlamydophila psittaci,* and *Campylobacter jejuni* for gastric, cutaneous, ocular adnexal, and small intestinal MALT lymphomas, respectively.[39–42]

To date, efforts to clearly identify infectious triggers implicated in SS pathogenesis and in SS-related lymphoproliferation have failed.

A role of viruses in the activation of B-cells in ectopic lymphoid structures of pSS glands and in lymphomagenesis has been hypothesized. Croia et al.[43] recently demonstrated a latent Epstein-Barr virus (EBV) infection in B cells and lytic EBV infection in plasma cells exclusively within inflammatory infiltrates of SS SG tissue, suggesting a potential EBV contribution to local growth and differentiation of self-reacting B cells. Furthermore, a high prevalence of *C. psittaci* subclinical infection has recently been shown in Italian patients with SS with a higher incidence of *C. psittaci* detection in MALT lymphoma, as compared with MESA or without SS patients without a lymphoproliferative disease.[44]

An important example of chronic antigen-driven overstimulation of B cells is represented by HCV-related lymphoproliferation. Epidemiology studies showed a higher risk of NHL in patients with chronic HCV infection compared with healthy subjects.[45] Importantly, HCV is a sialotropic virus and is linked to both SG chronic lymphocytic inflammation and sicca syndrome. SS and HCV infection share also other features: the association with cryoglobulinemia and serum RF positivity, and profound similarities in immunoglobulin gene usage and hypervariable sequences by the expanded B cell clones, with genetic homology with RF sequences. Therefore HCV-related sicca syndrome, especially when positive for anti-Ro/SSA and anti-La/SSB antibodies, can be considered as a particular subset of SS both from a clinical and biologic perspective, associated with a well-recognized infectious trigger, ie, HCV.[46–50]

## 4.4 Rheumatoid Factor Specificity of Sjögren's Syndrome–Related Lymphomas

SS-related lymphomas, and also a fraction of B-cell lymphomas related to infection, appear to derive from B cells which employ Ig genes associated with autoantibody production.[51,52] The expansion of anti-Ro/SSA and anti-La/SSB and RF-positive clones in SS SGs is well known. In MESA and in SS-lymphomas, the expanded clones often show a biased *VH* and *Vk* gene usage (eg, *VH1-69, VH3-7, VH4-59, Kv325,* and *Kv328*), particular *VDJ* combinations (eg, *VH1-69/DP10-D-JH4, VH3/ DP54-DH21/9-JH3,* and *VH4/DP71-D2-JH2*), and similarity with RF database sequences.[51,53–57] Interestingly, these sequences are similar to those detected in HCV-related lymphomas.[48]

In 1986, Fox et al. found a CRI in RF of SS patients, detected by a monoclonal antibody (MoAb 17.109). Interestingly, this CRI was also expressed on the B cells infiltrating the SGs of SS, and was present in RF paraproteins from patients affected by lymphoma but not in healthy subjects, suggesting the involvement of 17.109-positive B cells in the transition from clonal B-cell expansion to B-cell neoplastic transformation in SS.[58]

Both MESA (fully benign or with lymphoproliferation) and lymphomatous B clones show a strong similarity in *CDR3* sequences, even when derived from different patients, indicating the antigen-based selection of specific B clones. Homology with RF sequences was highlighted by molecular studies in 1997.[51] Subsequently, Martin et al.[55] demonstrated that SS-related lymphoma B cells may indeed produce Igs with RF activity.

Bende et al.,[59] comparing *IgVH-CDR3* of B-cell NHLs with *CDR3* database sequences, also found that SG MALT lymphomas expressed B-cell antigen receptor-Ig with strong *CDR3* homology to RFs and that MALT lymphoma–derived antibodies showed a strong RF reactivity in vitro.

Therefore a pathogenic model of SS lymphomagenesis, in which SS lymphoma could develop from expanded mRF-producing B cells rather than from clones producing more SS-specific autoantibodies, ie, anti-Ro/SSA and anti-La/SSB, has been proposed.[55,60] According to this model, in SS-inflamed SGs, a sustained production of Igs in response to different exogenous antigens and/or to autoantigens, together with additional proliferative stimuli provided by the local molecular and cellular milieu of ectopic lymphoid glandular tissue (see Section 4.9), could induce a continuous stimulation of RF-positive B cells that are more prone to mutational events leading to malignant transformation. Somatic mutations may lead to changes in antibody affinity/specificity.

## 4.5 Why Cryoglobulinemia Develops: Information From HCV-Related Cryoglobulinemia

In HCV-related CV, HCV infection triggers the expansion of RF-positive clones. Why this event preferentially occurs in the course of HCV infection, compared with other chronic infections, remains unclear. One study demonstrated that RFs in HCV-related cryoglobulins also recognize the HCV epitope NS3, and the same study reported a murine model where the response elicited in the mouse by the NS3 HCV peptide induced the production of an anti-HCV antibody also reacting against IgG, thus being an RF.[50] Therefore a possible mechanism of infection triggering autoimmunity, ie, by a double antibody reactivity or by molecular mimicry, may be postulated.

In SS, cryoglobulinemia is closely linked to lymphoma and is a red flag for it, if not diagnosed; about one-half of SS patients with lymphoma have positive serum cryoglobulins, despite the fact that HCV infection is lacking. The possibility that in SS, triggers which are different from HCV may, in any case, lead to pathogenic events in part similar to those occurring in HCV-related cryoglobulinemia, deserves additional study.

## 4.6  Cryoglobulinemic Vasculitis in Sjögren's Syndrome: The Clinical Picture

Formally developed classification criteria for CV were recently published[61] and then validated,[62] showing a sensitivity of 88.5% (CI 95%, 84.3–92.8) and a specificity of 93.6% (CI 95%, 89.5–97.7).[61] Serum mixed cryoglobulinemia, ie, serum positivity of mixed cryoglobulins, occurs in about 10% to 15% patients with SS, whereas a frank clinical CV is less common, although it greatly affects the SS-related morbidity.[22] However, the biological, and, to some extent, also the clinical, characteristics of HCV-unrelated CV may be different from HCV-related CV.

A subanalysis of the sensitivity and the specificity of the CV classification criteria was then performed in 55 SS patients carrying serum cryoglobulins with or without the clinical picture of CV (CwV), because SS represented the largest subgroup within the HCV-negative cases of cryoglobulinemia.[63] The sensitivity and specificity of the classification criteria for CV in SS patients were high: 88.9% (CI 95%, 76.5–100) and 91.3% (CI 95%, 79.2–100), respectively.[63] No differences between SS-CV and SS-CwV patients were observed in common clinical features of lymphoproliferation (lymphadenopathy, splenomegaly, SG swelling, lachrymal gland swelling, and B symptoms), although the prevalence of a lymphoproliferative disorder was more common in CV than in CvW (nonmalignant lymphoproliferative disorder in 13/29 in CV vs 4/26 in CwV, P = 0.02; malignant lymphoma in 10/29 CV vs 3/26 CwV, P = 0.046). Furthermore, type II cryoglobulinemia was more common in SS-CV as compared with SS-CwV. Overall, in SS, CV is more associated with monoclonal type II cryoglobulins and with NHL if compared with the single presence of serum cryoglobulins without vasculitis.[64]

Skin vasculitis in the course of SS was thoroughly investigated by the Italian collaborative network, Italian Study Group of SS. A total of 652 SS patients were studied, and cryoglobulinemic purpura was well differentiated from hypergammaglobulinemic purpura. Peripheral neuropathy, low C4, leukopenia, serum monoclonal component, and the presence of anti-La/SSB antibodies characterized CV, whereas RF, leukopenia, serum monoclonal component, and anti-Ro/SSA antibodies were significantly associated with hypergammaglobulinemic purpura. Lymphoma was associated only with CV. Thus whereas hypergammaglobulinemic purpura is a cutaneous vasculitis related to a benign B-cell proliferation in SS, CV is a systemic immune complex-mediated vasculitis with a higher risk of lymphoma. CV, but not hypergammaglobulinemic purpura, is like a prelymphomatous condition in SS.[65]

## 4.7  Cryoglobulinemia Is More Related to MALT Lymphoproliferation in Sjögren's Syndrome

B-cell NHL is a well-known complication of the usual subset of CV, ie, CV secondary to HCV infection (80% to 90% of cases of CV).[66] However, CV may also be HCV-negative, and one common case is HCV-negative CV in SS. Thus two different diseases (ie, CV HCV-related and SS with CV, HCV-unrelated) are both associated with mixed cryoglobulinemia and both predispose to B-cell NHL.

Whereas lymphomas complicating the course of HCV-related CV usually involve the bone marrow,[66,67] B-cell NHL complicating the course of SS usually involves the MALT sites.[4,14,31,68] Cryoglobulinemia appears to be linked to MALT lymphoproliferation in SS, and then shows a different biologic background when compared with cryoglobulinemia linked to HCV infection. Recently, three different approaches have better addressed this issue.[69] First, molecular analyses of B-cell clonal expansion were performed in the bone marrow from consecutive SS cases with mixed cryoglobulinemia, HCV-unrelated, and compared with classical HCV-related CV patients without SS. A polyclonal pattern was more prevalent in SS patients with type II or type III mixed cryoglobulinemia. In contrast, a clonal pattern was demonstrated in the majority of bone marrow biopsies from HCV-related CV patients. Thus a pattern of B-cell oligoclonal/monoclonal expansion is much less common in SS-related cryoglobulinemia. Secondly, a bone marrow involvement by lymphoma detected by biopsy, was rarely found in SS-related lymphomas also when associated with cryoglobulinemia. Overall, the bone marrow appears to be rarely involved in SS-related lymphomas with cryoglobulinemia, which is consistent with the hypothesis of a primary role of chronic inflammation and lymphoproliferation somewhere else, ie, salivary MALT, as a predisposing factor to lymphoma in SS.[69,70] Finally, in one patient with SS, CV, and parotid B-cell NHL of MALT, bilateral parotidectomy with a lack of any additional treatment was soon followed by a decrease of serum RF and cryoglobulins, implying a crucial role of salivary MALT for the production of cryoglobulins.[69]

## 4.8 B-Cell Clonality in MALT Lymphoproliferation of Sjögren's Syndrome

B-cell hyperactivity and clonal expansion are well-recognized hallmarks of SS. Although SS-related B lymphomas are monoclonal diseases, the detection of B-cell oligoclonality or monoclonality is not unusual in SS salivary lesions, occurring also in the absence of malignant lymphoproliferation. Therefore monoclonality is not synonymous with malignancy and it cannot be used as a diagnostic criterion for lymphoma in difficult cases.

Analyzing both synchronous and metachronous tissue biopsies (mainly of the parotid glands) from SS patients with distinct lymphoproliferative MALT lesions, different subsets of B-cell clonal expansion have been found: polyclonal, oligoclonal, or monoclonal expansion; localized or disseminated; and with or without clonal persistence. Molecular analyses of B-cell clonality, together with an accurate pathological evaluation and adequate clinical correlations, are useful for a better definition of specific subsets of SS patients with a higher risk of lymphoma development. In detail, the expansion of a single dominant B-cell clone, localized or disseminated, and in metachronous lesions, could be related to more advanced stages of disease and to a higher progression toward B-cell malignancy. Conversely, the detection of different dominant clones in different synchronous and metachronous biopsies indicates a fluctuating rather than an established monoclonal B disorder, and a polyclonal or small oligoclonal B-cell expansion in fully benign pathological lesions could be considered of minor clinical relevance in terms of risk of malignant transformation.[51,53,68,71]

## 4.9 Ectopic Germinal Center–Like Structures and Chemokines in Sjögren's Syndrome Salivary Glands

Ectopic germinal center (GC)–like structures have been identified in SS, suggesting that the chronic inflammation continuously promotes the maintenance and organization of these structures.[72,73]

In SGs of SS patients, ectopic GCs have a proper architectural organization, eg, lacking afferent lymph vessels and a capsulated structure, and show molecular and cellular networks that differ from the classical structure of GCs found in secondary lymphoid organs (SLOs), such as the nodes and the spleen.[74]

B-cells in ectopic GCs of SS patients express a phenotype (CD20++, CD21++, CD23++, IgM++, and IgD++) closer to that of transitional type II B lymphocytes and marginal zone–like B cells rather than that harbored from centroblasts and centrocytes in classical SLOs.[75–77] Despite this, these structures show functional activity, with somatic hypermutation (SHM) and class switch recombination (CSR) processes resembling those of classical GCs. Follicular dendritic cells are present and express the activation-induced cytidine deaminase (AID) that is responsible for both SHM and CSR. Therefore these ectopic lymphoid structures possess the complete machinery for B-cell differentiation and clonal expansion. Notably, AID expression was also demonstrated in lymphoma complicating SS.[78]

Interestingly, whereas B-cells normally undergo negative selection and autoreactive lymphocytes are not allowed to colonize or are deleted in classical GCs of SLOs, autoreactive B cells persist in ectopic GCs in pSS and are able to bypass traditional tolerance checkpoint controls.[77,79] One mechanism may be represented by the expression of Toll-like receptor (TLR) 9, that provides an additional signal, allowing B-cell survival and protecting self-reactive clones against negative selection. Thus these structures in inflamed SGs in SS represent the optimal milieu for a severe dysregulation of immune tolerance to occur, allowing an abnormal antigen-driven B-cell activation and proliferation.[80]

It has been demonstrated that some chemokines may play an important role in the organization of ectopic lymphoid structures and lymphoproliferation in pSS.

Pitzalis and coworkers, investigating the SG expression of chemokines involved in lymphoma, such as *CXCL13*, *CCL21*, and *CXCL12*, found a distinct distribution of these chemokines in different histological subsets of lymphoproliferative lesions in SS.[81] Increased *CXCL13* and *CCL21* were found in lymphoepithelial lesions; conversely *CXCL12* was expressed by infiltrating B cell of MALT lymphoma. Based on these findings, they speculated that *CXCL13* and *CCL21* could mainly play a role in organizing the ectopic GC-like structures, whereas *CXCL12* would exert a more specific role in enhancing B-cell proliferation.

Interestingly, polymorphisms of the *CXCR5* gene that codify for the receptor of *CXCL12* have been associated both with pSS and SS-unrelated NHL.[82,83]

Recently, Theander and coworkers[70] found that the detection of GC-like structures in SGs of SS patients was significantly related to NHL development. Of the seven cases of NHL in a total of 175 pSS patients evaluated retrospectively, six (86%) had GCs in the biopsy performed at the time of pSS diagnosis, with a median of 7 years between this biopsy and the occurrence of lymphoma (range 2–12 years). Only one patient was negative for GCs in SG biopsy, and in this case the subsequent malignant lymphoma was located in a tear gland. The negative predictive value for lymphoma development of the presence of GCs in baseline minor SG biopsy was 99%, but on the other hand, the positive predictive value was 16%, indicating that the sole formation of GCs is likely necessary, but not sufficient, for lymphoma development.

When considering that there is a positive association between GCs and lymphocytic focus score (LFS; the number of lymphocyte foci per 4 mm$^2$ of tissue, where *focus* is an aggregate of 50 lymphocytes) on SG biopsies, the observation by Risselada et al.,[84] who found that the mean LFS was significantly higher in patients developing NHL in SS ($3.0 \pm 0.894$ vs $2.25 \pm 1.086$; $p=0.021$), is of major interest. An LFS ≥3 contributed significantly to NHL development, with the threshold of ≥3 showing again a negative predictive value of 98%, and a positive predictive value of 16% for lymphoma development, as in the study by Theander[70] dealing with GCs.

In the end, routinely performing SG biopsy is important not only for its diagnostic value, but also to better evaluate the risk of malignant lymphoproliferation in pSS.

## 4.10 Molecular and Cellular Network in Salivary Glands With Lymphoproliferation

The SG ECs are able to promote inflammation and lymphoproliferation in SS.[85] Through the expression of costimulatory molecules and the production of cytokines and chemokines, ECs regulate the migration and activation of both innate and adaptive immune system cells, and orchestrate the organization of ectopic lymphoid GC-like structures in SGs of SS.[3,86–88]

During chronic stimulation driven by exogenous antigens and/or autoantigens, ECs display antigen-presenting cell–like ability and produce a potent B-cell activating factor, also known as *BAFF* or *BLyS*.[76] ECs also induce plasmocytoid dendritic cells to produce interferon (IFN)-α, which acts on myeloid dendritic cells (mDCs) stimulating both their cooperation with T cells and the activation of B-cell proliferation via an additional, IFN-α–dependent, BAFF production.[89–92]

BAFF is a member of the TNF family that promotes B-cell activation and survival.[93,94] It binds BAFF receptor 3, mainly expressed by B lymphocytes. The biological sources of BAFF are macrophages, dendritic cells (DCs), ECs, stromal-derived bone marrow cells, activated T cells, and finally also B cells themselves,[95] which both produce and respond to BAFF in an autocrine loop of stimulation.[91,96] The BAFF transgenic mice display a hyperactivity of B cells leading to a tissue and blood lymphoid proliferation in a picture resembling SS and SLE and resulting in an overt marginal zone lymphoma after many years.[97,98]

Cumulative data show that BAFF contributes in the pathogenesis of SS and NHL. High levels of BAFF are found in saliva, sera, and affected tissues of SS patients.[91,99–101] Furthermore a pathogenetic role of BAFF in SS is also supported by genetic studies, and, indirectly, by the efficacy of anti-BAFF therapy with belimumab in pSS.[102,103] Polymorphisms in the BAFF gene have been associated to both several types of NHL development[104] and many diseases of the immune system, including SS,[105] SLE,[106] and CV.[107,108] Moreover, the mutation His159Tyr of the BAFF receptor was shown in patients with NHL, and a significantly increased prevalence of the same mutation was observed in SS patients complicated with lymphoma, particularly in younger patients.[28]

Quartuccio et al.[109] found that serum BAFF levels were increased to a greater level in pSS patients with lymphoma or prelymphomatous conditions, such as MESA and CV, if compared with SS patients without lymphoproliferation lesions. They also demonstrated an association between higher levels of BAFF with clonal B-cell expansion and with European League Against Rheumatism Disease Activity Index (ESSDAI) in SS. These data further underscore the existence of a link between the overexpression of BAFF and lymphoproliferation in SS, and that this link is particularly evident in the advanced phases of lymphoproliferation and in patients with greater disease activity.

Also other cytokine pathways have been associated with lymphoma development in pSS, including interleukin (IL)-4, IL-6, IL-10, IL-12,[110,111] and, more recently, the IL-22 axis and Fms-like tyrosine kinase three (Flt-3)–mediated signal.

The IL-22/IL-22R1 axis is implicated in the pathogenesis of B- and T-cell lymphomas, with an aberrant expression of IL-22R1 on the surface of lymphomatous cells. Ciccia et al.[112] showed an overexpression of IL-22R1 in pSS-related lymphoma on the surface of infiltrating B cells and tissue macrophages and found a colocalization of this receptor with an enhanced expression and activity of pSTAT3 within the same cells. They also showed that the IL-22 axis activation was correlated with IL-18, found overexpressed in pSS lymphoma.

Flt-3 ligand (Flt-3L) is a cytokine, acting on lymphocyte ontogenesis in bone marrow and blood that stimulates hematopoietic progenitor growth through activation of the specific receptor Flt-3.[113] Tobòn et al.[114] demonstrated that serum levels of Flt-3L were higher in pSS compared with controls. They also showed that infiltrating B cells expressed Flt-3 in the SG, and that ECs were able to produce Flt-3L, suggesting a possible reverberating loop of B-cell activation. High levels of Flt-3L were also associated with an increased risk of lymphoma development in SS.

A schematic picture summarizing B-cell expansion and lymphomagenesis in SS is shown by Fig. 6.1.

## 5. BIOPSY AND IMAGING FOR AN IMPROVED EVALUATION OF LYMPHOPROLIFERATION IN SJÖGREN'S SYNDROME

Imaging is important for the assessment of lymphoma in SS, but tissue biopsy remains crucial for diagnosis. A complete assessment of SS always includes SG biopsy. An accurate pathologic evaluation is important for both the diagnosis and the prognosis of SS. When integrated with clinical and molecular findings, different stages of lymphoproliferation may be dissected, related to a different risk of lymphoma evolution.[31] Biopsy is requested for the final diagnosis of malignant lymphoma, and some SS patients with persistent parotid swelling may indeed exhibit an indolent parotid lymphoma.[70,84] For this reason, parotid biopsy should be performed whenever possible when persistent parotid/glandular swelling occurs in SS.

In the past few years, many efforts have been devoted to identifying a sensitive imaging method to reveal parenchymal changes in SS SGs, in particular to detect lymphoma. Data concerning ultrasonography (US), magnetic resonance imaging (MRI), and, more recently, 18F-fluorodeoxyglucose positron emission tomography (FDG PET) has been published.

By US, a parotid lymphomatous process often appears as a hypoechoic mass because of the arrangement of lymphoma cells providing very few acoustic interfaces to generate internal echoes. The presence of a parotid hypoechoic area with a "cobblestone-like" inhomogeneity pattern may raise the suspicion of lymphoma. US does not provide, however, decisive information; in particular, an indolent MALT lymphoma may be not distinguished from nonmalignant lymphoproliferative lesions. Furthermore, US is not able to provide the evaluation of the whole parotid gland, detecting only parenchymal gland changes limited to the superficial parotid lobe (that takes account of 80% of the gland), whereas scanning the deep lobe proves difficult or impossible. US is, in any case, a useful technique for a rapid, repeatable, and noninvasive evaluation without any discomfort for the patient.[115,116]

MRI appears to be superior to US in the diagnosis of both benign and malignant parotid diseases. In SS, "salt-and-pepper" or "honeycombing" images indicate glandular inhomogeneity. The lymphoma MRI picture, conversely, has a homogeneous signal intensity, characterized by a low signal in the T1-weighted and a high intensity in T2-weighted sequences. However, even if this MRI pattern is highly suggestive of lymphoma, correlation studies between MRI and

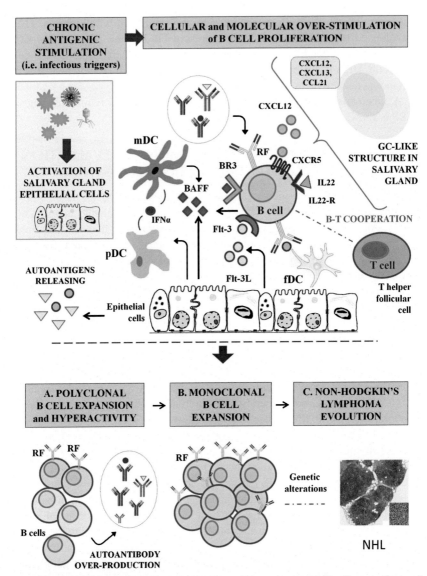

**FIGURE 6.1  Schematic model of Sjögren's syndrome–associated B-cell expansion and lymphomagenesis.** *BAFF*, B-cell activating factor; *BR3*, B-cell activating factor receptor 3; *fDC*, follicular dendritic cell; *Flt-3*, Fms-like tyrosine kinase 3; *Flt-3L*, Fms-like tyrosine kinase 3 ligand; *GC*, germinal center; *IFNα*, interferon α; *IL-22*, interleukin 22; *IL-22R*, interleukin 22 receptor; *mDC*, myeloid dendritic cell; *NHL*, non-Hodgkin lymphoma; *pDC*, plasmocytoid dendritic cell; *RF*, rheumatoid factor.

histological features indicate that MRI is not able to distinguish between a localized lymphatic benign infiltrate and an early stage malignant lymphoma. On the other hand, MRI, for its excellent soft-tissue analysis, is helpful for surgical assessment and before parotid biopsy.[115]

Finally, recent studies highlight the role of FDG PET to detect lymphoma in SS. Although data are still limited, they are encouraging. Cohen et al.[117] found that the majority of pSS patients had significantly higher FDG uptake in SGs, lymph nodes, and lungs compared with controls and, importantly, the maximum standard uptake value($SUV_{max}$) was higher in SS patients with lymphoma that in those without lymphoma. Moreover, the authors demonstrated that $SUV_{max}$ does not correlate with disease activity measured by the ESSDAI, and developed a PET/computed tomography (CT) activity score correlating with disease activity.

A potential role of FDG PET in the posttherapy assessment of SG lymphomas in SS has recently been reported by Poulou et al.[118] An association between $SUV_{max}$ and histological findings was found with regards to minor SG biopsies but not with parotid volumes. Of interest, an $SUV_{max}$ <3.0 practically excluded residual lymphoma.

## 6. TREATMENT

Treatment of lymphoma in SS should be individualized to the patient, taking into account, besides the lymphoma histotype and stage, the concomitant autoimmune disease, comorbidities, and many other individual factors including age, work, and patient expectations, preferences, and opinions.

Two large studies[12,119] have evaluated the management of SS-related lymphoma obtaining similar results. A therapeutic algorithm approach to different subgroups of MALT lymphoma, the most common lymphoma histotype in SS. For localized extranodal MALT lymphoma without bone marrow dissemination or lymphadenopathy, often asymptomatic, and with an International Prognostic Index score (based on five items: age, stage, extranodal involvement, performance status, and lactate dehydrogenase serum levels) between 0 and 1, a "wait and see" policy can be adopted, although patients need to undergo frequent and regular staging procedures including clinical examination, CT, digestive endoscopy, and bone marrow biopsy.

Depending on other factors, however, treatment can be considered. A younger age is important. Parotidectomy appears to be effective only in the short term,[69] and lymphomatous parotid swelling may soon relapse also after local radiotherapy. This is not unexpected, because the affected tissue may regenerate, and, importantly, the malignant B-cell clone may be only apparently confined to the parotid gland, while being disseminated to other MALT sites, such as other major and minor SGs, the stomach, and the lung.[68,120]

Furthermore, especially in younger women, it is logical to consider the possible efficacy of the currently available B-cell depleting therapies, in view of the lack of oncogenetic alternatives. Even a reduction of the B-cell lymphoproliferative disorder, if not a complete response, may be beneficial. Rituximab appears, at present, a possible option, and it is probably the best currently available treatment when cryoglobulinemia is accompanied by a CV.[121,122] The subsequent repeated or maintenance treatment with rituximab may be considered.[123] If cryoglobulinemia is absent, however, rituximab may prove effective in MALT lymphomas in SS, although this appears more controversial.[124] The local overproduction of BAFF in MALT sites such as the parotid glands may represent one important cause of tissue resistance to B-cell depletion by rituximab monotherapy.[125,126] The murine model clearly supported this notion.[127] Indeed, that the anti-CD20 therapy with rituximab might not deplete the B-cell infiltrate in the SS salivary tissue was highlighted as long as 14 years ago,[128] and has been confirmed since then, although repeated treatments might possibly be more effective.

A sequential therapy with anti-BAFF medication followed an anti-CD20 drug (or possibly a combined therapy) could prove successful.[129] Importantly, only when sequential therapy with rituximab was shortly preceded by therapy with belimumab (rituximab or belimumab alone being previously ineffective) was the regression of low-grade parotid lymphoma of MALT and of CV recently observed in an SS patient. This shows that an effective therapy for lymphoproliferation, lacking direct oncogenetic properties, is possible in SS, and indicates the relevance of the optimal use of targeted treatments. Furthermore, being effective on MALT infiltrates, the sequential or combined use of anti-BAFF and anti-CD20 therapy might prove effective not only for lymphoproliferation in SS, but also for sicca manifestations; a trial including this approach has recently been planned.

For disseminated MALT lymphoma, potentially related to a higher risk of transformation into more aggressive subtypes, the most employed and effective scheme reported is a combination of rituximab and chemotherapy agents such as cyclophosphamide, fludarabine, or, more recently, bendamustine.[130–132]

Finally, for the treatment of high-grade DLBCL, the standard of care is currently a CHOP (ie, cyclophosphamide, hydroxydaunomycin [doxorubicin], Oncovin [vincristine], and prednisone) regimen combined to rituximab.[133] When chemotherapy is used with an oncohematological approach, the hematologist or oncologist becomes the key reference medical figure for the patient. Sicca, however, remains, despite aggressive chemotherapy.[134]

## REFERENCES

1. Zintzaras E, Voulgarelis M, Moutsopoulos HM. The risk of lymphoma development in auto-immune diseases: a meta-analysis. *Arch Intern Med* 2005;**165**:2337–44.
2. Smedby KE, Hjalgrim H, Askling J, Chang ET, Gregersen H, Porwit-MacDonald A, et al. Autoimmune and chronic inflammatory disorders and risk of non-Hodgkin lymphoma by sub-type. *J Natl Cancer Inst* 2006;**98**:51–60.
3. Mitsias DI, Kapsogeorgou EK, Moutsopoulos HM. The role of epithelial cells in the initia-tion and perpetuation of autoimmune lesions: lessons from Sjögren's syndrome (autoimmune epithelitis). *Lupus* 2006;**15**:255–61.

4. Anderson LG, Talal N. The spectrum of benign to malignant lymphoproliferation in Sjögren's syndrome. *Clin Exp Immunol* 1972;**10**:199–221.

5. Jaffe ES, Harris NL, Vardiman JW. *Pathology and genetics of tumours of haematopoietic and lymphoid tissues.* Lyon, France: IARC Press; 2001.

6. Wang SS, Vajdic CM, Linet MS, Slager SL, Voutsinas J, Nieters A, et al. Associations of non-Hodgkin lymphoma (NHL) risk with autoimmune conditions according to putative NHL loci. *Am J Epidemiol* 2015;**181**:406–21.

7. Ekstrom Smedby K, Vajdic CM, Falster M, Engels EA, Martinez-Maza O, Turner J, et al. Autoimmune disorders and risk of non-Hodgkin lymphoma subtypes: a pooled analysis within the InterLymph Consortium. *Blood* 2008;**111**:4029–38.

8. Nishishinya MB, Pereda CA, Munoz-Fernandez S, Pego-Reigosa JM, Rua-Figueroa I, Andreu JL, et al. Identification of lymphoma predictors in patients with primary Sjögren's syndrome: a systematic literature review and meta-analysis. *Rheumatol Int* 2015;**35**:17–26.

9. Theander E, Henriksson G, Ljungberg O, Mandl T, Manthorpe R, Jacobsson LT. Lymphoma and other malignancies in primary Sjögren's syndrome: a cohort study on cancer incidence and lymphoma predictors. *Ann Rheum Dis* 2006;**65**:796–803.

10. Kassan SS, Thomas TL, Moutsopoulos HM, Hoover R, Kimberly RP, Budman DR, et al. Increased risk of lymphoma in sicca syndrome. *Ann Intern Med* 1978;**89**:888–92.

11. De Re V, De Vita S, Sansonno D, Toffoli G. Mixed cryoglobulinemia syndrome as an additional autoimmune disorder associated with risk for lymphoma development. *Blood* 2008;**111**:5760.

12. Voulgarelis M, Ziakas PD, Papageorgiou A, Baimpa E, Tzioufas AG, Moutsopoulos HM. Prognosis and outcome of non-Hodgkin lymphoma in primary Sjögren syndrome. *Med Baltim* 2012;**91**:1–9.

13. Royer B, Cazals-Hatem D, Sibilia J, Agbalika F, Cayuela JM, Soussi T, et al. Lymphomas in patients with Sjögren's syndrome are marginal zone B-cell neoplasms, arise in diverse extra-nodal and nodal sites, and are not associated with viruses. *Blood* 1997;**90**:766–75.

14. Voulgarelis M, Dafni UG, Isenberg DA, Moutsopoulos HM. Malignant lymphoma in primary Sjögren's syndrome: a multicenter, retrospective, clinical study by the European concerted action on Sjögren's syndrome. *Arthritis Rheum* 1999;**42**:1765–72.

15. Zucca E, Conconi A, Mughal TI, Sarris AH, Seymour JF, Vitolo U, et al. Patterns of outcome and prognostic factors in primary large-cell lymphoma of the testis in a survey by the International Extranodal Lymphoma Study Group. *J Clin Oncol* 2003;**21**:20–7.

16. Deutsch AJ, Aigelsreiter A, Staber PB, Beham A, Linkesch W, Guelly C, et al. MALT lymphoma and extranodal diffuse large B-cell lymphoma are targeted by aberrant somatic hypermutation. *Blood* 2007;**109**:3500–4.

17. Skopouli FN, Dafni U, Ioannidis JP, Moutsopoulos HM. Clinical evolution, and morbidity and mortality of primary Sjögren's syndrome. *Semin Arthritis Rheum* 2000;**29**:296–304.

18. Theander E, Manthorpe R, Jacobsson LT. Mortality and causes of death in primary Sjögren's syndrome: a prospective cohort study. *Arthritis Rheum* 2004;**50**:1262–9.

19. Tzioufas AG, Boumba DS, Skopouli FN, Moutsopoulos HM. Mixed monoclonal cryoglobulinemia and monoclonal rheumatoid factor cross-reactive idiotypes as predictive factors for the development of lymphoma in primary Sjögren's syndrome. *Arthritis Rheum* 1996;**39**:767–72.

20. Ioannidis JP, Vassiliou VA, Moutsopoulos HM. Long-term risk of mortality and lymphoproliferative disease and predictive classification of primary Sjögren's syndrome. *Arthritis Rheum* 2002;**46**:741–7.

21. Brito-Zeron P, Ramos-Casals M, Bove A, Sentis J, Font J. Predicting adverse outcomes in primary Sjögren's syndrome: identification of prognostic factors. *Rheumatology (Oxford)* 2007;**46**:1359–62.

22. Baimpa E, Dahabreh IJ, Voulgarelis M, Moutsopoulos HM. Hematologic manifestations and predictors of lymphoma development in primary Sjögren syndrome: clinical and pathophysiologic aspects. *Med Baltim* 2009;**88**:284–93.

23. Ramos-Casals M, Brito-Zeron P, Yague J, Akasbi M, Bautista R, Ruano M, et al. Hypocomplementaemia as an immunological marker of morbidity and mortality in patients with primary Sjögren's syndrome. *Rheumatology (Oxford)* 2005;**44**:89–94.

24. Solans-Laque R, Lopez-Hernandez A, Bosch-Gil JA, Palacios A, Campillo M, Vilardell-Tarres M. Risk, predictors, and clinical characteristics of lymphoma development in primary Sjögren's syndrome. *Semin Arthritis Rheum* 2011;**41**:415–23.

25. Quartuccio L, Isola M, Baldini C, Priori R, Bartoloni Bocci E, Carubbi F, et al. Biomarkers of lymphoma in Sjögren's syndrome and evaluation of the lymphoma risk in prelymphomatous conditions: results of a multicenter study. *J Autoimmun* 2014;**51**:75–80.

26. Vitali C, Bombardieri S, Jonsson R, Moutsopoulos HM, Alexander EL, Carsons SE, et al. Classification criteria for Sjögren's syndrome: a revised version of the European criteria proposed by the American-European Consensus Group. *Ann Rheum Dis* 2002;**61**:554–8.

27. Quartuccio L, Baldini C, Bartoloni E, Priori R, Carubbi F, Corazza L, et al. Anti-SSA/SSB-negative Sjögren's syndrome shows a lower prevalence of lymphoproliferative manifestations, and a lower risk of lymphoma evolution. *Autoimmun Rev* 2015;**14**:1019–22.

28. Papageorgiou A, Mavragani CP, Nezos A, Zintzaras E, Quartuccio L, De Vita S, et al. A BAFF receptor His159Tyr mutation in Sjögren's syndrome-related lymphoproliferation. *Arthritis Rheumatol* 2015;**67**:2732–41.

29. Tzioufas AG. B-cell lymphoproliferation in primary Sjögren's syndrome. *Clin Exp Rheumatol* 1996;**14**(Suppl. 14):S65–70.

30. Campo E, Swerdlow SH, Harris NL, Pileri S, Stein H, Jaffe ES. The 2008 WHO classification of lymphoid neoplasms and beyond: evolving concepts and practical applications. *Blood* 2011;**117**:5019–32.

31. De Vita S, De Marchi G, Sacco S, Gremese E, Fabris M, Ferraccioli G. Preliminary classification of nonmalignant B cell proliferation in Sjögren's syndrome: perspectives on pathobiology and treatment based on an integrated clinico-pathologic and molecular study approach. *Blood Cells Mol Dis* 2001;**27**:757–66.

32. Wotherspoon AC, Doglioni C, Isaacson PG. Low-grade gastric B-cell lymphoma of mucosa-associated lymphoid tissue (MALT): a multifocal disease. *Histopathology* 1992;**20**:29–34.

33. Burke JS. Are there site-specific differences among the MALT lymphomas: morphologic, clinical? *Am J Clin Pathol* 1999;**111**:S133–43.

34. Joao C, Farinha P, da Silva MG, Martins C, Crespo M, Cabecadas J. Cytogenetic abnormalities in MALT lymphomas and their precursor lesions from different organs: a fluorescence in situ hybridization (FISH) study. *Histopathology* 2007;**50**:217–24.

35. Musone SL, Taylor KE, Nititham J, Chu C, Poon A, Liao W, et al. Sequencing of *TNFAIP3* and association of variants with multiple autoimmune diseases. *Genes Immun* 2011;**12**:176–82.

36. Chanudet E, Huang Y, Zeng N, Streubel B, Chott A, Raderer M, et al. *TNFAIP3* abnormalities in MALT lymphoma with autoimmunity. *Br J Haematol* 2011;**154**:535–9.

37. Nocturne G, Tarn J, Boudaoud S, Locke J, Miceli-Richard C, Hachulla E, et al. Germline variation of *TNFAIP3* in primary Sjögren's syndrome-associated lymphoma. *Ann Rheum Dis* 2015.

38. Zucca E, Bertoni F, Vannata B, Cavalli F. Emerging role of infectious etiologies in the pathogenesis of marginal zone B-cell lymphomas. *Clin Cancer Res* 2014;**20**:5207–16.

39. Ponzoni M, Ferreri AJ, Guidoboni M, Lettini AA, Cangi MG, Pasini E, et al. Chlamydia infection and lymphomas: association beyond ocular adnexal lymphomas highlighted by multiple detection methods. *Clin Cancer Res* 2008;**14**:5794–800.

40. Lecuit M, Abachin E, Martin A, Poyart C, Pochart P, Suarez F, et al. Immunoproliferative small intestinal disease associated with *Campylobacter jejuni*. *N Engl J Med* 2004;**350**: 239–48.

41. Schollkopf C, Melbye M, Munksgaard L, Smedby KE, Rostgaard K, Glimelius B, et al. Borrelia infection and risk of non-Hodgkin lymphoma. *Blood* 2008;**111**:5524–9.

42. Wotherspoon AC, Ortiz-Hidalgo C, Falzon MR, Isaacson PG. *Helicobacter pylori*–associated gastritis and primary B-cell gastric lymphoma. *Lancet* 1991;**338**:1175–6.

43. Croia C, Astorri E, Murray-Brown W, Willis A, Brokstad KA, Sutcliffe N, et al. Implication of Epstein-Barr virus infection in disease-specific autoreactive B cell activation in ectopic lymphoid structures of Sjögren's syndrome. *Arthritis Rheumatol* 2014;**66**:2545–57.

44. Fabris M, Dolcetti R, Pasini E, Quartuccio L, Pontarini E, Salvin S, et al. High prevalence of *Chlamydophila psittaci* subclinical infection in Italian patients with Sjögren's syndrome and parotid gland marginal zone B-cell lymphoma of MALT-type. *Clin Exp Rheumatol* 2014;**32**:61–5.

45. Negri E, Little D, Boiocchi M, La Vecchia C, Franceschi S. B-cell non-Hodgkin's lymphoma and hepatitis C virus infection: a systematic review. *Int J Cancer* 2004;**111**:1–8.

46. Mariette X. Lymphomas complicating Sjögren's syndrome and hepatitis C virus infection may share a common pathogenesis: chronic stimulation of rheumatoid factor B cells. *Ann Rheum Dis* 2001;**60**:1007–10.

47. De Vita S, Damato R, De Marchi G, Sacco S, Ferraccioli G. True primary Sjögren's syndrome in a subset of patients with hepatitis C infection: a model linking chronic infection to chronic sialadenitis. *Isr Med Assoc J* 2002;**4**:1101–5.

48. De Re V, De Vita S, Gasparotto D, Marzotto A, Carbone A, Ferraccioli G, et al. Salivary gland B cell lymphoproliferative disorders in Sjögren's syndrome present a restricted use of antigen receptor gene segments similar to those used by hepatitis C virus-associated non-Hodgkins's lymphomas. *Eur J Immunol* 2002;**32**:903–10.

49. De Re V, De Vita S, Marzotto A, Rupolo M, Gloghini A, Pivetta B, et al. Sequence analysis of the immunoglobulin antigen receptor of hepatitis C virus-associated non-Hodgkin lymphomas suggests that the malignant cells are derived from the rheumatoid factor-producing cells that occur mainly in type II cryoglobulinemia. *Blood* 2000;**96**:3578–84.

50. De Re V, Sansonno D, Simula MP, Caggiari L, Gasparotto D, Fabris M, et al. HCV-NS3 and IgG-Fc crossreactive IgM in patients with type II mixed cryoglobulinemia and B-cell clonal proliferations. *Leukemia* 2006;**20**:1145–54.

51. De Vita S, Boiocchi M, Sorrentino D, Carbone A, Avellini C, Dolcetti R, et al. Characterization of prelymphomatous stages of B cell lymphoproliferation in Sjögren's syndrome. *Arthritis Rheum* 1997;**40**:318–31.

52. De Vita S, Pivetta B, Ferraccioli GF, Marzotto A, De Re V, Dolcetti R, et al. Immunoglobulin gene usage and somatic mutations in primary Sjögren's syndrome–associated monoclonal B-cell lymphoproliferation prelymphomatous and frankly malignant. *J Rheumatol* 1997;**24**:36 (abstract).

53. Bahler DW, Swerdlow SH. Clonal salivary gland infiltrates associated with myoepithelial sialadenitis (Sjögren's syndrome) begin as nonmalignant antigen-selected expansions. *Blood* 1998;**91**:1864–72.

54. Miklos JA, Swerdlow SH, Bahler DW. Salivary gland mucosa–associated lymphoid tissue lymphoma immunoglobulin V(H) genes show frequent use of V1-69 with distinctive CDR3 features. *Blood* 2000;**95**:3878–84.

55. Martin T, Weber JC, Levallois H, Labouret N, Soley A, Koenig S, et al. Salivary gland lymphomas in patients with Sjögren's syndrome may frequently develop from rheumatoid factor B cells. *Arthritis Rheum* 2000;**43**:908–16.

56. Anderson LG, Cummings NA, Asofsky R, Hylton MB, Tarpley Jr TM, Tomasi Jr TB, et al. Salivary gland immunoglobulin and rheumatoid factor synthesis in Sjögren's syndrome: natural history and response to treatment. *Am J Med* 1972;**53**:456–63.
57. Kipps TJ, Tomhave E, Chen PP, Fox RI. Molecular characterization of a major autoantibody-associated cross-reactive idiotype in Sjögren's syndrome. *J Immunol* 1989;**142**:4261–8.
58. Fox RI, Chen P, Carson DA, Fong S. Expression of a cross-reactive idiotype on rheumatoid factor in patients with Sjögren's syndrome. *J Immunol* 1986;**136**:477–83.
59. Bende RJ, Aarts WM, Riedl RG, de Jong D, Pals ST, van Noesel CJ. Among B cell non-Hodgkin's lymphomas, MALT lymphomas express a unique antibody repertoire with frequent rheumatoid factor reactivity. *J Exp Med* 2005;**201**:1229–41.
60. Roosnek E, Lanzavecchia A. Efficient and selective presentation of antigen-antibody complexes by rheumatoid factor B cells. *J Exp Med* 1991;**173**:487–9.
61. De Vita S, Soldano F, Isola M, Monti G, Gabrielli A, Tzioufas A, et al. Preliminary classification criteria for the cryoglobulinaemic vasculitis. *Ann Rheum Dis* 2011;**70**:1183–90.
62. Quartuccio L, Isola M, Corazza L, Ramos-Casals M, Retamozo S, Ragab GM, et al. Validation of the classification criteria for cryoglobulinaemic vasculitis. *Rheumatology (Oxford)* 2014;**53**:2209–13.
63. Quartuccio L, Isola M, Corazza L, Maset M, Monti G, Gabrielli A, et al. Performance of the preliminary classification criteria for cryoglobulinaemic vasculitis and clinical manifestations in hepatitis C virus-unrelated cryoglobulinaemic vasculitis. *Clin Exp Rheumatol* 2012;**30**:S48–52.
64. Quartuccio L, Corazza L, Monti G, Gabrielli A, Tzioufas A, Ferri G, et al. Lymphoma prevalence in patients with serum cryoglobulins with or without cryoglobulinemic vasculitis: data extrapolated from the cryoglobulinemic vasculitis classification criteria database. *Arthritis Rheum* 2011;**63**:1529.
65. Quartuccio L, Isola M, Baldini C, Priori R, Bartoloni E, Carubbi F, et al. Clinical and biological differences between cryoglobulinaemic and hypergammaglobulinaemic purpura in primary Sjögren's syndrome: results of a large multicentre study. *Scand J Rheumatol* 2015;**44**:36–41.
66. Monti G, Pioltelli P, Saccardo F, Campanini M, Candela M, Cavallero G, et al. Incidence and characteristics of non-Hodgkin lymphomas in a multicenter case file of patients with hepatitis C virus-related symptomatic mixed cryoglobulinemias. *Arch Intern Med* 2005;**165**:101–5.
67. Mazzaro C, De Re V, Spina M, Dal Maso L, Festini G, Comar C, et al. Pegylated-interferon plus ribavirin for HCV-positive indolent non-Hodgkin lymphomas. *Br J Haematol* 2009;**145**:255–7.
68. Gasparotto D, De Vita S, De Re V, Marzotto A, De Marchi G, Scott CA, et al. Extrasalivary lymphoma development in Sjögren's syndrome: clonal evolution from parotid gland lymphoproliferation and role of local triggering. *Arthritis Rheum* 2003;**48**:3181–6.
69. De Vita S, Quartuccio L, Salvin S, Corazza L, Zabotti A, Fabris M. Cryoglobulinaemia related to Sjögren's syndrome or HCV infection: differences based on the pattern of bone marrow involvement, lymphoma evolution and laboratory tests after parotidectomy. *Rheumatology (Oxford)* 2012;**51**:627–33.
70. Theander E, Vasaitis L, Baecklund E, Nordmark G, Warfvinge G, Liedholm R, et al. Lymphoid organisation in labial salivary gland biopsies is a possible predictor for the development of malignant lymphoma in primary Sjögren's syndrome. *Ann Rheum Dis* 2011;**70**:1363–8.
71. Dong L, Masaki Y, Takegami T, Jin ZX, Huang CR, Fukushima T, et al. Clonality analysis of lymphoproliferative disorders in patients with Sjögren's syndrome. *Clin Exp Immunol* 2007;**150**:279–84.

72. Pitzalis C, Jones GW, Bombardieri M, Jones SA. Ectopic lymphoid-like structures in infection, cancer and autoimmunity. *Nat Rev Immunol* 2014;**14**:447–62.

73. Amft N, Curnow SJ, Scheel-Toellner D, Devadas A, Oates J, Crocker J, et al. Ectopic expression of the B cell-attracting chemokine BCA-1 *(CXCL13)* on endothelial cells and within lymphoid follicles contributes to the establishment of germinal center-like structures in Sjögren's syndrome. *Arthritis Rheum* 2001;**44**:2633–41.

74. Aloisi F, Pujol-Borrell R. Lymphoid neogenesis in chronic inflammatory diseases. *Nat Rev Immunol* 2006;**6**:205–17.

75. Daridon C, Pers JO, Devauchelle V, Martins-Carvalho C, Hutin P, Pennec YL, et al. Identification of transitional type II B cells in the salivary glands of patients with Sjögren's syndrome. *Arthritis Rheum* 2006;**54**:2280–8.

76. Mackay F, Groom JR, Tangye SG. An important role for B-cell activation factor and B cells in the pathogenesis of Sjögren's syndrome. *Curr Opin Rheumatol* 2007;**19**:406–13.

77. Le Pottier L, Devauchelle V, Fautrel A, Daridon C, Saraux A, Youinou P, et al. Ectopic germinal centers are rare in Sjögren's syndrome salivary glands and do not exclude autoreactive B cells. *J Immunol* 2009;**182**:3540–7.

78. Bombardieri M, Barone F, Humby F, Kelly S, McGurk M, Morgan P, et al. Activation-induced cytidine deaminase expression in follicular dendritic cell networks and interfollicular large B cells supports functionality of ectopic lymphoid neogenesis in autoimmune sialoadenitis and MALT lymphoma in Sjögren's syndrome. *J Immunol* 2007;**179**:4929–38.

79. Fauchais AL, Martel C, Gondran G, Lambert M, Launay D, Jauberteau MO, et al. Immunological profile in primary Sjögren syndrome: clinical significance, prognosis and long-term evolution to other auto-immune disease. *Autoimmun Rev* 2010;**9**:595–9.

80. Guerrier T, Le Pottier L, Youinou P, Pers JO, Jamin C. Importance of Toll-like receptors for B lymphocyte survival in primary Sjögren's syndrome. *Bull Group Int Rech Sci Stomatol Odontol* 2013;**52**:e1–6.

81. Barone F, Bombardieri M, Rosado MM, Morgan PR, Challacombe SJ, De Vita S, et al. *CXCL13, CCL21,* and *CXCL12* expression in salivary glands of patients with Sjögren's syndrome and MALT lymphoma: association with reactive and malignant areas of lymphoid organization. *J Immunol* 2008;**180**:5130–40.

82. Lessard CJ, Li H, Adrianto I, Ice JA, Rasmussen A, Grundahl KM, et al. Variants at multiple loci implicated in both innate and adaptive immune responses are associated with Sjögren's syndrome. *Nat Genet* 2013;**45**:1284–92.

83. Song H, Tong D, Cha Z, Bai J. C-X-C chemokine receptor type 5 gene polymorphisms are associated with non-Hodgkin lymphoma. *Mol Biol Rep* 2012;**39**:8629–35.

84. Risselada AP, Kruize AA, Goldschmeding R, Lafeber FP, Bijlsma JW, van Roon JA. The prognostic value of routinely performed minor salivary gland assessments in primary Sjögren's syndrome. *Ann Rheum Dis* 2014;**73**:1537–40.

85. Tzioufas AG, Kapsogeorgou EK, Moutsopoulos HM. Pathogenesis of Sjögren's syndrome: what we know and what we should learn. *J Autoimmun* 2012;**39**:4–8.

86. Dimitriou ID, Kapsogeorgou EK, Moutsopoulos HM, Manoussakis MN. CD40 on salivary gland epithelial cells: high constitutive expression by cultured cells from Sjögren's syndrome patients indicating their intrinsic activation. *Clin Exp Immunol* 2002;**127**:386–92.

87. Manoussakis MN, Kapsogeorgou EK. The role of intrinsic epithelial activation in the pathogenesis of Sjögren's syndrome. *J Autoimmun* 2010;**35**:219–24.

88. Hillen MR, Ververs FA, Kruize AA, Van Roon JA. Dendritic cells, T-cells and epithelial cells: a crucial interplay in immunopathology of primary Sjögren's syndrome. *Expert Rev Clin Immunol* 2014;**10**:521–31.

89. Farkas A, Tonel G, Nestle FO. Interferon-alpha and viral triggers promote functional maturation of human monocyte-derived dendritic cells. *Br J Dermatol* 2008;**158**:921–9.

90. Lavie F, Miceli-Richard C, Ittah M, Sellam J, Gottenberg JE, Mariette X. B-cell activating factor of the tumour necrosis factor family expression in blood monocytes and T cells from patients with primary Sjögren's syndrome. *Scand J Immunol* 2008;**67**:185–92.

91. Daridon C, Devauchelle V, Hutin P, Le Berre R, Martins-Carvalho C, Bendaoud B, et al. Aberrant expression of BAFF by B lymphocytes infiltrating the salivary glands of patients with primary Sjögren's syndrome. *Arthritis Rheum* 2007;**56**:1134–44.

92. Ittah M, Miceli-Richard C, Eric Gottenberg J, Lavie F, Lazure T, Ba N, et al. B cell-activating factor of the tumor necrosis factor family (BAFF) is expressed under stimulation by interferon in salivary gland epithelial cells in primary Sjögren's syndrome. *Arthritis Res Ther* 2006;**8**:R51.

93. Moisini I, Davidson A. BAFF: a local and systemic target in autoimmune diseases. *Clin Exp Immunol* 2009;**158**:155–63.

94. Schneider P, MacKay F, Steiner V, Hofmann K, Bodmer JL, Holler N, et al. BAFF, a novel ligand of the tumor necrosis factor family, stimulates B cell growth. *J Exp Med* 1999;**189**:1747–56.

95. Thompson JS, Schneider P, Kalled SL, Wang L, Lefevre EA, Cachero TG, et al. BAFF binds to the tumor necrosis factor receptor-like molecule B cell maturation antigen and is important for maintaining the peripheral B cell population. *J Exp Med* 2000;**192**:129–35.

96. Groom J, Kalled SL, Cutler AH, Olson C, Woodcock SA, Schneider P, et al. Association of BAFF/BLyS overexpression and altered B cell differentiation with Sjögren's syndrome. *J Clin Invest* 2002;**109**:59–68.

97. Mackay F, Woodcock SA, Lawton P, Ambrose C, Baetscher M, Schneider P, et al. Mice transgenic for BAFF develop lymphocytic disorders along with autoimmune manifestations. *J Exp Med* 1999;**190**:1697–710.

98. Batten M, Fletcher C, Ng LG, Groom J, Wheway J, Laabi Y, et al. TNF deficiency fails to protect BAFF transgenic mice against autoimmunity and reveals a predisposition to B cell lymphoma. *J Immunol* 2004;**172**:812–22.

99. Cheema GS, Roschke V, Hilbert DM, Stohl W. Elevated serum B lymphocyte stimulator levels in patients with systemic immune-based rheumatic diseases. *Arthritis Rheum* 2001;**44**:1313–9.

100. Mariette X, Roux S, Zhang J, Bengoufa D, Lavie F, Zhou T, et al. The level of BLyS (BAFF) correlates with the titre of autoantibodies in human Sjögren's syndrome. *Ann Rheum Dis* 2003;**62**:168–71.

101. Mumcu G, Bicakcigil M, Yilmaz N, Ozay H, Karacayli U, Cimilli H, et al. Salivary and serum B-cell activating factor (BAFF) levels after hydroxychloroquine treatment in primary Sjögren's syndrome. *Oral Health Prev Dent* 2013;**11**:229–34.

102. Mariette X, Seror R, Quartuccio L, Baron G, Salvin S, Fabris M, et al. Efficacy and safety of belimumab in primary Sjögren's syndrome: results of the BELISS open-label phase II study. *Ann Rheum Dis* 2015;**74**:526–31.

103. De Vita S, Quartuccio L, Seror R, Salvin S, Ravaud P, Fabris M, et al. Efficacy and safety of belimumab given for 12 months in primary Sjögren's syndrome: the BELISS open-label phase II study. *Rheumatology (Oxford)* 2015;**54**(12):2249–56.

104. Novak AJ, Slager SL, Fredericksen ZS, Wang AH, Manske MM, Ziesmer S, et al. Genetic variation in B-cell-activating factor is associated with an increased risk of developing B-cell non-Hodgkin lymphoma. *Cancer Res* 2009;**69**:4217–24.

105. Nezos A, Papageorgiou A, Fragoulis G, Ioakeimidis D, Koutsilieris M, Tzioufas AG, et al. B-cell activating factor genetic variants in lymphomagenesis associated with primary Sjögren's syndrome. *J Autoimmun* 2014;**51**:89–98.

106. Zayed RA, Sheba HF, Abo Elazaem MA, Elsaadany ZA, Elmessery LO, Mahmoud JA, et al. B-cell activating factor promoter polymorphisms in Egyptian patients with systemic lupus erythematosus. *Ann Clin Lab Sci* 2013;**43**:289–94.

107. Gragnani L, Piluso A, Giannini C, Caini P, Fognani E, Monti M, et al. Genetic determinants in hepatitis C virus–associated mixed cryoglobulinemia: role of polymorphic variants of BAFF promoter and Fc gamma receptors. *Arthritis Rheum* 2011;**63**:1446–51.

108. Ayad MW, Elbanna AA, Elneily DA, Sakr AS. Association of BAFF -871C/T promoter polymorphism with hepatitis C-related mixed cryoglobulinemia in a cohort of Egyptian patients. *Mol Diagn Ther* 2015;**19**:99–106.

109. Quartuccio L, Salvin S, Fabris M, Maset M, Pontarini E, Isola M, et al. BLyS upregulation in Sjögren's syndrome associated with lymphoproliferative disorders, higher ESSDAI score and B-cell clonal expansion in the salivary glands. *Rheumatology (Oxford)* 2013;**52**: 276–81.

110. De Vita S, Dolcetti R, Ferraccioli G, Pivetta B, De Re V, Gloghini A, et al. Local cytokine expression in the progression toward B cell malignancy in Sjögren's syndrome. *J Rheumatol* 1995;**22**:1674–80.

111. Ferraccioli GF, De Vita S. Cytokine expression in the salivary glands of Sjögren's syndrome patients in relation to tissue infiltration and lymphoepithelial lesions. *Arthritis Rheum* 1997;**40**:987–90.

112. Ciccia F, Guggino G, Rizzo A, Bombardieri M, Raimondo S, Carubbi F, et al. Interleukin (IL)-22 receptor 1 is over-expressed in primary Sjögren's syndrome and Sjögren-associated non-Hodgkin lymphomas and is regulated by IL-18. *Clin Exp Immunol* 2015;**181**:219–29.

113. Ray RJ, Paige CJ, Furlonger C, Lyman SD, Rottapel R. Flt3 ligand supports the differentiation of early B cell progenitors in the presence of interleukin-11 and interleukin-7. *Eur J Immunol* 1996;**26**:1504–10.

114. Tobon GJ, Renaudineau Y, Hillion S, Cornec D, Devauchelle-Pensec V, Youinou P, et al. The Fms-like tyrosine kinase 3 ligand, a mediator of B cell survival, is also a marker of lymphoma in primary Sjögren's syndrome. *Arthritis Rheum* 2010;**62**:3447–56.

115. Makula E, Pokorny G, Kiss M, Voros E, Kovacs L, Kovacs A, et al. The place of magnetic resonance and ultrasonographic examinations of the parotid gland in the diagnosis and follow-up of primary Sjögren's syndrome. *Rheumatology (Oxford)* 2000;**39**:97–104.

116. De Vita S, Lorenzon G, Rossi G, Sabella M, Fossaluzza V. Salivary gland echography in primary and secondary Sjögren's syndrome. *Clin Exp Rheumatol* 1992;**10**:351–6.

117. Cohen C, Mekinian A, Uzunhan Y, Fauchais AL, Dhote R, Pop G, et al. 18F-fluorodeoxyglucose positron emission tomography/computer tomography as an objective tool for assessing disease activity in Sjögren's syndrome. *Autoimmun Rev* 2013;**12**:1109–14.

118. Poulou LS, Ziakas P, Papageorgiou A, Papanikolaou M, Kapsogeorgou E, Tzioufas A, et al. FDG-PET/CT in the post-therapy evaluation of salivary gland lymphomas in Sjögren's syndrome: a prospective study. *Eur Congr Radiol. (C-0344 d)* 2013.

119. Pollard RP, Pijpe J, Bootsma H, Spijkervet FK, Kluin PM, Roodenburg JL, et al. Treatment of mucosa-associated lymphoid tissue lymphoma in Sjögren's syndrome: a retrospective clinical study. *J Rheumatol* 2011;**38**:2198–208.

120. De Vita S, Ferraccioli G, Avellini C, Sorrentino D, Dolcetti R, Di Loreto C, et al. Widespread clonal B-cell disorder in Sjögren's syndrome predisposing to *Helicobacter pylori*–related gastric lymphoma. *Gastroenterology* 1996;**110**:1969–74.

121. De Vita S, Quartuccio L, Isola M, Mazzaro C, Scaini P, Lenzi M, et al. A randomized controlled trial of rituximab for the treatment of severe cryoglobulinemic vasculitis. *Arthritis Rheum* 2012;**64**:843–53.

122. Quartuccio L, Isola M, Masolini P, Scaini P, Zani R, Tavoni A, et al. Health-related quality of life in severe cryoglobulinaemic vasculitis and improvement after B-cell depleting therapy. *Clin Exp Rheumatol* 2013;**31**:S9–14.

123. Quartuccio L, Zuliani F, Corazza L, Scaini P, Zani R, Lenzi M, et al. Retreatment regimen of rituximab monotherapy given at the relapse of severe HCV-related cryoglobulinemic vasculitis: long-term follow up data of a randomized controlled multicentre study. *J Autoimmun* 2015;**63**:88–93.

124. Quartuccio L, Fabris M, Salvin S, Maset M, De Marchi G, De Vita S. Controversies on rituximab therapy in Sjögren syndrome-associated lymphoproliferation. *Int J Rheumatol* 2009:424935.

125. Quartuccio L, Fabris M, Moretti M, Barone F, Bombardieri M, Rupolo M, et al. Resistance to rituximab therapy and local BAFF overexpression in Sjögren's syndrome–related myoepithelial sialadenitis and low-grade parotid B-cell lymphoma. *Open Rheumatol J* 2008;**2**:38–43.

126. Pers JO, Devauchelle V, Daridon C, Bendaoud B, Le Berre R, Bordron A, et al. BAFF-modulated repopulation of B lymphocytes in the blood and salivary glands of rituximab-treated patients with Sjögren's syndrome. *Arthritis Rheum* 2007;**56**:1464–77.

127. Gong Q, Ou Q, Ye S, Lee WP, Cornelius J, Diehl L, et al. Importance of cellular microenvironment and circulatory dynamics in B cell immunotherapy. *J Immunol* 2005;**174**:817–26.

128. De Vita S, De Marchi G, Sacco S, Zaja F, Scott CA, Ferraccioli G. Treatment of B-cell disorders of MALT in Sjögren's syndrome with anti-CD20 monoclonal antibody. In: *Proceedings of the 8th International Symposium on Sjögren's Syndrome Kanazawa, Japan*. 2002. p. 51. P8-2.

129. De Vita S, Quartuccio L, Salvin S, Picco L, Scott CA, Rupolo M, et al. Sequential therapy with belimumab followed by rituximab in Sjögren's syndrome associated with B-cell lymphoproliferation and overexpression of BAFF: evidence for long-term efficacy. *Clin Exp Rheumatol* 2014;**32**:490–4.

130. Rummel MJ, Niederle N, Maschmeyer G, Banat GA, von Grunhagen U, Losem C, et al. Bendamustine plus rituximab versus CHOP plus rituximab as first-line treatment for patients with indolent and mantle-cell lymphomas: an open-label, multicentre, randomised, phase 3 non-inferiority trial. *Lancet* 2013;**381**:1203–10.

131. Saadoun D, Pineton de Chambrun M, Hermine O, Karras A, Choquet S, Jego P, et al. Using rituximab plus fludarabine and cyclophosphamide as a treatment for refractory mixed cryoglobulinemia associated with lymphoma. *Arthritis Care Res (Hoboken)* 2013;**65**:643–7.

132. Zucca E, Conconi A, Laszlo D, Lopez-Guillermo A, Bouabdallah R, Coiffier B, et al. Addition of rituximab to chlorambucil produces superior event-free survival in the treatment of patients with extranodal marginal-zone B-cell lymphoma: 5-year analysis of the IELSG-19 randomized study. *J Clin Oncol* 2013;**31**:565–72.

133. Voulgarelis M, Giannouli S, Tzioufas AG, Moutsopoulos HM. Long term remission of Sjögren's syndrome associated aggressive B cell non-Hodgkin's lymphomas following combined B cell depletion therapy and CHOP (cyclophosphamide, doxorubicin, vincristine, prednisone). *Ann Rheum Dis* 2006;**65**:1033–7.

134. Ferraccioli G, Damato R, De Vita S, Fanin R, Damiani D, Baccarani M. Haematopoietic stem cell transplantation (HSCT) in a patient with Sjögren's syndrome and lung malt lymphoma cured lymphoma not the autoimmune disease. *Ann Rheum Dis* 2001;**60**:174–6.

Chapter 7

# Spontaneous and Inducible Animal Models of Sjögren's Syndrome

E. Astorri, D. Lucchesi, C. Pitzalis, M. Bombardieri

*Barts and The London School of Medicine and Dentistry, London, United Kingdom*

## 1. SPONTANEOUS MODELS

Most of the information from animal models of (Sjögren's syndrome) SS derives from studies of inbred mouse strains or mice carrying specific genetic defects that spontaneously develop autoimmune sialadenitis.[1] These included New Zealand black (NZB), NZB/New Zealand white (NZW),[2] and the Murphy Roths large (MRL) with its substrains.[3] In these models, SS-like pathology is mostly associated with other autoimmune phenomena typical of systemic lupus erythematosus (SLE) and they are thus more reminiscent of secondary SS in humans. An SS-like pathology has also been described in nonobese diabetic (NOD) mice,[4] a model also of insulin-dependent diabetes mellitus (IDDM) and in its variants such as the NOD.H2$^{h4}$ substrain, which is protected from IDDM. Finally, sialadenitis also developed in NFS/sld[a] and IQI/Jic[b] mice. In the context of this chapter, among the spontaneous models of SS, we will mostly focus on the description of the NOD strain and substrains, as these are the most robust models of SS because they mirror many of the typical features of the human condition, including salivary gland immune cell infiltration with focal lymphocytic sialadenitis, exocrine dysfunction, extraglandular manifestations, female predominance, and presence of autoantibodies.

### 1.1 NOD Mice

The NOD mouse strain is an excellent model of organ-specific autoimmune diseases and an important tool for dissecting tolerance mechanisms. The strength of this mouse strain is that it develops spontaneous autoimmune sialadenitis,[5] which shares

---

a. NFS inbred strain carrying the sublingual glands differentiation arrest (sld) mutation.
b. An inbred mouse strain maintained at the Central Institute for Experimental Animals, Japan.

Sjögren's Syndrome. http://dx.doi.org/10.1016/B978-0-12-803604-4.00007-1

many similarities to human SS, including the presence of specific autoantibodies, autoreactive CD4+ and CD8+ T cells, and genetic linkage to disease similar to that found in humans. NOD mice are also prone to developing other autoimmune syndromes, including autoimmune diabetes, which shares many similarities to autoimmune diabetes [type 1 diabetes (T1D)] in human subjects; autoimmune thyroiditis; and autoimmune peripheral polyneuropathy,[6] an SLE–like disease that develops if mice are exposed to killed *Mycobacterium*; and prostatitis (in male mice).

### 1.1.1 NOD Strain Origins and Characteristics

Makino and colleagues[7] originally developed the NOD strain in Japan during the selection of a cataract-prone strain derived from the outbred Jcl:ICR[c] line of mice. During the selection of this cataract-prone strain, the NOD strain was established, through repetitive brother–sister mating, as a subline that spontaneously developed diabetes. The incidence of spontaneous diabetes in the NOD mouse is 60% to 80% in females and 20% to 30% in males.[8] Diabetes onset typically occurs at 12–14 weeks of age in female mice and slightly later in male mice. Histological studies have shown that few immune cell infiltrates are noted in islets until approximately 3–4 weeks of age, when both male and female mice begin to demonstrate mononuclear infiltrates that surround the islet (periinsulitis). These infiltrates progress and invade the islets (insulitis) over the subsequent few weeks, such that most mice demonstrate severe insulitis by 10 weeks of age.[9] The finding that the reduced incidence in male mice occurs in spite of similar levels of early insulitis suggests that late regulatory events control disease progression. Thus the autoimmune process in the pancreas of NOD mice includes two checkpoints: checkpoint 1, or insulitis, which is completely penetrant; and checkpoint 2, or overt diabetes, which is not completely penetrant.[10] Autoimmune sialadenitis in NOD mice has an incidence similar to insulitis, being more common in female as compared with male NOD mice. Conversely, dacryoadenitis develops more often in male mice. Initial immune cell infiltrates in NOD submandibular glands are observed around 10 weeks of age in females, several weeks after the development of the insulitis. Importantly, decrease in exocrine secretory function follows the inflammatory process and is evident normally after 16 weeks of age with reduced salivary flow. This feature is unique of NOD mice in comparison with other animal models of SS, in which autoimmune sialadenitis is not followed by reduction of exocrine function of the salivary glands. Thus NOD mice offer the possibility to investigate not only the mechanisms leading to breach of tolerance and autoimmunity, but also to understand the events that link chronic inflammation in the target organ to reduction of exocrine function. Interestingly, the incidence of disease is highest when mice are maintained in a relatively germ-free environment but dramatically decreases when mice are maintained in conventional "dirty" housing facilities.[11,12] The basis for this effect is unclear, but it has been suggested that it reflects the fine

---

c. An inbred albino mouse strain originally distributed by the Institute of Cancer Research (ICR) in the USA and distributed by CLEA, Japan (Jcl).

tuning of the immune system that occurs during exposure to foreign proteins and protects the individual from allergy, autoimmunity, and other diseases of immune dysregulation.[13] In addition to the classical NOD mice, a congenic NOD strain, the NOD.H2$^{h4}$, has been developed and is characterized by almost complete protection from insulitis but a high incidence of sialadenitis.[14] In keeping with the classical NOD strain, female, but not male, NOD.H2$^{h4}$ mice develop lymphocytic infiltration of the salivary glands and autoantibodies against Ro and La, although this process is generally delayed compared with NOD mice.[15] Interestingly, the NOD.H2$^{h4}$ strain also develops iodine-induced autoimmune thyroiditis, another organ-specific autoimmune disease which is often associated with SS in humans.[16]

### 1.1.2 NOD Genetics

Multiple loci control the genetic susceptibility to diabetes in this mouse. NOD mice harbor a unique major histocompatibility complex (MHC) haplotype, termed H-2g7, that is essential and is the highest genetic contributor for disease susceptibility.[17,18] This MHC haplotype does not express an I-E molecule because of a defective Eα locus. Moreover, the unique I-A molecule contains a nonaspartic acid substitution at position 57 of the β chain that substantially alters the repertoire of MHC binding peptides presented by this allele. Strikingly, this substitution is also seen in human T1D MHC susceptibility loci in the DQ β chain.[19] Several studies that examine the MHC requirement in NOD mice for the development of insulitis and diabetes conclude that homozygosity of the H-2g7 haplotype may be necessary for diabetes development and that dominant protection may be provided by some MHC manipulations, including introducing a functional I-E or non–I-Ag7 allele but not others.[20,21] The major contributor to autoimmune diseases susceptibility is the MHC class II molecule itself. Its unique structure, its ability to bind an array of low affinity peptides, and its shared structural features in humans susceptible to autoimmune disease suggests that targeting this gene product, both in terms of genetic screening and potential therapy, remains a high priority. Finally, it should be noted that multiple genes are encoded within the MHC loci, many of which have been associated with immune functions. Possibly, the high susceptibility endowed by the H-2g7 MHC may be caused, in part, by polymorphisms in other genes, such as tumor necrosis factor (TNF)-α, encoded within this chromosomal segment.

In addition to the MHC locus, many other loci contribute to disease development and are termed *insulin-dependent diabetes (Idd) loci.* To date, over 20 potential Idd loci have been identified,[18,22] but in most cases the exact structural or regulatory elements that lie within these loci still await identification. Interestingly, different loci have been associated with the development of diabetes and sialadenitis, with the Idd3 and Idd5 intervals, on chromosomes 3 and 1 respectively, being more strongly involved in conferring susceptibility to SS-like disease. This suggests that the autoimmune process in the pancreas and in the salivary glands of NOD mice occur independently. These two NOD genetic regions, designated *Aec2* and *Aec1,* are necessary and sufficient to recapitulate

SS-like disease in nonsusceptible C57 black 6 (C57BL/6) mice.[23] Interestingly, a bioinformatics-based approach applied to the C57BL/6.NOD-*Aec1Aec2* strain demonstrated that loci-dependent aberrations in innate immune responses affecting salivary gland homeostasis precede the onset of overt disease.[24]

Researchers have discovered some clues about the nature of some of these genetic susceptibilities. In the case of the Idd5 locus (which may encode two regulatory elements), a unique polymorphism in the *ctla-4* gene was determined that affects gene splicing. Interestingly, *CTLA-4* is also a candidate gene in humans susceptible to a variety of autoimmune diseases, although the structural basis for *CTLA-4* dysfunction is distinct.[25] Candidate genes have been suggested in other Idd loci as well. *VAV3* polymorphisms may account for Idd18, *CD101* for Idd10, and the interleukin (IL)-2 or IL-21 genes for Idd3.

Overall, differently from other mouse strains in which autoimmunity is driven by single genetic defects (ie, MRL/lpr), NOD mice represent a more reliable model of the immune dysregulation that leads to human autoimmunity and chronic inflammation in the target organs. In particular, the existence of multiple susceptibility loci in the NOD strain again highlights the inherent complexity of the autoimmune process and supports the hypothesis that multiple tolerance networks are defective and interact in this strain. In fact, the spontaneous incidence of autoimmunity in the NOD mouse strain is likely to be a consequence of the absence of protective genes, as well.

### 1.1.3 Lessons From Gene Knockout in NOD Mice: The Role of Cytokines in NOD Mouse Sialadenitis

Knockout or transgenic mice in the NOD background represented a valid model to evaluate the specific role of single cytokines in the disease pathogenesis. More recently, the use of cytokine blocking compounds has provided further insight into the complex networks of proinflammatory and antiinflammatory mediators regulating salivary gland inflammation. It is important to underline that because of the redundancy of the cytokine system, with the differential and often paradoxical role of cytokines in different phases of the immune responses, a full understanding of the pathogenic relevance of each cytokine system in NOD sialadenitis is extremely difficult. In this contest it is also interesting to underline the differences in terms of disease development and progression in the sialadenitis and the diabetes in the NOD mice transgenic or knockout for specific cytokines.

NOD.IFNγ−/− do not develop inflammatory infiltrates in the salivary glands and do not present loss of salivary flow. Conversely, these animals develop diabetes and dacryoadenitis with lachrymal gland dysfunction with similar incidence and severity as in the NOD original strain.[26] This data suggests that interferon (IFN) γ may exert differential roles in the diverse anatomical districts, possibly in combination with local factors. In this regard, IFNγ has been shown to be able to directly activate ductal epithelial cells to produce proinflammatory cytokines and express class II MHC in NOD mice.[27] Whether these events occur in an early phase of the salivary gland disease process, as suggested,[28] and to what extent they are able to influence the development of the sialadenitis, is still unclear.

Despite IL-4, messenger RNA (mRNA) has not been detected by traditional reverse transcription polymerase chain reaction (PCR) in the salivary glands of NOD mice. NOD.*IL-4−/−* do not show secretory loss, although inflammatory infiltrates in the salivary glands still develop with B-/T-cell infiltration similar to the original strain.[29] This effect is possibly related to the systemic and local reduction in (auto)antibody production influenced by the absence of IL-4.

The role of IL-10 in sialadenitis has been originally investigated by transgenic expression of the murine IL-10 gene under the salivary amylase promoter in C57BL/6 mice. In these mice, IL-10 induced apoptosis of glandular epithelial cells via up-regulation of *FasL* expression on T lymphocytes.[30] Accordingly, NOD mice deficient for IL-10 develop normal disease progression.[28] Conversely, administration of an adeno-associated virus expressing IL-10 via retrograde cannulation of submandibular glands in NOD mice resulted in reduced glandular inflammation and preservation of the salivary flow. Similarly controversial results have been described in the insulitis of NOD mice where IL-10 exerts a proinflammatory role in early phases,[31] whereas treatment with IL-10/Fc fusion protein protects mice from developing diabetes.[32] Thus it is likely that IL-10 may exert different net effects depending on different phases of the autoimmune process and diverse local milieu of cytokine expression.

### 1.1.4 Histological and Functional Characteristics of the Immune Cell Infiltrates in NOD Salivary Glands: Formation of Ectopic Germinal Centers

The immune cells infiltrating the submandibular glands of NOD mice are organized in focal aggregates similar to the ones observed in the human salivary glands. Most often these aggregates surround a central ductal structure or a blood vessel. Inflammatory foci in early stages are mainly composed of CD4+ T cells with a minority of B220+ B cells and CD8+ cytotoxic T cells. Interestingly, an organization of T and B cells in separate and distinct areas within the gland has been demonstrated, similar to human SS.[33] Furthermore, we and others have shown that in NOD salivary glands and pancreatic islets, a true phenomenon of ectopic lymphoid neogenesis takes place, with presence of follicular dendritic cell networks, ectopic expression of the lymphoid chemokines (*CXL13, CCL21,* and *CCL21*)/lymphotoxin (LT) pathway, formation of functional germinal center–like structures with GL7+ B cells, and in situ production of autoantibodies.[9,34–36] Of relevance, pharmacological blockade of LTβ using a LTβR-immunoglobulin (Ig) fusion protein was able to prevent and ameliorate both sialadenitis and dacryoadenitis in NOD mice, resulting in reduced ectopic expression of lymphoid chemokines, blockade of the lymphoneogenetic process, and preservation of exocrine function.[34,35] Similarly to NOD mice, female NOD.H2$^{h4}$ mice also develop ectopic germinal centers spontaneously in the salivary glands. Interestingly, whereas these mice display circulating anti-Ro and anti-La autoantibodies before the formation of ectopic follicles in the salivary glands (but in concomitance with germinal center formation in the spleen), the production of anti-double stranded DNA antibodies is delayed and coincides with the formation of ectopic follicles.[37]

The formation of an ectopic germinal center strongly suggests that an in situ antigen-driven process involving the adaptive arm of the immune system takes place within the target tissue. In this regard, evidence that T cells may be activated in an antigen-driven process within the submandibular glands of NOD mice has been provided by the demonstration that lesional T cells isolated from NOD salivary glands display a preferential and restricted T-cell receptor Vβ usage (similarly to the human counterpart), with predominance of Vβ6 and Vβ8 expression by focal T lymphocytes.[38] In addition, dendritic cells and activated macrophages have been described in NOD submandibular glands, suggesting the possibility that local antigen presentation is taking place within focal inflammatory infiltrates.

Tissue expression of various cytokines and chemokines in NOD salivary glands have been described as a result of local activation of immune cells. On the other hand, the aberrant production of these molecules results in the continuous recruitment and activation of inflammatory cells in an amplificatory loop resulting in disease chronicization. Normally, increase in local expression of proinflammatory cytokines in NOD mice is observed in parallel with the development of initial focal infiltrates around 10–12 weeks of age. Conversely, expression of Th2-related cytokines, such as IL-4 and IL-5, is normally absent in the target organ of NOD mice. The pattern of cytokine expression in NOD sialadenitis is reminiscent of that observed in salivary glands of SS patients and related to a T helper cell (Th1)–mediated inflammation. Accordingly, high levels of mRNA of TNFα, IL-1β, IFNγ, IL-2, IL-6, IL-10, and IL-12 have been detected in NOD submandibular glands.[38,39] Finally, the expression of B-cell activating factor (BAFF), a strong B-cell survival and activating factor which is a member of the TNF superfamily, together with that of other molecules related to B-cell activation has been reported by microarray analysis in salivary glands of 8–12 week-old NOD mice, further supporting that the salivary gland microenvironment is sufficient to promote local B-cell activation.[46]

### 1.1.5 Autoreactive B-Cell Activation and Autoantibody Production in NOD Mice

B-cell activation and autoantibody production is one of the hallmarks of human SS. NOD mice display features of B-cell abnormalities that share several characteristics with human SS. Hypergammaglobulinemia has been described in the serum of female and male NOD mice with approximately a 1.5-fold increase of circulating IgG as compared to control BALB/c[d] mice. Around 70% of diabetic NOD females aged >25 weeks also display antinuclear reactivity with indirect immunofluorescence on Hep-2 cells, a similar prevalence as compared with human SS.[40] Conversely, anti-Ro52 autoantibodies are uncommonly observed in the sera of NOD mice, with a prevalence of around 10%. Anti-Ro60 and anti-La antibodies are undetectable.[41] More recently, NOD mouse sera have been

---

d. Albino mice first isolated by H. Bagg (Bagg ALBino), the "/c" was added in 1932 by Snell.

demonstrated to react with a described neo-autoantigen of SS: the $\alpha$-fodrin, a nonerythroid spectrin that becomes antigenic after the cleavage by calpains to a 120-kD protein that occurs during the apoptosis process. Serum anti–$\alpha$-fodrin antibodies are detectable by western blot in NOD mice as early as 12 weeks of age, and their levels seem to correlate with salivary gland inflammation until 30 weeks of age.[42] Anti–$\alpha$-fodrin B-cell reactivity is likely to represent a T-cell–dependent antigen-driven process with splenic Th1 lymphocytes responding to antigenic challenge with recombinant $\alpha$-fodrin (as assessed by T-cell proliferation and Th1-related cytokine expression).[42] The possibility that the source of antigenic $\alpha$-fodrin resides within the salivary gland microenvironment is suggested by the demonstration that ductal epithelial cells in NOD mice, but not control mice, express the 120-Kd fragment of $\alpha$-fodrin. However, evidence that a population of antigen-specific anti–$\alpha$-fodrin T cells localizes within NOD salivary glands has not been provided. Finally, another important autoantigen in NOD mice that acts as a target of humoral immune response is muscarinic receptor M3; these antibodies have been suggested to be the more important antibody specificity in mediating exocrine dysfunction in submandibular glands in NOD mice.[40]

NOD.Igμ$^{null}$ mice, which lack B lymphocytes, do not develop decrease in salivary flow despite the presence of focal lymphocytic infiltrates in the submandibular glands. Moreover, transfer of human IgG from SS patients into NOD.Igμ$^{null}$ mice is able to induce secretory loss.[43] Similarly, transfer of IgG from old NOD mice into young NOD mice in the absence of focal salivary glands infiltrates resulted in impaired secretory function.[44] All together these data strongly implicate autoantibody production in the development of salivary hypofunction and secretory loss in NOD mice. Thus a better understanding of the mechanism behind the production of these autoantibodies would represent an important step toward the treatment of this disease in humans.

### 1.1.6 Aberrant Apoptosis in NOD Salivary Glands

As with human SS, apoptosis of acinar and ductal salivary gland epithelial cells is an important feature of the autoimmune process in the sialadenitis of NOD mice, although to what extent increased epithelial cell apoptosis is relevant in mediating exocrine dysfunction in NOD mice is still unclear. Increased levels of apoptotic ductal and acinar epithelial cells in submandibular glands have been reported as early as week 8 in NOD mice.[45] Interestingly, NOD-scid mice, which lack functional T and B cells and thus inflammatory infiltrates in the salivary glands, display enhanced epithelial cell apoptosis. This would suggest that apoptosis in NOD salivary glands occurs at a very early stage and even before the development of cellular infiltrates. Early apoptotic events, possibly as a result of abnormal salivary gland homeostasis developing before or concomitant to the onset of immune cell infiltrates, are also believed to induce break of tolerance toward salivary gland–associated antigens and trigger the autoimmune exocrinopathy in NOD mice.[46]

As further evidence that abnormal apoptosis of epithelial cells is an important feature of NOD sialadenitis, increased activation of proapoptotic molecules involved in triggering and regulating the apoptotic process, such as caspases and proteins of the *bcl-2* family, can be observed in both NOD and NOD-scid mice. An altered balance between proapoptotic (ie, *Bax*) and antiapoptotic (*bcl-2* and *bcl-xL*) members of the *bcl-2* family has been described in epithelial cells of submandibular glands of old NOD and young and old NOD-scid mice.[47] Conversely, infiltrating lymphocytes strongly express *bcl-2* and *bcl-xL* but not *Bax* and are likely to be resistant from apoptosis. Downstream molecules in the apoptotic cascade such as caspases are also activated in NOD submandibular glands; ie, caspases 3 and 8 are strongly expressed by acinar cells of both NOD and NOD-scid mice but not control mice.[47] More recent evidence suggests that genetic abnormalities profoundly influence altered salivary gland apoptosis of epithelial cells in NOD mice. Microarray analysis of C57BL/6 mice carrying two NOD genetic intervals (*Idd3* and *Idd5*) that confer susceptibility toward autoimmune exocrinopathy (C57BL/6.NOD-Aec1Aec2) showed dysregulated expression of several caspases and *bcl-2* family members before the onset of the sialadenitis at as early as 8 weeks of age.[48]

Activation of the Fas/FasL pathway is likely to play a central upstream role in mediating early and late apoptotic events in NOD salivary glands. Progressive over-expression of *Fas/FasL* mRNA and protein levels has been demonstrated in submandibular glands of NOD mice from 5 to 20 weeks of age.[45,49] Interestingly, increased protein expression of *Fas* and *FasL* by acinar and ductal epithelial cells has been reported as early as the first week of age in NOD mice,[49] suggesting that activation of the *Fas/FasL* pathway is a very early event in NOD exocrinopathy. However, higher epithelial expression of *Fas* and *FasL* was observed in old vs young NOD mice and in NOD vs NOD-scid mice,[49] suggesting that further activation of the *Fas/FasL* pathway is dependent on the presence of immune cell infiltrates and chronic inflammation. Accordingly, a close correlation between the amount of epithelial cells undergoing apoptosis and the magnitude of mononuclear cell infiltration could be observed in NOD submandibular glands.[38] In contrast, although aberrant apoptotic events have been observed very early in NOD-scid mice, these mice do not develop salivary and lacrimal hypofunction, possibly because of increased expression of antiapoptotic proteins such as *bcl-2*.[49] This may suggest that, at early stages, low-level apoptosis is dependent on disrupted salivary gland homeostasis and possibly leads to breach of tolerance and autoimmunity in NOD mice. Conversely, when a chronic inflammatory infiltrate develops, Fas/FasL-triggered apoptosis of ductal and acinar epithelial cells is dependent on local immune cell activation with release of soluble mediators, with cytokines likely to play a pivotal role.

## 1.2 Other Spontaneous Models of SS: NZB and NZB/NZW F1, NFS/sld, IQI/Jic and MRL/+ and MRL/lpr Mice

The NFS/sld mouse provides a model for primary SS, in which aberrant immune responses against α-fodrin is facilitated.[50] A defect in salivary gland development leads to the cleavage of a structural protein (fodrin) by caspases. Subsequent to neonatal thymectomy, the 3d-Tx NFS/sld mouse develops T-cell infiltrates reactive to the fodrin 125-kD in the salivary and lacrimal glands. Sera from patients with SS recognized autoantibodies to fodrin 125-kD[42]; however, the specificity of these autoantibodies for SS was found not to be as strong as originally thought. In addition to SS-like disease, the 3d-Tx NFS/sld mice developed severe autoimmune lesions involving arthritis and interstitial pneumonia with aging.

Kallikrein (Klk)-13 has been suggested to play a role as an autoantigen in the disease development in IQI/Jic mice.[51] Focal infiltration of lymphocytes with parenchymal destruction was noted in both lacrimal and salivary glands. Sialadenitis was more prominent in females than in males. Interestingly, the lymphocytes in small foci were CD4+ cells, whereas in larger lesions, the majority of infiltrating cells were B cells (B220+). As in a subpopulation of patients with primary SS, the IQI/Jic mouse develops inflammatory lesions in multiple organs such as the lung, pancreas, and kidney.[52]

MRL mice were first reported to present periductal lymphocytic infiltrates in salivary glands in 1982.[3,53] MRL/+ and MRL/lpr mice differ with respect to a mutation involving the *Fas* gene,[54] a cell surface receptor transducing apoptotic signals. Cellular turnover of immune cells, including apoptosis, has been found to be crucial in the process of negative and positive selection, as well as in the regulation of immune responses. Defective apoptosis related to the *lpr* mutation induces increasing susceptibility and severity of the disease, most likely by accelerating the disease course. Immunohistochemical analyses attempting to characterize T cells in MRL/lpr mice have suggested local activation of T cells.[55] Interestingly, the T-cell response at the site of inflammation is not completely polyclonal, indicating the presence of T-cell clones, which might be strongly associated with the pathogenesis, a fact confirmed by T-cell transfer experiments.[56]

A differentiated pattern of cytokine expression has been suggested to influence the development and progression of the autoimmune sialadenitis in MRL/lpr mice.[57] The genes for the inflammatory cytokines IL-1β and TNF were expressed in the salivary glands before the onset of sialadenitis. IL-6 mRNA expression was detected at the time of onset of salivary gland inflammation and up-regulated with advancing age. Despite female predominance and presence of anti-Ro antibodies in a subset of mice, hyposalivation, which is the main clinical hallmark of defective glandular secretion, is absent in this model. Nonetheless, the MRL/lpr mouse should be considered as a valuable model when studying the implication of *Fas* and altered cytokine expression in relation to specific disease symptoms. Although deficient cytokine regulation alone cannot cause autoimmunity, it may certainly imbalance tolerance mechanisms, hence facilitating the development of autoimmune diseases.

In NZB/NZW F1 mice, a model of lupus, which also develops progressive focal sialadenitis,[58] glandular involvement is more pronounced in females compared with males, a phenomenon generally being less apparent in NZB mice.[2]

## 2. INDUCIBLE MODELS OF SS-LIKE SIALADENITIS AND AUTOIMMUNITY

The possibility of using inducible models of sialadenitis would offer the opportunity to overcome intrinsic limitations (ie, frequent incomplete penetrance, variable and often delayed onset, and difficulties of gene targeting) which hinder the use of spontaneous models in order to precisely dissect the pathogenic mechanisms underlying the development of autoimmunity, immune cell infiltration in the salivary glands, and exocrine dysfunction typical of SS.

Several approaches in the attempt to induce experimental SS have been undertaken. Historically, animals have been immunized according to standard immunization protocols using salivary gland extracts or putative autoantigens. However, unlike experimental animal models which successfully mimic other chronic inflammatory/autoimmune conditions (ie, collagen-induced arthritis for rheumatoid arthritis or experimental autoimmune encephalomyelitis in the case of multiple sclerosis), in general this approach has not proven very effective in consistently reproducing the classical features of SS. As such, they will be described very briefly here.

More recently, viral-induced models of sialadenitis have been developed, either via systemic infection with murine viruses displaying tropism for the salivary glands or via direct retrograde cannulation of viruses into salivary gland excretory ducts, which have provided very significant insights into the mechanisms leading to the development of focal lymphocytic sialadenitis, breach of self-tolerance, and the development of autoimmune traits.

### 2.1 Immunization Methods to Induce Sialadenitis

Experimental sialadenitis can be induced by immunization of PL/J$^e$ mice with carbonic anhydrase II (CAII),[59] the cytoplasmic isoform of a family of enzymes that catalyze the reversible hydration of carbon dioxide to bicarbonate and hydrogen ions. Within tissues, CAII is highly expressed by transporting epithelial cells, such as in ducts present in salivary glands, the pancreas, the biliary tract, and kidneys.[60] In view of the fact that a significant percentage of patients with SS had autoantibodies to CAII,[61] PL/J mice with different H-2 haplotypes were immunized with purified CAII. Compared with control and untreated mice, CAII-immunized mice showed a significant increase in the number and size of mononuclear cell infiltrates in the salivary glands. Among several mouse strains with different H-2 haplotypes, strains bearing H-2s and H-2u were particularly susceptible to CAII-induced sialadenitis.[61]

It was later reported that repeated immunizations (ie, a minimum of two) of mice with homologous salivary gland extracts in association with *Klebsiella* O3 lipopolysaccharides as an adjuvant were able to induce an experimental autoimmune sialadenitis characterized by perivascular accumulation of a predominant

---

e. "Princeton Leukemia" strain maintained by Jackson laboratories.

T-cell infiltrate associated with loss of acinar structures and development of organ-specific autoantibodies directed against a series of putative autoantigens.[62]

More recently, an experimental model of autoimmune sialadenitis was described in mice immunized with the ribonucleoprotein Ro60, which together with Ro52 and La48 is one of the major autoantigens in SS, with circulating autoantibodies that can be detected in up to 75% of patients with SS.[63] Immunization experiments using Ro60 peptides revealed certain sequences capable of inducing autoantibody production resembling Ro and La autoimmunity in humans.[64] When repetitively administered intraperitoneally in BALB/c mice, this immunization strategy was able to induce a disease resembling several aspects of SS. In particular, these mice showed SS-like histopathology, decreased salivary gland function, and production of anti-Ro/SSA and anti-La/SSB.[64] Although of high interest, this model also presents several drawbacks such as (1) it is quite laborious, because after the initial immunization, 4 more rounds of immunizations up to day 63 are required for disease development; (2) the disease develops slowly and over the course of 38 weeks, which makes this model expensive and time-consuming to run; and (3) the disease penetrance is low, with fewer than 50% of the mice developing SS-like focal lymphocytic infiltrates in the salivary glands. As such, it remains a valid model but not amenable to a widespread use as an inducible model of SS.

## 2.2 Virus-Induced Experimental Sialadenitis

### 2.2.1 Murine Cytomegalovirus

Around 70% to 90% of the world population has encountered human cytomegalovirus (CMV). Given the tropism of CMV for the salivary glands in humans, this virus has been considered a putative etiological agent of SS. Investigations of the presence of the CMV genome in the salivary glands of SS patients and nonimmune sicca patients invariably, and not surprisingly, lead to the detection of the viral genome in both groups, possibly suggesting that it is not the presence of the virus itself, but the interaction with the host immune system which is needed to trigger an SS-like sialadenitis.[65] In keeping with this hypothesis, the infection of mice with murine CMV (MCMV) is capable of inducing different and progressive features of SS depending on the strains used and their genetic background. To elaborate the role of a viral etiology, four different strains of mice (C57Bl/6 [B6]-+/+, *Fas*-deficient B6-lpr/lpr, *TNFRI*-deficient B6-*tnfr1(0/0)*, and B6-*tnfr1(0/0)*-lpr/lpr mice) were infected intraperitoneally with murine cytomegalovirus (MCMV) (Table 7.1).[66] All mice developed acute sialadenitis by day 28 and chronic sialadenitis from 100 days of age onward. Interestingly, murine CMV in C57Bl/6 wild type and lpr/lpr mice lead to the development of acute sialadenitis and salivary gland infiltration in both genotypes (albeit more sever in the presence of the lpr mutation), but in the lpr/lpr animals it also lead to the development of anti-Ro and anti-La antibodies, the most typical autoantibodies associated to SS. It is worth noting that, in contrast to the MRL/lpr strain previously described in this chapter (in Section 1 dedicated to the spontaneous models of SS), the lpr/lpr mutation on a C57Bl/6

**TABLE 7.1 Main Characteristics of Commonly Used Murine Models of Sjögren's Syndrome**

| | Mouse Strain | Focal Sialadenitis | Anti-Ro/SSA | Exocrine Dysfunction | Associated Autoimmunity |
|---|---|---|---|---|---|
| Spontaneous | NOD | Yes | Yes (>10 <50%) | Yes | IDDM, autoimmune thyroiditis |
| | NOD.H2[h4] | Yes | Yes (same as NOD but delayed) | Yes | Autoimmune thyroiditis |
| | NZB/W F1 | Yes | Yes | No | SLE |
| | MRL/lpr | Yes | Yes (<10%) | No | SLE |
| | NFS/sld | Yes | No | No | Arthritis and interstitial pneumonia |
| | IQI/Jic | Yes | No | No | Inflammatory lesions in multiple organs (lung, pancreas, and kidney) |
| Inducible | Immunization with CAII in PL/J mice | Yes | No | No | No |
| | Immunization with Ro60 in BALB/c | Yes | Yes | Yes | No |
| | Infection with MCMV in multiple strains | Yes | Yes | Yes | No |
| | Infection with AdV5 in C57BL/6 mice | Yes | No | Yes | No |

*AdV5*, Adenoviruses 5; *CAII*, carbonic anhydrase II; *IDDM*, insulin-dependent diabetes mellitus; *MCMV*, murine cytomegalovirus; *NOD*, nonobese diabetes; *SLE*, systemic lupus erythematosus.

background induces only a mild autoimmunity late in the animals' life, mainly involving kidneys but not the salivary glands. It has been suggested that both *Fas* and *TNFRI*-mediated apoptosis contribute to the clearance of MCMV-infected cells in the salivary glands,[66] as apoptotic cells were detected during the acute, but not the chronic, phase of inflammation. Indeed, defects in these molecules may lead to a postinfectious chronic inflammation resembling the histopathology of SS. In keeping with this hypothesis, salivary gland–specific correction of the *Fas* defect via local overexpression of *FasL* in C57Bl/6-lpr/lpr mice was able to reduce the severity of MCMV-induced sialadenitis.[67] Finally, very recent evidence suggested that natural killer (NK) cells play a fundamental role in regulating the fine balance between the control of viral infection and the onset of autoimmunity. Specifically, NK cells expressing *TRAIL* (TNF-related apoptosis inducing ligand) were shown to be able to eliminate autoreactive CD4 T cells and limit the onset of SS-like sialadenitis and autoimmunity in the MCMV-induced model of SS, although at the expenses of a less-efficient viral clearance, leading to chronic MCMV infection in the salivary glands.[68]

### 2.2.2 Adenovirus-Induced Sialadenitis

Adenoviruses (AdV) 5 have been commonly used for gene transfer experiments given their ability to infect a wide group of different cell types and the capacity to harbor large genes in their genome incorporated via homologous recombination techniques. Typically, AdV used for this scope are engineered as replication-defective vectors, ie, lacking the *E1-E3* genes encoding for viral structural proteins, and are thus unable to finalize their life cycle and expand the infection to other cells after new rounds of replications.

Initial work with AdV suggested that the delivery, via retrograde cannulation of the excretory submandibular gland ducts, of proinflammatory mediators such as IL-17A encoded by replication-deficient AdV5 vectors was necessary to induce sialadenitis and autoimmunity in nonautoimmune-prone mice.[69] However, we have recently described a novel model of SS-like disease whereby focal lymphocytic sialadenitis is triggered by the direct delivery in the submandibular glands of wild-type C57Bl/6 mice of an AdV5 simply harboring a reporter gene (used for validation purposes but not causing a proinflammatory effect per se).[70] A threshold effect was observed, in which the delivery of high doses of viral particles (ie, >$10^7$ cfu) was required for the induction of focal lymphocytic sialadenitis. One single administration of AdV5 (independently from the reporter gene used) was sufficient to induce immune cell infiltration, which progressed from a diffuse innate immune cell invasion within the first week to a progressive accumulation of cells of the adaptive immune arm (ie, CD4 T cells and B cells). In turn, by 3 weeks post–AdV delivery, the inflammatory infiltrate was extremely reminiscent not only of the periductal inflammatory foci observed in SS patients (Fig. 7.1), but also recapitulated the formation of ectopic follicles which were characterized by distinct B- and T-cell areas and development of high endothelial venules. Interestingly, before the onset of a high degree of

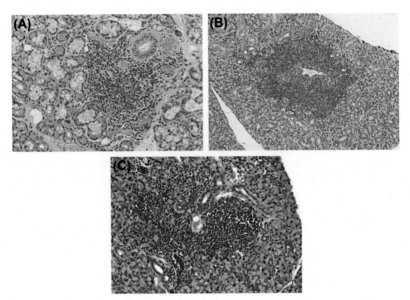

**FIGURE 7.1**   Development of periductal focal lymphocytic sialoadenitis in submandibular glands of animal models of SS showing high resemblance with the typical inflammatory lesions observed in SS patients. (A) SS patient, (B) Female NOD mouse at 20 weeks, (C) AdV-injected C57BL/6 mouse after 3 weeks.

lymphoid organization and segregation, an up-regulation of lymphoid chemokines *CXCL13, CCL19,* and *CCL21* and their receptor was observed. The lymphoid chemokine *CXCL13* was selectively expressed in the B cell–rich areas, whereas *CCL21* was exclusively produced in association with high endothelial cells in the T-cell areas of the foci. This pattern is highly reminiscent of the distribution of these chemokines in secondary lymphoid tissue such as lymph nodes. Moreover, markers of germinal center functionality were detected in the injected salivary glands, including follicular dendritic cell network development in the B-cell area, expression of GL7 (a protein expressed by germinal center B cells in murine secondary lymphoid organs) by B cells within the aggregates and detectable transcripts of activation-induced cytidine deaminase, the enzyme responsible for somatic hypermutation and class-switch recombination of the immunoglobulin genes.

In addition to the development of the typical focal lymphocytic sialadenitis, this model also recapitulated other essential features of SS such as (1) exocrine dysfunction with significant reduction in salivary flow, and (2) breach of self-tolerance with the development of antinuclear antibodies in 75% of the animals by 3 weeks after AdV delivery.[70] Notably, however, these mice did not develop anti-Ro and/or anti-La antibodies.

Interestingly, in this model, viral particles were efficiently cleared from most of the salivary gland parenchyma as early as the first week post–AdV delivery, but persisted in ductal epithelial cells, where viral infection could be detected by immunofluorescence and/or PCR methods up to 4 weeks after infection. This observation is highly relevant to the human disease because ductal epithelial cells, particularly in striated ducts, do not efficiently clear viruses and represent privileged sites for immune evasion and viral persistence, as also demonstrated in human salivary glands.[71]

Although this model presents some intrinsic limitations and lacks some important features of the human disease, namely the absence of chronicity and the development of a full-blown autoimmune disease, it also offers unique opportunities to study the mechanisms which regulate the development of SS-like focal lymphocytic sialadenitis in the salivary glands, the formation of ectopic germinal centers, and the breach of self-tolerance. In particular, this AdV-induced model has not only the benefit of being highly reproducible and developing within few weeks from viral infection, but also offers the significant advantage of being inducible in nonautoimmune-prone strains such as C57Bl/6 and 129, which are amenable for direct gene targeting without the need of extensive, time-consuming, and costly backcrossing. As an example, a recent study using this inducible model conducted in collaboration with the University of Birmingham was able to demonstrate that *Il-22*[−/−] mice are impaired in their capacity to form focal lymphocytic foci in response to viral infection. This deficiency is due to the inability, in the absence of IL-22, to trigger the production of lymphoid chemokines *CXCL13* and *CXCL12* in stromal and epithelial cells, respectively. In addition, *Il-22*[−/−] mice were protected from the development of autoantibodies, suggesting that local IL-22 production by cells of the mucosal innate immunity is critical in controlling the cellular and molecular interactions which lead from mucosal infection to focal sialadenitis, B-cell recruitment and humoral autoimmunity.[72]

## REFERENCES

1. van Blokland SC, Versnel MA. Pathogenesis of Sjögren's syndrome: characteristics of different mouse models for autoimmune exocrinopathy. *Clin Immunol* 2002;**103**:111–24.
2. Kessler HS. A laboratory model for Sjögren's syndrome. *Am J Pathol* 1968;**52**:671–85.
3. Hoffman RW, Alspaugh MA, Waggie KS, Durham JB, Walker SE. Sjögren's syndrome in MRL/l and MRL/n mice. *Arthritis Rheum* 1984;**27**:157–65.
4. Miyagawa J, Hanafusa T, Miyazaki A, Yamada K, Fujino-Kurihara H, Nakajima H, et al. Ultrastructural and immunocytochemical aspects of lymphocytic submandibulitis in the non-obese diabetic (NOD) mouse. *Virchows Arch B Cell Pathol Incl Mol Pathol* 1986;**51**:215–25.
5. Constantopoulos SH, Tsianos EV, Moutsopoulos HM. Pulmonary and gastrointestinal manifestations of Sjögren's syndrome. *Rheum Dis Clin North Am* 1992;**18**:617–35.
6. Sorrentino D, Ferraccioli GF, Labombarda A, De Vita S, Avellini C, Beltrami CA, et al. *Helicobacter pylori*, gastric MALT and B-cell clonality. *Clin Exp Rheumatol* 1996; **14**(Suppl. 14):S51–4.
7. Makino S, Kunimoto K, Muraoka Y, Mizushima Y, Katagiri K, Tochino Y. Breeding of a non-obese, diabetic strain of mice. *Jikken Dobutsu* 1980;**29**:1–13.

8. Kikutani H, Makino S. The murine autoimmune diabetes model: NOD and related strains. *Adv Immunol* 1992;**51**:285–322.

9. Astorri E, Bombardieri M, Gabba S, Peakman M, Pozzilli P, Pitzalis C. Evolution of ectopic lymphoid neogenesis and in situ autoantibody production in autoimmune nonobese diabetic mice: cellular and molecular characterization of tertiary lymphoid structures in pancreatic islets. *J Immunol* 2010;**185**:3359–68.

10. Andre I, Gonzalez A, Wang B, Katz J, Benoist C, Mathis D. Checkpoints in the progression of autoimmune disease: lessons from diabetes models. *Proc Natl Acad Sci USA* 1996;**93**:2260–3.

11. Bowman MA, Leiter EH, Atkinson MA. Prevention of diabetes in the NOD mouse: implications for therapeutic intervention in human disease. *Immunol Today* 1994;**15**:115–20.

12. Singh B, Rabinovitch A. Influence of microbial agents on the development and prevention of autoimmune diabetes. *Autoimmunity* 1993;**15**:209–13.

13. Bach JF. The effect of infections on susceptibility to autoimmune and allergic diseases. *N Engl J Med* 2002;**347**:911–20.

14. Weatherall D, Sarvetnick N, Shizuru JA. Genetic control of diabetes mellitus. *Diabetologia* 1992;**35**(Suppl. 2):S1–7.

15. Cihakova D, Talor MV, Barin JG, Baldeviano GC, Fairweather D, Rose NR, et al. Sex differences in a murine model of Sjögren's syndrome. *Ann N Y Acad Sci* 2009;**1173**:378–83.

16. Rose NR, Saboori AM, Rasooly L, Burek CL. The role of iodine in autoimmune thyroiditis. *Crit Rev Immunol* 1997;**17**:511–7.

17. Tisch R, McDevitt H. Insulin-dependent diabetes mellitus. *Cell* 1996;**85**:291–7.

18. Wicker LS, Todd JA, Peterson LB. Genetic control of autoimmune diabetes in the NOD mouse. *Annu Rev Immunol* 1995;**13**:179–200.

19. Todd JA, Bell JI, McDevitt HO. *HLA-DQ* β gene contributes to susceptibility and resistance to insulin-dependent diabetes mellitus. *Nature* 1987;**329**:599–604.

20. Nishimoto H, Kikutani H, Yamamura K, Kishimoto T. Prevention of autoimmune insulitis by expression of I-E molecules in NOD mice. *Nature* 1987;**328**:432–4.

21. Bohme J, Schuhbaur B, Kanagawa O, Benoist C, Mathis D. MHC-linked protection from diabetes dissociated from clonal deletion of T cells. *Science* 1990;**249**:293–5.

22. Todd JA, Wicker LS. Genetic protection from the inflammatory disease type 1 diabetes in humans and animal models. *Immunity* 2001;**15**:387–95.

23. Brayer J, Lowry J, Cha S, Robinson CP, Yamachika S, Peck AB, et al. Alleles from chromosomes 1 and 3 of NOD mice combine to influence Sjögren's syndrome–like autoimmune exocrinopathy. *J Rheumatol* 2000;**27**:1896–904.

24. Delaleu N, Nguyen CQ, Tekle KM, Jonsson R, Peck AB. Transcriptional landscapes of emerging autoimmunity: transient aberrations in the targeted tissue's extracellular milieu precede immune responses in Sjögren's syndrome. *Arthritis Res Ther* 2013;**15**:R174.

25. Ueda H, Howson JM, Esposito L, Heward J, Snook H, Chamberlain G, et al. Association of the T-cell regulatory gene *CTLA4* with susceptibility to autoimmune disease. *Nature* 2003;**423**:506–11.

26. Trembleau S, Penna G, Gregori S, Chapman HD, Serreze DV, Magram J, et al. Pancreas-infiltrating Th1 cells and diabetes develop in IL-12-deficient nonobese diabetic mice. *J Immunol* 1999;**163**:2960–8.

27. Hamano H, Haneji N, Yanagi K, Ishimaru N, Hayashi Y. Expression of *HLA-DR* and cytokine genes on interferon-gamma-stimulated human salivary gland cell line. *Pathobiology* 1996;**64**:255–61.

28. Cha S, Peck AB, Humphreys-Beher MG. Progress in understanding autoimmune exocrinopathy using the non-obese diabetic mouse: an update. *Crit Rev Oral Biol Med* 2002;**13**:5–16.

29. Wang B, Gonzalez A, Hoglund P, Katz JD, Benoist C, Mathis D. Interleukin-4 deficiency does not exacerbate disease in NOD mice. *Diabetes* 1998;**47**:1207–11.

30. Saito I, Haruta K, Shimuta M, Inoue H, Sakurai H, Yamada K, et al. *Fas* ligand-mediated exocrinopathy resembling Sjögren's syndrome in mice transgenic for IL-10. *J Immunol* 1999;**162**:2488–94.

31. Wogensen L, Lee MS, Sarvetnick N. Production of interleukin 10 by islet cells accelerates immune-mediated destruction of beta cells in nonobese diabetic mice. *J Exp Med* 1994;**179**:1379–84.

32. Zheng XX, Steele AW, Hancock WW, Stevens AC, Nickerson PW, Roy-Chaudhury P, et al. A noncytolytic IL-10/Fc fusion protein prevents diabetes, blocks autoimmunity, and promotes suppressor phenomena in NOD mice. *J Immunol* 1997;**158**:4507–13.

33. Anderson MS, Venanzi ES, Klein L, Chen Z, Berzins SP, Turley SJ, et al. Projection of an immunological self shadow within the thymus by the AIRE protein. *Science* 2002;**298**:1395–401.

34. Gatumu MK, Skarstein K, Papandile A, Browning JL, Fava RA, Bolstad AI. Blockade of lymphotoxin-beta receptor signaling reduces aspects of Sjögren's syndrome in salivary glands of non-obese diabetic mice. *Arthritis Res Ther* 2009;**11**:R24.

35. Fava RA, Kennedy SM, Wood SG, Bolstad AI, Bienkowska J, Papandile A, et al. Lymphotoxin-beta receptor blockade reduces *CXCL13* in lacrimal glands and improves corneal integrity in the NOD model of Sjögren's syndrome. *Arthritis Res Ther* 2011;**13**:R182.

36. Hjelmstrom P. Lymphoid neogenesis: de novo formation of lymphoid tissue in chronic inflammation through expression of homing chemokines. *J Leukoc Biol* 2001;**69**:331–9.

37. Karnell JL, Mahmoud TI, Herbst R, Ettinger R. Discerning the kinetics of autoimmune manifestations in a model of Sjögren's syndrome. *Mol Immunol* 2014;**62**:277–82.

38. Robinson CP, Cornelius J, Bounous DE, Yamamoto H, Humphreys-Beher MG, Peck AB. Characterization of the changing lymphocyte populations and cytokine expression in the exocrine tissues of autoimmune NOD mice. *Autoimmunity* 1998;**27**:29–44.

39. Yamano S, Atkinson JC, Baum BJ, Fox PC. Salivary gland cytokine expression in NOD and normal BALB/c mice. *Clin Immunol* 1999;**92**:265–75.

40. Humphreys-Beher MG, Brinkley L, Purushotham KR, Wang PL, Nakagawa Y, Dusek D, et al. Characterization of antinuclear autoantibodies present in the serum from nonobese diabetic (NOD) mice. *Clin Immunol Immunopathol* 1993;**68**:350–6.

41. Skarstein K, Wahren M, Zaura E, Hattori M, Jonsson R. Characterization of T cell receptor repertoire and anti-Ro/SSA autoantibodies in relation to sialadenitis of NOD mice. *Autoimmunity* 1995;**22**:9–16.

42. Haneji N, Nakamura T, Takio K, Yanagi K, Higashiyama H, Saito I, et al. Identification of alpha-fodrin as a candidate autoantigen in primary Sjögren's syndrome. *Science* 1997;**276**:604–7.

43. Robinson CP, Brayer J, Yamachika S, Esch TR, Peck AB, Stewart CA, et al. Transfer of human serum IgG to nonobese diabetic Igμ$^{null}$ mice reveals a role for autoantibodies in the loss of secretory function of exocrine tissues in Sjögren's syndrome. *Proc Natl Acad Sci USA* 1998;**95**:7538–43.

44. Esch TR, Taubman MA. Autoantibodies in salivary hypofunction in the NOD mouse. *Ann N Y Acad Sci* 1998;**842**:221–8.

45. Kong L, Robinson CP, Peck AB, Vela-Roch N, Sakata KM, Dang H, et al. Inappropriate apoptosis of salivary and lacrimal gland epithelium of immunodeficient NOD-scid mice. *Clin Exp Rheumatol* 1998;**16**:675–81.

46. Robinson CP, Yamamoto H, Peck AB, Humphreys-Beher MG. Genetically programmed development of salivary gland abnormalities in the NOD (nonobese diabetic)-scid mouse in the absence of detectable lymphocytic infiltration: a potential trigger for sialoadenitis of NOD mice. *Clin Immunol Immunopathol* 1996;**79**:50–9.

47. Masago R, Aiba-Masago S, Talal N, Zuluaga FJ, Al-Hashimi I, Moody M, et al. Elevated pro-apoptotic *Bax* and caspase 3 activation in the NOD.scid model of Sjögren's syndrome. *Arthritis Rheum* 2001;**44**:693–702.

48. Killedar SJ, Eckenrode SE, McIndoe RA, She JX, Nguyen CQ, Peck AB, et al. Early pathogenic events associated with Sjögren's syndrome (SjS)-like disease of the NOD mouse using microarray analysis. *Lab Invest* 2006;**86**:1243–60.

49. Van Blokland SC, Van Helden-Meeuwsen CG, Wierenga-Wolf AF, Tielemans D, Drexhage HA, Van De Merwe JP, et al. Apoptosis and apoptosis-related molecules in the submandibular gland of the nonobese diabetic mouse model for Sjögren's syndrome: limited role for apoptosis in the development of sialoadenitis. *Lab Invest* 2003;**83**:3–11.

50. Haneji N, Hamano H, Yanagi K, Hayashi Y. A new animal model for primary Sjögren's syndrome in NFS/sld mutant mice. *J Immunol* 1994;**153**:2769–77.

51. Takada K, Takiguchi M, Konno A, Inaba M. Autoimmunity against a tissue kallikrein in IQI/Jic Mice: a model for Sjögren's syndrome. *J Biol Chem* 2005;**280**:3982–8.

52. Takada K, Takiguchi M, Konno A, Inaba M. Spontaneous development of multiple glandular and extraglandular lesions in aged IQI/Jic mice: a model for primary Sjögren's syndrome. *Rheumatology* 2004;**43**:858–62.

53. Hang L, Theofilopoulos AN, Dixon FJ. A spontaneous rheumatoid arthritis-like disease in MRL/l mice. *J Exp Med* 1982;**155**:1690–701.

54. Watanabe-Fukunaga R, Brannan CI, Copeland NG, Jenkins NA, Nagata S. Pillars article: lymphoproliferation disorder in mice explained by defects in *Fas* antigen that mediates apoptosis. 1992. *J Immunol* 2012;**189**:5101–4.

55. Skarstein K, Nerland AH, Eidsheim M, Mountz JD, Jonsson R. Lymphoid cell accumulation in salivary glands of autoimmune MRL mice can be due to impaired apoptosis. *Scand J Immunol* 1997;**46**:373–8.

56. Skarstein K, Johannessen AC, Holmdahl R, Jonsson R. Effects of sialadenitis after cellular transfer in autoimmune MRL/lpr mice. *Clin Immunol Immunopathol* 1997;**84**:177–84.

57. Hamano H, Saito I, Haneji N, Mitsuhashi Y, Miyasaka N, Hayashi Y. Expressions of cytokine genes during development of autoimmune sialadenitis in MRL/lpr mice. *Eur J Immunol* 1993;**23**:2387–91.

58. Jonsson R, Tarkowski A, Backman K, Klareskog L. Immunohistochemical characterization of sialadenitis in NZB X NZW F1 mice. *Clin Immunol Immunopathol* 1987;**42**:93–101.

59. Nishimori I, Bratanova T, Toshkov I, Caffrey T, Mogaki M, Shibata Y, et al. Induction of experimental autoimmune sialoadenitis by immunization of PL/J mice with carbonic anhydrase II. *J Immunol* 1995;**154**:4865–73.

60. Heming TA, Geers C, Gros G, Bidani A, Crandall ED. Effects of dextran-bound inhibitors on carbonic anhydrase activity in isolated rat lungs. *J Appl Physiol* 1986;**61**:1849–56.

61. Inagaki Y, Jinno-Yoshida Y, Hamasaki Y, Ueki H. A novel autoantibody reactive with carbonic anhydrase in sera from patients with systemic lupus erythematosus and Sjögren's syndrome. *J Dermatol Sci* 1991;**2**:147–54.

62. Mu MM, Chakravortty D, Takahashi K, Kato Y, Sugiyama T, Koide N, et al. Production of experimental autoimmune sialadenitis in mice immunized with homologous salivary gland extract and *Klebsiella* O3 lipopolysaccharide. *J Autoimmun* 2001;**16**:29–36.

63. Garberg H, Jonsson R, Brokstad KA. The serological pattern of autoantibodies to the Ro52, Ro60, and La48 autoantigens in primary Sjögren's syndrome patients and healthy controls. *Scand J Rheumatol* 2005;**34**:49–55.

64. Scofield RH, Asfa S, Obeso D, Jonsson R, Kurien BT. Immunization with short peptides from the 60-kDa Ro antigen recapitulates the serological and pathological findings as well as the salivary gland dysfunction of Sjögren's syndrome. *J Immunol* 2005;**175**:8409–14.

65. Maitland N, Flint S, Scully C, Crean SJ. Detection of cytomegalovirus and Epstein–Barr virus in labial salivary glands in Sjögren's syndrome and non-specific sialadenitis. *J Oral Pathol Med* 1995;**24**:293–8.

66. Fleck M, Kern ER, Zhou T, Lang B, Mountz JD. Murine cytomegalovirus induces a Sjögren's syndrome-like disease in C57Bl/6-lpr/lpr mice. *Arthritis Rheum* 1998;**41**:2175–84.

67. Fleck M, Zhang HG, Kern ER, Hsu HC, Muller-Ladner U, Mountz JD. Treatment of chronic sialadenitis in a murine model of Sjögren's syndrome by local *FasL* gene transfer. *Arthritis Rheum* 2001;**44**:964–73.

68. Schuster IS, Wikstrom ME, Brizard G, Coudert JD, Estcourt MJ, Manzur M, et al. *TRAIL+* NK cells control CD4+ T cell responses during chronic viral infection to limit autoimmunity. *Immunity* 2014;**41**:646–56.

69. Nguyen CQ, Yin H, Lee BH, Carcamo WC, Chiorini JA, Peck AB. Pathogenic effect of interleukin-17A in induction of Sjögren's syndrome–like disease using adenovirus-mediated gene transfer. *Arthritis Res Ther* 2010;**12**:R220.

70. Bombardieri M, Barone F, Lucchesi D, Nayar S, van den Berg WB, Proctor G, et al. Inducible tertiary lymphoid structures, autoimmunity, and exocrine dysfunction in a novel model of salivary gland inflammation in C57BL/6 mice. *J Immunol* 2012;**189**:3767–76.

71. Campbell AE, Cavanaugh VJ, Slater JS. The salivary glands as a privileged site of cytomegalovirus immune evasion and persistence. *Med Microbiol Immunol* 2008;**197**:205–13.

72. Barone F, Nayar S, Campos J, Cloake T, Withers DR, Toellner KM, et al. IL-22 regulates lymphoid chemokine production and assembly of tertiary lymphoid organs. *Proc Natl Acad Sci USA* August 18, 2015;**112**(35):11024–9.

Chapter 8

# Genetics, Genomics, Gene Expression Profiling, and Epigenetics in Sjögren's Syndrome

**S.J. Bowman, B.A. Fisher**

*University of Birmingham, Birmingham, United Kingdom; University Hospitals Birmingham NHS Trust, Birmingham, United Kingdom*

## 1. HISTORICAL BACKGROUND

Henrik Sjögren, a Swedish ophthalmologist, described the condition that bears his name in 1933.[1] He coined the term *keratoconjunctivitis sicca* to distinguish the ocular surface features from those seen in vitamin-A deficiency (xerophthalmia). The term *xerostomia* is, however, used to describe oral dryness. Henri Gougerot, a French dermatologist, had already described three patients with sicca syndrome and salivary gland atrophy in 1925.[2] Jan Mikulicz-Radecki, an Austro-Polish surgeon described the histological features in 1892.[3]

The distinction between primary Sjögren's syndrome (pSS) and secondary Sjögren's syndrome (SS) was set out in the 1960s.[4] Also in the 1960s, the link with mucosa-associated lymphoid tissue (MALT) B-cell lymphoma was reported,[5] Chisholm and Mason described their scoring system for the histological features of salivary gland biopsies in pSS,[6] and the anti-Ro/SSA and anti-La/SSB antibodies were first identified.[7] Subsequently these antibodies were shown to be associated with *HLA-DR3* and other human leukocyte antigen (HLA) haplotypes[8] and the neonatal lupus syndrome.[9]

The glandular features and management of pSS and secondary SS are generally regarded as being similar, although fibrosis, for example, is a more typical feature in scleroderma-related secondary SS. Unless otherwise stated, this chapter will focus on pSS.

Sjögren's Syndrome. http://dx.doi.org/10.1016/B978-0-12-803604-4.00008-3
**119**

## 2. EPIDEMIOLOGY, PREVALENCE, AND CLASSIFICATION CRITERIA

Sjögren's syndrome is a worldwide disease with a strong female bias that traditionally reported as 9:1 but is possibly as high as13:1.[10] Typically, pSS presents in the fifth or sixth decade but can present at any age including, rarely, in childhood.

Initial research into the prevalence of pSS came up with widely differing estimates as low as 0.08% (1 in 1250) using the San Diego (CA) criteria,[11] or as high as 3% of the adult female population in a community-based study in the United Kingdom.[12] One explanation for this variation was the use of different, more permissive classification criteria in the latter study.

The most widely used classification criteria for pSS are the American-European Consensus Group (AECG) criteria.[13] These require a combination of oral and/or ocular dryness symptoms/signs, and at least one positive test for anti-Ro/SSA and anti-La/SSB antibodies, and/or a minor labial salivary gland biopsy with features of focal periductal lymphocytic sialadenitis. More recent studies using the AECG criteria have estimated the community prevalence at 0.1% to 0.4%[14] and 0.04% to 0.05% in the hospital setting.[15]

More recently, a preliminary American College of Rheumatology criteria set requires two out of three components, including positive autoantibodies (also including antinuclear antibody [ANA] ≥1:320 and a positive rheumatoid factor), a positive minor labial salivary gland biopsy, and/or an abnormal Ocular Staining Score ≥3.[16] In interpreting genetic and other research studies, it is essential to have agreed classification criteria so that there is confidence that participants in a study have the specified condition. At the present time an international group of experts is bringing these criteria together to produce American College of Rheumatology–European League Against Rheumatism consensus criteria.

## 3. IMMUNOPATHOLOGY OF SJÖGREN'S SYNDROME

A detailed description of the immunopathology of pSS is beyond the scope of this review. In order to place the genetic data in context it is helpful, however, to be aware of the broad themes underpinning potential pathogenetic mechanisms. The triggering factor for pSS is unknown. One dominant hypothesis is that of "autoimmune epitheliitis."[17] In this hypothesis, an unknown trigger upregulates HLA class II expression and costimulatory factors on the ductal epithelial cells in secretory glands along with stimulating production of proinflammatory cytokines and other molecules. The HLA molecules present an unknown set of antigens to T cells, thus further upregulating the immune response, which then becomes chronic through the development of focal lymphocyte aggregation and the production of chemokines and other molecules that maintain these structures, resulting in persistent nonresolving inflammation. In some patients these lymphoid aggregates take on features similar to those seen in secondary lymphoid organs, with marked B-cell expansion and fully formed germinal centers (GCs) with light and dark zones thought capable of supporting the development of high-affinity, somatically mutated B cells.[18] The presence of GCs may indicate a greater likelihood of subsequent B-cell lymphoma development,[19] likely resulting from the genetic instability associated with DNA hypermutation (see above). Systemic B-cell activation with autoantibody production and hypergammaglobulinemia is also a hallmark of pSS (see above). The role of both T- and B-cell immunity would place genes encoding molecules involved in a broad range of adaptive immune responses, including HLA, but also antigen processing, cytokines, chemokines, B-cell and T-cell regulation, and receptor molecules as potential candidates for susceptibility to pSS.

Along with T cells and B cells, another key theme is of upregulation of the innate immune system. This "first line of defense" is triggered by, for example, common bacterial lipopolysaccharides and other highly conserved pathogen-associated molecular patterns and molecules released from damaged cells (danger-associated molecular patterns, also referred to as *alarmins*) to quickly upregulate the immune system in a non-HLA, non–antigen-specific manner while waiting for the adaptive antigen-driven immune response, which may take days or weeks to mature. Pattern recognition receptors such as the Toll-like receptors (TLRs) recognize these molecules, leading to upregulation of type I and type II interferons that have a broad and rapid stimulatory effect on the immune system affecting T-cells, B-cells, and also natural killer cells.[20] An upregulated "interferon (IFN) signature" has been recognized for some time in conditions such as pSS, systemic lupus erythematosus (SLE) and other connective tissue diseases.[21,22] We will review how studies of genetics and epigenetics, transcriptomics, proteomics, and metabolomics have informed, or have the potential to inform, our understanding of pSS. Hypothetical relationships between these "-omics" and the etiology of complex traits are illustrated in Fig. 8.1.

## 4. "TRADITIONAL" GENETICS: HUMAN LEUKOCYTE ANTIGENS

In the late 1950s and 1960s the HLAs were identified as key components of transplant rejection.[23] To summarize two decades of research that established our knowledge of the basic components of the immune system, Class I HLAs are found on the surface of almost all cells, whereas class II HLAs are found predominantly on cells of the immune system. The genes encoding the human HLA proteins are found on chromosome 6. There are three main HLA Class I gene loci (*HLA-A*, *HLA-B*, and *HLA-C*), and three main Class II HLA gene loci (*HLA-DR*, *HLA-DQ*, and *HLA-DP*), but there are over 200 other genes in this region of chromosome 6. The proximity of these loci to each other mean that certain combinations such as the *HLA-A1*, *B8*, *DR3*, *DQ2* combination (haplotype) are typically inherited as a "block" together (linkage disequilibrium). Class I molecules typically present antigens derived from inside cells to cytotoxic (killer) T cells.

**(A)**

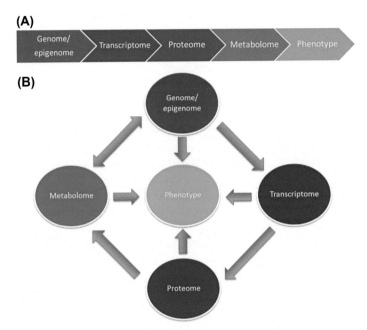

FIGURE 8.1 Two hypotheses of the relationship between "-omic" levels and phenotype: a linear hierarchical process (A), or phenotype arising as a result of the interaction of variation at all levels (B). Environmental effects might influence multiple "-omic" levels. *Adapted from Ritchie MD, Holzinger ER, Li R, Pendergrass SA, Kim D. Methods of integrating data to uncover genotype– phenotype interactions. Nat Rev Genet 2015;16:85–97.*

In virally infected cells, this allows the cytotoxic T cells to recognize infected cells and destroy them. Class II molecules are typically found on antigen-presenting cells and present antigens originally from outside of cells (although they are then internalized and processed before presentation on the cell surface by HLA class II molecules), such as bacterial antigens, to helper T cells that then stimulate B cells to support antibody production that recognizes the bacterial molecules and facilitates their removal by the immune system.

The HLA proteins were found to have multiple variants at each locus (eg, *HLA-DR1, DR2, DR3*, etc.). This was originally characterized by antibody reactivity analysis (serotyping) but subsequently, after the discovery of the polymerase chain reaction (PCR), by genotyping. Although the genotyping approach is more precise, serotyping can identify antigenic specificities that are common to several genotypes.

The identification of the HLA antigens was followed by the discovery that certain autoimmune diseases were linked to particular HLA types. Rheumatoid arthritis (RA) was found to be associated with *HLA-DR4* in Caucasian populations and *HLA-DR1* in other ethnic groups,[24] leading to the idea of the "shared epitope" hypothesis.[25,26] These findings in turn led to a number of other key developments for our understanding of autoimmune disease.

One of these is the development of statistical methods that examine the concordance of disease in identical and nonidentical twins or between parents and children or siblings to calculate how much of the risk of developing an autoimmune disease such as RA is attributed to genes and how much to the environment,[27] as well as understanding how much of the genetic element was caused by HLA region or other non-HLA region genes. In addition, these findings of HLA associations with disease or particular autoantibodies associated with disease have generated a dominant model of autoimmunity in which a particular antigen or set of antigens presented by particular HLA molecule(s) play a critical role in triggering the condition.

There have been no large-scale monozygotic versus dizygotic twin studies, or large multiplex family studies in pSS.[28] Based on case reports and small studies, the estimated concordance rate for SS is low and the sibling prevalence likewise, suggesting that the heritability of SS is low and environmental factors play a greater role.[29–31] In practical terms, this would suggest that in the absence of a preexisting family history, the likelihood of the child of a patient with pSS developing pSS as well is likely to be only modestly greater than the general population. In contrast, however, a recent study by Kuo et al.[32] researching the Taiwanese National Health Insurance Research Database suggests that half the phenotypic variance in pSS can be explained by familial factors.

PSS has been closely linked to the presence of particular genes of the human major histocompatibility complex (MHC) that encodes HLA proteins. A meta-analysis found that the HLA class II alleles *DRB1\*03:01, DQA1\*05:01*, and *DQB1\*02:01* were associated with an increased risk, and *DQA1\*02:01, DQA1\*03:01*, and *DQB1\*05:01* with a lower risk, although it should be noted that there was some heterogeneity in the classification criteria used for pSS.[33] These links are principally between the HLA types and the presence of anti-Ro/SSA and anti-La/SSB autoantibodies rather than with the disease per se. Patients with high levels of both anti-Ro/SSA and anti-La/SSB antibodies have a very high (~90%) likelihood of being *HLA DR3 DQ2* positive (typically associated with the *DRB1\*03-DQB1\*02-DQA1\*0501* extended haplotype), whereas pSS patients who have high levels of anti-Ro/SSA antibody only and are negative for anti-La/SSB antibodies have an increased frequency of *DR2(15)* and *DQ6* (typically associated with the *DRB1\*1501-DQA1\*0102-DQB1\*0602* extended haplotype).[34] Conversely, secondary SS in patients with RA is associated with *HLA-DR4*,[35] emphasizing that the clinical and histopathological similarities between pSS and secondary SS do not extend into identical genetic backgrounds.

Another issue to consider is that genetic susceptibility can differ between disease subsets within a single disease, or overlap between different autoimmune diseases with common features, both clinical and serological.[28] RA is an example of a disease where serology (anti-cyclic citrullinated peptide [CCP] antibodies), the environment (smoking status), and genetics (*HLA* and *PTPN22*) interact in a complex manner (Fig. 8.2).[36]

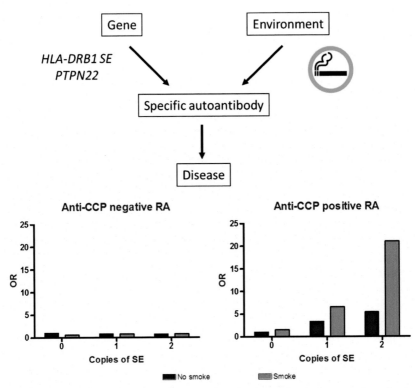

**FIGURE 8.2**   Example of a proposed gene–environment interaction in the generation of auto-antibody positive rheumatoid arthritis. Data from Klareskog et al. shows that smoking confers an increased risk for anti-CCP antibody positive rheumatoid arthritis in the presence of the *HLA-DRB1* shared epitope (SE), and suggests a gene–environment interaction that is specific for the autoanti-body positive subgroup in this population. Such gene–environment interactions are likely to apply to other autoimmune diseases. *CCP*, Cyclic citrullinated peptide; *RA*, rheumatoid arthritis; *OR*, odds ratio; *SE*, shared epitope. *Data from Klareskog L, Stolt P, Lundberg K, Källberg H, Bengtsson C, Grunewald J, et al. A new model for an etiology of rheumatoid arthritis: smoking may trigger HLA-DR (shared epitope)-restricted immune reactions to autoantigens modified by citrullination.* Arthritis Rheum *January, 2006;54(1):38–46; See also Mahdi H, Fisher BA, Källberg H, Plant D, Malmström V, Rönnelid J, et al. Specific interaction between genotype, smoking and autoimmunity to citrullinated alpha-enolase in the etiology of rheumatoid arthritis.* Nat Genet *2009;41:1319–24.*

Celiac disease, pSS, and autoimmune thyroid disease are recognized disease associations.[37] Celiac disease is an HLA-associated condition with *DQA1\*05* and *DQB1\*02* either on the same or separate chromosomes found in 90% of patients[38] and these also form part of the extended *HLA-DR3 DQ2* haplotype associated with pSS, perhaps at least in part explaining this association. It is not clear whether having two copies of a susceptible *HLA* gene is associated with particular clinical features such as lymphoma.

Another observation from HLA studies is that the susceptibility alleles vary in different population groups.[33,39] Women with anti-Ro/SSA and anti-La/SSB antibodies in Japan (irrespective of current disease status with regard to SLE or pSS) are more likely to have the *DRB1\*08032* allele or the associated haplotype[40] rather than the *DRB1\*03* in Caucasian populations. *DRB1\*0803* has also been associated with pSS in Chinese populations.[41]

Despite several decades of research into HLA associations with disease the precise reasons for these associations remains largely speculative.[42] There was hope, for example, that if the precise details of the HLA association were known, including the key HLA peptide binding pockets that this could be used to identify the disease-specific antigens or otherwise explain the nature of the HLA association. Alternatively, it was proposed that candidate antigens could be identified by their ability to stimulate patient T cells when presented on appropriately HLA-restricted antigen-presenting cells.[34] Although these studies have yielded results of interest, to date they have not identified specific antigens associated with pSS.

## 5. CANDIDATE GENE ANALYSIS

Candidate gene analysis is a powerful tool to examine genetic contribution to disease. Using PCR technology, the incidence of a particular gene variant in a patient population can be compared to the incidence among population controls. It does require a hypothesis to decide which genes to examine.

Lessard et al.[43] have summarized in detail the results of a large number of candidate gene studies in pSS. Not surprisingly, the themes underpinning the search for genes of interest outside of classical HLA molecules derive from our understanding of immunopathology, namely genes coding for molecules involved in the innate immune system and IFN-related genes (eg, *IRF5* and *STAT4*); cytokine genes (eg, for interleukin (IL)-10, IL-1 family, IL-6); MHC-related genes such as *TAP*, lymphotoxin β and TNF, and the Ro/La autoantigens themselves; and B-cell related genes (eg, *BLK*, *EBF1*, and *BAFF*).[29,30,44,45]

Gorr et al.[46] have performed a literature search in PubMed of genes and proteins that have been associated with pSS (excluding gene expression and proteomic studies) as a useful and updated resource for researchers.

## 6. GENOME-WIDE ASSOCIATION STUDIES

In the last decade, technology has made large strides in relation to searching the genome for locations that have some association with complex diseases or traits without the potential "bias" of a particular hypothesis.

Microsatellite analysis was one initial approach that could also be used to dissect whether a candidate gene or a nearby area was more closely linked to a particular condition or trait. A microsatellite consists of a tract of tandemly repeated (ie, adjacent) DNA motifs that range in length from two to five nucleotides, and are typically repeated 5–50 times. They are distributed throughout the genome and can be amplified for identification by PCR, using the unique sequences of flanking regions as primers. Microsatellites can therefore be used in genetic linkage analysis to locate a gene or a mutation associated with a given trait or disease.

In general, however, it is another related technology, that of single nucleotide polymorphisms (SNPs) which have been more widely used in preference to microsatellite analysis as high-resolution markers in gene mapping related to diseases or normal traits such as in genome-wide association studies (GWASs). A SNP is a DNA sequence variation occurring commonly within a population (eg, 1%) in which a single nucleotide (A, T, C, or G) differs between individuals. They occur widely (although not entirely homogenously) throughout the genome and can be detected by PCR techniques.

As well as examining disease associations, it is also possible to examine subsets of patients through SNP analyses. Reksten et al.[47] identified two SNPs in *CCL11* (eotaxin) associated with GC-like structures in salivary glands of pSS patients. Suggestive associations were also found in SNPs in the B-cell activation and/or GC-formation related genes *AICDA*, *BANK1*, and *BCL2*, and to a lesser extent in SNPs in *IL17A*, *ICA1*, *PKN1*, and the nuclear factor (NF)-κB pathway genes *CARD8*, *IKBKE*, and *TANK*.

Online genome maps and registries, statistical software, and microarray genechips such as those produced by Affymetrix (Santa Clara, California) and Illumina (San Diego, California) can be used to screen the genome for particular locations linked to disease or traits.[48] These studies usually require many thousands of patients and controls in both the discovery and validation cohorts. Unlike candidate gene analysis, GWASs do not start with any a priori hypotheses.

In pSS, SLE, and some other autoimmune disorders, one current theme, across a range of studies, is the overexpression of IFN-inducible genes including Toll-like receptors, *STAT4*, *IRF5*, *BAFF*, and *MECP2*.[49,50] IFN is typically upregulated by viruses and this may provide a link between the "disease trigger" in these disorders and subsequent pathogenic processes.

In a GWAS by Lessard et al. in 2013 using Illumina microarray technology of four datasets totaling 4337 patient samples and 12,459 control samples, the HLA region at 6p21 demonstrated the strongest association with the peak at *HLA-DQB1*. Other risk loci included *IRF5*, *STAT4*, *IL-12A*, *BLK*, *CXCR5*, and *TNIP1*[51] (Fig. 8.3).

*IRF5* is a transcription factor mediating type 1 IFN responses; *STAT4* is a transcription factor for cellular responses initiated by type 1 IFNs and can be induced by IL-12 in some circumstances. In other words, these all participate in type 1 IFN pathway signaling. *BLK* is a nonreceptor Src family tyrosine kinase involved in B-cell receptor signaling and B-cell development, whereas *CXCR5* is a receptor for the chemokine *CXCL13* (also known as B-lymphocyte chemoattractant, *BLC*). *IL-12* can induce *CXCR5* expression, potentially linking the two themes of type 1 IFNs and B-cell activation. The function of *TNIP1* is not fully described but is involved in NF-κB regulation. In a study of SNPs in 1105 patients and 4460 controls, an association was found between antibody-positive primary SS and two SNPs in *TNIP1*.[52]

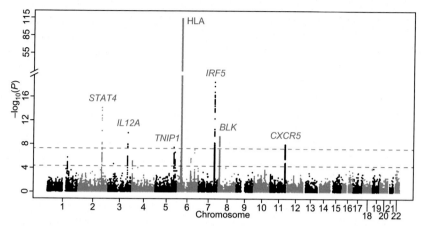

**FIGURE 8.3** Summary of genome-wide association (GWAS) results for 27,501 variants overlapping between DS1 and DS2 after imputation and meta-analysis. The $-\log_{10}(P)$ for each variant is plotted according to chromosome and base pair position. A total of seven loci (in *red font*) exceeded the genome-wide significance threshold of $P_{meta} < 5 \times 10^{-8}$ (*red-dashed line*). Suggestive threshold ($P_{meta} < 5 \times 10^{-5}$) is indicated by a *blue-dashed line. Reproduced with kind permission from Lessard CJ, Li H, Adrianto I, Ice JA, Rasmussen A, Grundahl KM, et al. Variants at multiple loci implicated in both innate and adaptive immune responses are associated with Sjögren's syndrome.* Nat Genet *2013;45:1284–92.*

In a GWAS in a Chinese population,[53] the associations with *STAT4*, *TNFAIP3*, and the MHC reported from European Caucasian patients was also seen, but in addition, a novel association with the transcription factor GTF2I SNP rs117026326 was reported and confirmed in another study.[54]

## 7. EPIGENETICS

### 7.1 Gene Methylation and Other Processes

An area of genetics that is currently of considerable interest and research is that of "epigenetics," ie, how factors outside of the genetic code alter the expression of genes in time and place. Such factors include nutritional, chemical, and physical environmental exposures which operate through processes, such as DNA methylation or histone acetylation.[55]

Although the resulting gene expression changes do not entail alterations in the DNA sequence, they are potentially inheritable,[56] with data showing they can persist for one or two subsequent generations.[57] They can control gene expression patterns during cell development, the cell cycle, and biological/environmental changes. Disease-associated epigenetic alterations of gene expression could therefore theoretically contribute to pathogenesis of inflammatory diseases such as pSS.

Chromatin is found in the cell nucleus and is a nucleoprotein complex consisting of DNA wrapped around a core made of histone proteins along with enzymes and transcription complexes. The positive charge of histones partly counters the negative charge of DNA and therefore allows the DNA to coil compactly, making up the chromosome structure.

Euchromatin describes loosely packaged chromatin, associated with high concentrations of genes and active transcription, whereas heterochromatin describes densely packaged chromatin with inactive genes. Switching between these states can therefore activate or inactivate gene expression of relevance to immunopathogenetic states.

There are a number of processes that can affect nucleosome dynamics and therefore gene expression by modulating the packaging of DNA in the nucleus and/or the binding of transcription factors. Posttranslational histone methylation is the most commonly described process but others include acetylation, phosphorylation, ubiquitination, sumoylation, adenosine diphosphate, ribosylation, deamination, citrullination, protein conjugation, β-N-azcetylglucosamination, and ion/protein binding to DNA. These processes are typically reversible. DNA methylation occurring on the five position of the pyrimidine ring of cytosines in the context of the dinucleotide sequence CpG forms one of the most important mechanisms controlling gene expression through altering chromatin structure.

Thabet et al.[58] evaluated global DNA methylation within salivary gland epithelial cells (SGECs), peripheral T cells, and B cells from SS patients. Global DNA methylation was reduced in SGECs from SS patients, whereas no difference was observed in T and B cells. SGEC demethylation in SS patients was associated with a sevenfold decrease in DNA methyl transferase (DNMT) 1 enzyme expression and a twofold increase in Gadd45-α expression. SGEC demethylation appeared to be at least partly related to the infiltrating B cells as demonstrated in salivary gland biopsies of patients treated with anti-CD20 antibodies to deplete B cells. This hypothesis was further evaluated using coculture experiments with human salivary gland cells and B cells and could be related to an alteration of the *PKCδ/ERK/DNMT1* pathway.

Altorok et al.[59] performed a genome-wide analysis of DNA methylation in peripheral blood-derived naive CD4+ T cells in pSS and identified 311 demethylated genes including lymphotoxin-α, type-I IFN pathway genes, and genes encoding for water channel proteins, and 115 hypermethylated gene regions including *RUNX1*, which may have a role in lymphoma predisposition.

A targeted approach was adopted by Gestermann et al.[60] With the data from genetic association studies demonstrating a role for genes of the innate immune system such as *STAT4* and *IRF5*,[51,61,62] they examined the methylation profile of the promoter region of *IRF5* in peripheral blood CD4+ T cells, B cells, monocytes, and cultured SGECs in patients with pSS and healthy controls. In this study they compared the methylation profile of the *IRF5* promoter region in patients and controls but found no difference despite the known genetic polymorphisms and upregulation of *IRF5* messenger RNA (mRNA) levels in pSS patients. Miceli-Richards et al.[63] compared the methylation profiles of peripheral blood B and T cells from pSS patients and found that most methylation alterations were in B cells, particularly in anti-Ro/SSA and anti-La/SSB positive patients and typically among IFN regulatory genes.

Salivary gland acinar cells in SS show altered attachment to the basal lamina and this may be linked to hypermethylation of the *BP230* gene promoter region and reduced *BP230* mRNA levels, and this may link to cell survival.[64] Other apoptosis related genes may also be differentially methylated.[65]

These and other studies demonstrate the potential for DNA methylation and other processes to modify inflammation in pSS.

## 7.2 Micro-RNAs

Another process involved in cellular regulation is generated by micro RNAs (miRNAs).[56] Micro RNAs are small, noncoding RNAs, 19–24 nucleotides in length. They are involved in degrading mRNAs and disruption/repression of translation. Other nontranslated regulatory RNA species include long intergenic noncoding RNAs and circular RNAs.[66] Approximately 1000 human miRNAs have been identified to date.[66] After being generated in the nucleus, they are transported to the cytoplasm where generally they bind to the 3′ untranslated region of the targeted mRNA to exert their effects. Micro RNAs are derived from primary miRNA (pri-miRNA) via approximately 70 nucleotide stem-loop precursor miRNAs (pre-miRNAs). Interestingly, the La antigen has recently been described as having a role in binding and stabilizing pre-miRNAs, so protecting them from ribonuclease mediates degradation.[67]

Alevizos et al.,[68] in a proof of concept study, used Agilent (Santa Clara, California) miRNA microarrays and real-time quantitative PCR to examine minor salivary glands of patients with pSS and controls. Two miRNAs showed differential expression. MiR-768-3p was associated with increased salivary gland inflammation and miR-574 inversely so. Kapsogeorgou et al.[69] also used comparative array analysis to demonstrate distinctive miRNA signatures in SS patients. Tandon et al.[70] identified six new miRNAs from minor salivary glands in SS patients.

One miRNA involved in regulation of inflammation in RA, SLE, and psoriasis is miR-146a. Pauley et al.[71] demonstrated increased miR-146a expression in the peripheral blood of 25 pSS patients, as well as in the salivary glands of a mouse model of pSS. Zilahi et al.[72] also found increased miR-146a (and miR-146b) expression by peripheral blood mononuclear cells. Micro RNA146a is thought to have a role in regulating *TRAF6* and *IRAK1*, which are involved in TLR and IFN signaling, among other processes,[73] thus potentially linking data on miRNAs to other features of inflammation in pSS derived from other data (see above).

## 8. FUNCTIONAL GENOMICS

### 8.1 Gene Expression Profiling: Interferon Signature

Gene expression profiling using microarray technology can help identify genes that are overexpressed or underexpressed in particular circumstances, which may be relevant to disease pathogenesis.[29] This is quite a different type of analysis from genetic studies looking at disease risk through genetic variation between populations of individuals with a disease and those without. In gene expression profiling, the levels of expression of particular genes are assessed by extracting and amplifying whole mRNA populations from a sample tissue and comparing the levels of expression of particular mRNA molecules to those in the same tissue from controls, or, for example, in the same person over time after an intervention such as a medication. Microarray technology uses arrays of oligonucleotide probes on a "gene-chip" that capture mRNA complementary sequences (cDNA) present in biological samples. They identify the presence and amounts of known mRNAs in the sample to be evaluated.

Hjelmervik et al.[74] performed gene expression analyses on minor salivary gland tissue from 10 pSS patients and controls and found upregulation of *CXCL13* and *CD3D*. Other up-regulated genes included lymphotoxin β, MHC genes, cytokines, lymphocyte activation factors, and type I IFN genes. The gene for carbonic anhydrase II, which is essential in saliva production and secretion, and the apoptosis regulator Bcl-2–like two were down-regulated in pSS patients.

Gottenberg et al.[75] examined gene expression in minor labial salivary glands from seven patients and seven controls. The expression of 23 genes in the IFN pathways, including two *TLRs* (TLR8 and TLR9), was significantly different between patients and controls. The expression of two IFN-inducible genes, *BAFF* and IFN-induced transmembrane protein 1, were also upregulated in ocular epithelial cells as shown by quantitative reverse transcription (RT)-PCR.

Hu et al.[76] evaluated whole saliva from 10 pSS patients and 8 controls for gene expression profiles using an Affymetrix human genome U133 Plus 2.0 array, which contains >54,000 probe sets representing >47,000 transcripts and variants, including approximately 38,500 well-characterized human genes. They validated the candidate biomarkers generated by microarray profiling using real-time quantitative RT-PCR on the same set of samples. There were 162 genes differentially expressed in pSS patients, 37 of which were involved in the IFN pathway. Other genes of interest included *GIP2*, a signaling molecule, major histocompatibility class I and $\beta_2$-microglobulin.

In a subsequent study by the same group examining salivary gland tissue from six patients with pSS and MALT lymphoma, nine with pSS without lymphoma, and eight controls, they identified upregulation of genes involved in immune/defense response, antigen presentation/processing, apoptosis and cell signaling, and oxidative stress.[77] Six genes distinguished pSS patients from controls (Calmodulin-like 5, MAP/microtubule affinity-regulating kinase 2, carbonic anhydrase 1, Hemoglobin β, EPS8-like 3, interferon, and α-inducible protein 6) and eight distinguished MALT lymphoma from pSS alone (growth factor receptor-bound protein 2, Rho GDP dissociation inhibitor β, CD40 molecule, TNF receptor superfamily member 5, proteasome subunit β type 9 [large multifunctional peptidase 2], aldolase A, fructose-bisphosphate, peroxiredoxin 5,

P53-associated parkin-like cytoplasmic protein, peptidylprolyl isomerase A [cyclophilin A]).

Khuder et al.[78] pooled the data from nine publicly available data sets of gene expression profiles from saliva or salivary gland tissue of patients with pSS and identified 19 genes with the highest classification accuracy for pSS (*EPSTI1, IFI44, IFI44L, IFIT1, IFIT2, IFIT3, MX1, OAS1, SAMD9L, PSMB9, STAT1, HERC5, EV12B, CD53, SELL, HLA-DQA1, PTPRC, B2M,* and *TAP2*).

Other studies have also been published on peripheral blood or minor labial salivary glands of pSS patients also supporting the general theme of upregulation of IFN-related gene pathways.[79,80]

Devauchelle-Pensec et al.[81] performed minor labial salivary gland gene expression profiling before and after treatment with rituximab on 15 patients. B-cell signaling pathway genes and IFN-related genes were most differentially expressed between responders and nonresponders before therapy.[81] A comparison of gene expression modification before and after treatment identified eight genes that were differentially expressed (*CDC42SE2* and *GBP2* were downregulated and six were upregulated (*CDS1, CYB5R1, H2AFJ, HEXB, NR2F6,* and *RUSC1*)). Lavie et al.[82] in a separate analysis of gene expression of salivary glands from patients receiving rituximab demonstrated upregulation of the B-cell activating factor *(BAFF)*.

## 8.2 Genomics and Transcriptomics

In recent years, "next-generation sequencing" or high-throughput DNA sequencing techniques have been used to sequence the entire genome of individuals either healthy or with disease using platforms such as those developed by Illumina, Roche 454 pyrosequencing, or other companies.[83] This technology has been used to compare different populations, evaluate changes in cancer cells, and sequence whole bacteria and plants. In the United Kingdom, the 100,000 genomes project aims to sequence the whole genomes of patients with cancer and rare diseases (http://www.genomicsengland.co.uk/the-100000-genomes-project/).

Another related technology is that of "transcriptomics" or RNA-sequencing, which examines the total population of mRNA present in a cell or population of cells at a particular time point. Instead of using microarray probes to measure gene expression, this approach typically reverse transcribes all the mRNA into cDNA and then uses next-generation sequencing and computational analysis to produce a complete dataset of all the mRNA present in the cell or cell population studies. It has been used in pSS to examine miRNAs[84] (see above).

## 8.3 Microbiome Analysis

Another area of interplay between genetics, environmental factors such as diet and lifestyle, and metabolomics is through the microbiome. *Microbiome* is a term used for the complete set of bacteria living within our bodies, for example within the gastrointestinal tract.

Using PCR technology and whole genome high-throughput sequencing techniques such as 16S rRNA gene-sequencing or 454-pyrosequencing, it is possible to get a detailed listing of the whole bacteria population in a sample and the relative incidences of each bacteria.[85] In RA there has been considerable interest in the interplay between smoking, anti-CCP antibodies, HLA, disease activity, periodontitis, and periodontal bacteria such as *Porphyromonas gingivalis*[85] and also in the potential role of oral bacteria (eg, *Prevotella* sp.) in early RA.[86] The presence of gut *Prevotella copri* was found to correlate with early RA in a study of 44 patients plus controls.[87] Although this particular finding was not confirmed in a larger recent Chinese study, the correlated oral and gut microbiomes were both altered in RA and partially restored after treatment.[88] Although the microbiome in patients with pSS has been evaluated through traditional microbial culture approaches of supragingival plaque[89] and through molecular mimicry of T-cell responses to Ro epitopes,[90] studies using modern molecular genetic sequencing studies are still awaited.

## 8.4 Proteomics

Proteomics, the study of disease-associated variation in protein and peptide levels in biological samples, is another promising area of interest in pSS.

Ryu et al.[91] used two-dimensional gel electrophoresis and mass spectrometry on parotid saliva and demonstrated significant increases in six proteins: β-2-microglobulin, lactoferrin, immunoglobulin (Ig) κ light chain, polymeric Ig receptor, lysozyme C, and cystatin C in all stages of SS. Two presumed proline-rich proteins, amylase and carbonic anhydrase VI, were reduced in the patient group.

Hu et al.[76] (see also above for gene expression data) used a combination of two-dimensional gel electrophoresis and liquid mass spectrometry to identify overexpressed and underexpressed peptides and proteins in whole saliva in 10 pSS patients and controls. Fructose-bisphosphate aldolase A and α-enolase were overproduced, whereas a number of mainly secretory proteins such as carbonic anhydrase were underexpressed, although how this relates to autoantigenicity is speculative.

Baldini et al.[92], using two-dimensional gel electrophoresis, mass spectrometry, and Western blotting carried out a larger study that identified six overexpressed proteins: calgranulin; β-2 microglobulin; epidermal fatty acid binding protein (E-FABP); Psoriasin; IGKC protein; and α-enolase; and six underexpressed proteins: α-amylases precursor; carbonic anhydrase; cystatin SN precursor; prolactin-inducible protein precursor; short palate, lung, and nasal epithelium clone 2 (SPLUNC-2); and glyceraldehydes-3-phosphate dehydrogenase (G3PDH). As with Hu et al.[76] the overexpressed proteins are, to some extent, involved in immune activation and underexpressed proteins in glandular secretion. Overall, this study found that α-amylase precursor, β-2 microglobulin, G3PDH, IGKC protein, E-FABP, carbonic anhydrase VI and SPLUNC-2 showed the most significant differences in comparison both to healthy volunteers and non-SS sicca syndrome and, therefore, appeared to be the most significant discriminatory biomarkers for SS.

Delaleu et al. used a multiplex immunoassay for 187 proteomic biomarkers to identify four-plex (clusterin, IL4, IL5, and FGF4) and 6-plex (clusterin, IL4, IL5, CRP, apolipoprotein A2, and pregnancy-associated plasma protein A) signals in whole saliva with at least 94% accuracy in separating PSS from controls.[93] It would be of interest to explore the association of these salivary proteomic panels with the extent of glandular inflammation in larger cohorts.

## 8.5 Metabolomics

Metabolomics seeks to understand the downstream effects of genes, proteins, and enzymes on energy and metabolite consumption and regulation.[94] This is performed through analysis of low molecular weight metabolite components of the target samples. The most commonly used techniques for this are nuclear magnetic resonance spectroscopy or mass spectrometry. Target samples can include cell-free material such as urine, plasma, fecal extracts, synovial fluid, tears, or saliva, or cell extracts once processed into a suitable solvent.

To give an example of the linkage between genes, inflammation, and metabolomics, CD4+ T cells exposed to hypoxia during inflammation show an increase in the expression of genes involved in metabolism and homeostasis.[95] Macrophages also accumulate at sites of inflammation and contribute to the upregulation of proinflammatory cytokines such as IL-1, IL-6, IFNɤ, and TNFα. In hypoxic circumstances, lactic acid, which is a waste-product of normal metabolism, cannot be easily converted to pyruvate and therefore accumulates. This can then be measured in such circumstances as an indirect marker of inflammation, for example in RA synovial fluid.[94] A large number of other metabolites and profiles of metabolites can be examined through these techniques, both in disease states and in mouse/rat models of disease, where, for example, particular cytokines have been chronically induced or conversely knocked out, or after the use of particular medications.[94] In a study of patients with inflammatory bowel disease reduced fecal levels of butyrate, acetate, methylamine, and trimethylamine were seen compared to controls.[96] By combining an analysis of this kind with an evaluation of the microbiome in the same patients, a whole-system biology approach can begin to be developed. To date, metabolomics has not yet been intensively studied in pSS but is now beginning to be an area of interest.[97]

## 9. CONCLUSIONS

Genetic analysis has made significant contributions to our understanding of pSS. The link to specific HLA types has been an important linchpin of antigen-driven hypotheses of etiopathogenesis, although to date a causative antigen or process remains elusive. Candidate gene analysis outside of classical HLA molecules and GWAS analyses have supported existing concepts around the role of B cells, T cells, and the innate immune system in the pathogenesis of pSS. Functional genetics such as gene expression profiling both in the disease steady state and after therapy is becoming a standard tool for stratification of patients and for assessing responses to therapy. New techniques such as high-throughput sequencing, if applied to pSS, will further expand our knowledge of genes, the transcriptome, and the microbiome over the next few years.

## ACKNOWLEDGMENTS

In the past year Professor Simon Bowman has consulted for Eli Lilly, Takeda Pharmaceuticals, UCB, Novartis, Glenmark, Celgene, Medimmune, GSK, and Ono, and is in receipt of an Arthritis Research UK grant to which Roche Pharmaceuticals is contributing rituximab without charge. Dr. Ben Fisher has consulted for Medimmune, Takeda, and Novartis.

## REFERENCES

1. Sjögren H. Zur kenntnis der keratoconjunctivitis sicca. *Acta Ophthalmol* 1933;**11**(Suppl. II): 1–151.
2. Gougerot H. Insuffisance progressive et atrophie des glandes salivarires et mugueuses de la bouche, des conjunctives (et parfois de muqueuses, nasale, laryngée, vulvaire) sécheresse de la bouche, des conjonctives. *Bull Med (Paris)* 1926;**40**:360–5.
3. Mikulicz J. Uber eine eigenartige symmetrische Erkrankung der Tranen- und Mundspeicheldrusen. In: Billroth GT, editor. *Beitr. Chir. Fortschr. Stuttgart.* 1892. p. 610–30.
4. Bloch KJ, Buchanan WW, Wohl MJ, Bunim JJ. Sjögren's syndrome: a clinical, pathological and serological study of sixty-two cases. *Medicine* 1965;**44**:187–231.
5. Talal N, Bunim JJ. The development of malignant lymphoma in the course of Sjögren's syndrome. *Am J Med* 1964;**36**:529–40.
6. Chisholm DM, Mason DK. Labial salivary gland biopsy in Sjögren's syndrome. *J Clin Pathol* 1968;**21**:656–60.
7. Clark G, Reichlin M, Tomasi TB. Characterization of a soluble cytoplasmic antigen reactive with sera from patients with systemic lupus erythematosus. *J Immunol* 1969;**102**:117–22.
8. Harley JB, Alexander EL, Bias WB, Fox OF, Provost TT, Reichlin M, et al. Anti-Ro(SSA) and anti-La(SSB) in patients with Sjögren's syndrome. *Arthritis Rheumatol* 1986;**29**:196–206.
9. Kephart DC, Hood AF, Provost TT. Neonatal lupus erythematosus: new serologic findings. *J Invest Dermatol* 1981;**77**:331–3.
10. Ramos-Casals M, Solans R, Rosas J, Camps MT, Gil A, Del Pino-Montes J, et al. Primary Sjögren's syndrome in Spain: clinical and immunologic expression in 1010 patients. *Medicine (Baltimore)* 2008;**87**:210–9.
11. Fox RI, Robinson C, Curd J, Michelson P, Bone R, Howell FV. First International symposium on Sjögren's syndrome: suggested criteria for classification of Sjögren's syndrome. *Scand J Rheumatol* 1986;**61**:28–30.
12. Thomas E, Hay EM, Hajeer A, Silman AJ. Sjögren's syndrome: a community-based study of prevalence and impact. *Br J Rheumatol* 1998;**37**:1069–76.

13. Vitali C, Bombardieri S, Jonsson R, Moutsopoulos HM, Alexander EL, Carsons SE, et al. Classification criteria for Sjögren's syndrome: a revised version of the European criteria proposed by the American European Consensus Group. *Ann Rheum Dis* 2002;**61**:554–8.

14. Bowman SJ, Ibrahim GH, Holmes G, Hamburger J, Ainsworth JR. Estimating the prevalence among Caucasian women of primary Sjögren's syndrome in two general practices in Birmingham, UK. *Scand J Rheumatol* 2004;**33**:39–43.

15. Cornec D, Chiche L. Is primary Sjögren's syndrome an orphan disease? A critical appraisal of prevalence studies in Europe. *Ann Rheum Dis* 2015;**74**:e25. http://dx.doi.org/10.1136/annrheumdis-2014-206860. Epub 2014 November 7.

16. Shiboski SC, Shiboski CH, Criswell L, Baer A, Challacombe S, Lanfranchi H, et al. American College of Rheumatology classification criteria for Sjögren's syndrome: a data-driven, expert consensus approach in the Sjögren's International Collaborative Clinical Alliance cohort. *Arthritis Care Res (Hob)* 2012;**64**:475–87.

17. Moutsopoulos HM. Sjögren's syndrome: autoimmune epitheliitis. *Clin Immunol Immunopathol* 1994;**72**:162–5.

18. Pitzalis C, Jones GW, Bombardieri M, Jones SA. Ectopic lymphoid-like structures in infection, cancer and autoimmunity. *Nat Rev Immunol* 2014;**14**:447–62.

19. Theander E, Henriksson G, Ljungberg O, Mandl T, Manthorpe R, Jacobsson LT. Lymphoma and other malignancies in primary Sjögren's syndrome: a cohort study on cancer incidence and lymphoma predictors. *Ann Rheum Dis* 2006;**65**:796–803.

20. Low HZ, Witte T. Aspects of innate immunity in Sjögren's syndrome. *Arthritis Res Ther* 2011;**13**:218.

21. Rönnblom L. The type I interferon system in the etiopathogenesis of autoimmune diseases. *Ups J Med Sci* 2011;**116**:227–37.

22. Mavragani CP, Crow MK. Activation of the type I interferon pathway in primary Sjögren's syndrome. *J Autoimmun* 2010;**35**:225–31.

23. Park I, Teresaki P. Origins of the first HLA specificities. *Hum Immunol* 2000;**61**:185–9.

24. Woodrow JC, Nichol FE, Zaphiropoulos G. DR antigens and rheumatoid arthritis: a study of two populations. *Br Med J* 1981;**283**:1287–8.

25. Gregersen PK, Silver J, Winchester RJ. The shared epitope hypothesis: an approach to understanding the molecular genetics of susceptibility to rheumatoid arthritis. *Arthritis Rheumatol* 1987;**30**:1205–13.

26. Deighton CM, Wentzel J, Cavanagh G, Roberts DF, Walker DJ. Contribution of inherited factors to rheumatoid arthritis. *Ann Rheum Dis* 1992;**51**:182–5.

27. Gregersen PK. Genetics of rheumatoid arthritis: confronting complexity. *Arthritis Res* 1999;**1**:37–44.

28. Cobb BL, Lessard CJ, Harley JB, Moser KL. Genes and Sjögren's syndrome. *Rheum Dis Clin North Am* 2008;**34**:847–68.

29. Segal BM, Nazmul-Hossain ANM, Patel K, Hughes P, Moser KL, Rhodus NL. Genetics and genomics of Sjögren's syndrome: research provides clues to pathogenesis and novel therapies. *Oral Surg Oral Med Oral Pathol Oral Radiol Endod* 2011;**111**:673–80.

30. Anaya J-M, Delgado-Vega AM, Castiblanco J. Genetic basis of Sjögren's syndrome. How strong is the evidence? *Clin Dev Immunol* 2006;**13**:209–22.

31. Anaya JM, Tobon GJ, Pineda-Tamayo R, Castiblanco J. Autoimmune disease aggregation in families of patients with primary Sjögren's syndrome. *J Rheumatol* 2006;**33**:2227–34.

32. Kuo C-F, Grainge MJ, Valdes AM, See L-C, Luo S-F, Yu K-H, et al. Familial risk of Sjögren's syndrome and co-aggregation of autoimmune diseases in affected families. *Arthritis Rheumatol* 2015;**67**:1904–12.

33. Cruz-Tapias P, Rojas-Villarraga A, Maier-Moore S, Anaya JM. HLA and Sjögren's syndrome susceptibility: a meta-analysis of worldwide studies. *Autoimmun Rev* 2012;**11**:281–7.

34. Davies ML, Taylor EJ, Gordon C, Young SP, Welsh K, Bunce M, et al. Candidate T cell epitopes of the human La/SSB autoantigen. *Arthritis Rheumatol* 2002;**46**:209–14.

35. Mann DL, Moutsopoulos HM. HLA DR alloantigens in different subsets of patients with Sjögren's syndrome and in family members. *Ann Rheum Dis* 1983;**42**:533–6.

36. Källberg H, Padyukov L, Plenge RM, Rönnelid J, Gregersen PK, van der Helm-van Mil AHM, et al. Epidemiological Investigation of Rheumatoid Arthritis (EIRA) study group: gene-gene and gene-environment interactions involving *HLA-DRB1*, *PTPN22* and smoking in two subsets of rheumatoid arthritis. *Am J Hum Genet* 2007;**80**:867–75.

37. Collin P, Reunala T, Pukkala E, Laippala P, Keyriläinen O, Pasternack A. Coeliac disease: associated disorders and survival. *Gut* 1994;**35**:1215–8.

38. Megiorni F, Pizzuti A. *HLA-DQA1* and *HLA-DQB1* in Coeliac disease predisposition: practical implications of the molecular DNA typing. *J Biomed Sci* 2012;**19**:88.

39. Bolstad AI, Jonsson R. Genetic aspects of Sjögren's syndrome. *Arthritis Res* 2002;**4**:353–9.

40. Miyagawa S, Shinohara K, Nakajima M, Kidoguchi K, Fujita T, Fukumoto T, et al. Polymorphisms of HLA class II genes and autoimmune responses to Ro/SS-A-La/SS-B among Japanese subjects. *Arthritis Rheumatol* 1998;**41**:927–34.

41. Huang R, Yin J, Chen Y, Deng F, Chen J, Gao X, et al. The amino acid variation within the binding pocket 7 and 9 of *HLA-DRB1* molecules are associated with primary Sjögren's syndrome. *J Autoimmun* 2015;**57**:53–9.

42. Holoshitz J. The quest for better understanding of HLA-disease association: scenes from a road less travelled by. *Discov Med* 2013;**16**:93–101.

43. Lessard CJ, Ice JA, Maier-Moore J, Montgomery CG, Scofield H, Moser KL. Genetics, genomics, and proteomics of Sjögren's syndrome. In: Ramos-Casals M, Stone JH, Moutsopoulos HM, editors. *Sjögren's syndrome; diagnosis and therapeutics.* London, Dordrecht, Heidelberg, New York: Springer; 2012. ISBN: 978-0-85729-946-8.

44. Bolstad AI, Le Hellard S, Kristjansdottir G, Vasaitis L, Kvarnstrom M, Sjowall C, et al. Association between genetic variants in the tumour necrosis factor/lymphotoxin α/lymphotoxin β locus and primary Sjögren's syndrome in Scandinavian samples. *Ann Rheum Dis* 2012;**71**:981–8.

45. Nordmark G, Kristjansdottir G, Theander E, Appel S, Eriksson P, Vasaitis L, et al. Association of *EBF1, FAM167A(C8orf13)-BLK* and *TNFSF4* gene variants with primary Sjögren's syndrome. *Genes Immun* 2011;**12**:100–9.

46. Gorr S-U, Wennblom TJ, Horvath S, Wong DTW, Michie SA. Text-mining applied to autoimmune disease research: the Sjögren's syndrome knowledge base. *BMC Musculoskelet Disord* 2012;**13**:119.

47. Reksten TR, Johnsen SJ, Jonsson MV, Omdal R, Brun JG, Theander E, et al. Genetic associations to germinal centre formation in primary Sjögren's syndrome. *Ann Rheum Dis* 2014;**73**:1253–8.

48. Spain SL, Barrett JC. Strategies for fine-mapping complex traits. *Hum Mol Gen* 2015;**24**(R1):R111–9. July 8. pii: ddv260. [Epub ahead of print].

49. Emamian ES, Leon JM, Lessard CJ, Grandits M, Baechler EC, Gaffney PM, et al. Peripheral blood gene expression profiling in Sjögren's syndrome. *Genes Immun* 2009;**10**:285–96.

50. Cobb BL, Fei Y, Jonsson R, Bolstad AI, Brun JG, Rischmueller M, et al. Genetic association between methyl-CpG binding protein 2 (MECP2) and primary Sjögren's syndrome. *Ann Rheum Dis* 2010;**69**:1731–2.

51. Lessard CJ, Li H, Adrianto I, Ice JA, Rasmussen A, Grundahl KM, et al. Variants at multiple loci implicated in both innate and adaptive immune responses are associated with Sjögren's syndrome. *Nat Genet* 2013;**45**:1284–92.

52. Nordmark G, Wang C, Vasaitis L, Eriksson P, Theander E, Kvarnström M, et al. UK primary Sjögren's syndrome registry: association of genes in the NF-κB pathway with antibody-positive primary Sjögren's syndrome. *Scand J Immunol* 2013;**78**:447–54.

53. Li Y, Zhang K, Chen H, Sun F, Xu J, Wu Z, et al. A genome-wide association study in Han Chinese identifies a susceptibility locus for primary Sjögren's syndrome at 7q11.23. *Nat Genet* 2013;**45**:1361–5.

54. Zheng J, Huang R, Huang Q, Deng F, Chen Y, Yin J, et al. The *GTF2I* rs117026326 polymorphism is associated with anti-SSA-positive primary Sjögren's syndrome. *Rheumatology (Oxford)* 2015;**54**:562–4.

55. González S, Aguilera S, Urzúa U, Quest AF, Molina C, Alliende C, et al. Mechanotransduction and epigenetic control in autoimmune diseases. *Autoimmun Rev* 2011;**10**:175–9.

56. Konsta OD, Thabet Y, Le Dantec C, Brooks WH, Tzioufas AG. The contribution of epigenetics in Sjögren's syndrome. *Front Genet* 2014vol. 5:p1–9. Article 71.

57. Varriale A. DNA methylation, epigenetics, and evolution in vertebrates: facts and challenges. *Int J Evol Biol* 2014;**2014**:7:475981. http://dx.doi.org/10.1155/2014/475981.

58. Thabet Y, Le Dantec C, Ghedira I, Devauchelle V, Cornec D, Pers JO, et al. Epigenetic dysregulation in salivary glands from patients with primary Sjögren's syndrome may be ascribed to infiltrating B cells. *J Autoimmun* 2013;**41**:175–81.

59. Altorok N, Coit P, Hughes T, Koelsch KA, Stone DU, Rasmussen A, et al. Genome-wide DNA methylation patterns in naive CD4+ T cells from patients with primary Sjögren's syndrome. *Arthritis Rheumatol* 2014;**66**:731–9.

60. Gestermann N, Koutero M, Belkhir R, Tost J, Mariette X, Miceli-Richard C. Methylation profile of the promoter region of *IRF5* in primary Sjögren's syndrome. *Eur Cytokine Netw* 2012;**23**:166–72.

61. Nordmark G, Kristjansdottir G, Theander E, Appel S, Eriksson P, Vasaitis L, et al. Additive effects of the major risk alleles of *IRF5* and *STAT4* in primary Sjögren's syndrome. *Genes Immun* 2009;**10**:68–76.

62. Miceli-Richard C, Gestermann N, Ittah M, Comets E, Loiseau P, Puechal X, et al. The CGGGG insertion/deletion polymorphism of the *IRF5* promoter is a strong risk factor for primary Sjögren's syndrome. *Arthritis Rheumatol* 2009;**60**:1991–7.

63. Miceli-Richard C, Wang-Renault SF, Boudaoud S, Busato F, Lallemand C, Bethune K, et al. Overlap between differentially methylated DNA regions in blood B lymphocytes and genetic at-risk loci in primary Sjögren's syndrome. *Ann Rheum Dis* 2015. http://dx.doi.org/10.1136/annrheumdis-2014-206998. July 16. pii: annrheumdis-2014-206998. [Epub ahead of print].

64. Gonzalez S, Aguilera S, Alliende C, Urzua U, Quest AFG, Herrera L, et al. Alterations in type I hemidesmosome components suggestive of epigenetic control in the salivary glands of patients with Sjögren's syndrome. *Arthritis Rheumatol* 2011;**63**:1106–15.

65. Lu Q, Renaudineau Y, Cha S, Ilei G, Brooks WH, Selmi C, et al. Epigenetics in autoimmune disorders: highlights of the 10th Sjogren's syndrome symposium. *Autoimmun Rev* 2010;**9**:627–30.

66. Jimenez SA, Piera-Velazquez S. Potential role of human-specific genes, human-specific microRNAs and human-specific non-coding regulatory RNAs in the pathogenesis of systemic sclerosis and Sjögren's syndrome. *Autoimmun Rev* 2013;**12**:1046–51.

67. Liang C, Xiong K, Szulwach KE, Zhang Y, Wang Z, Peng J, et al. Sjögren syndrome antigen B (SSB)/La promotes global microRNA expression by binding microRNA precursors through stem-loop recognition. *J Biol Chem* 2013;**288**:723–36.

68. Alevizos I, Alexander S, Turner RJ, Illei GG. MicroRNA expression profiles as biomarkers of minor salivary gland inflammation and dysfunction in Sjögren's syndrome. *Arthritis Rheumatol* 2011;**63**:535–44.

69. Kapsogeorgou EK, Gourzi VC, Manoussakis MN, Moutsopoulos HM, Tzioufas AG. Cellular microRNAs (miRNAs) and Sjögren's syndrome: candidate regulators of autoimmune response and autoantigen expression. *J Autoimmun* 2011;**37**:129–35.

70. Tandon M, Gallo A, Jang SI, Illei GG, Alevizos I. Deep sequencing of short RNAs reveals novel microRNAs in minor salivary glands of patients with Sjögren's syndrome. *Oral Dis* 2012;**18**:127–31.

71. Pauley KM, Stewart CM, Gauna AE, Dupre LC, Kuklani R, Chan AL, et al. Altered miR-146a expression in Sjögren's syndrome and its functional role in innate immunity. *Eur J Immunol* 2011;**41**:2029–39.

72. Zilahi E, Tarr T, Papp G, Griger Z, Sipka S, Zeher M. Increased microRNA-146a/b, *TRAF6* gene and decreased *IRAK1* gene expressions in the peripheral mononuclear cells of patients with Sjögren's syndrome. *Immunol Lett* 2012;**141**:165–8.

73. Taganov KD, Boldin MP, Chang KJ, Baltimore D. NF-κB-dependent induction of microRNA miR-146, an inhibitor targeted to signaling proteins of innate immune responses. *Proc Natl Acad Sci* 2006; August 15;**103**(33):12481–6. Epub 2006 Aug 2.

74. Hjelmervik TOR, Petersen K, Jonassen I, Jonsson R, Bolstad AI. Gene expression profiling of minor salivary glands clearly distinguishes primary Sjögren's syndrome patients from healthy control subjects. *Arthritis Rheumatol* 2005;**52**:1534–44.

75. Gottenberg JE, Cagnard N, Lucchesi C, Letourneur F, Mistou S, Lazure T, et al. Activation of IFN pathways and plasmacytoid dendritic cell recruitment in target organs of primary Sjögren's syndrome. *Proc Natl Acad Sci USA* 2006;**103**:2770–5.

76. Hu S, Wang J, Meijer J, Leong S, Xie Y, Yu T, et al. Salivary proteomic and genomic biomarkers for primary Sjögren's syndrome. *Arthritis Rheumatol* 2007;**56**:3588–600.

77. Hu S, Zhou M, Jiang J, Wang J, Elashoff D, Gorr S, et al. Systems biology analysis of Sjögren's syndrome and MALT lymphoma development in parotid glands. *Arthritis Rheumatol* 2009;**60**:81–92.

78. Khuder SA, Al-Hashimi I, Mutgi AB, Altorok N. Identification of potential genomic biomarkers for Sjögren's syndrome using data pooling of gene expression microarrays. *Rheumatol Int* 2015;**35**:829–36.

79. Brkic A, Maria NI, van Helden-Meeuwsen CG, van der Merwe J, van Daele PL, Dalm VA, et al. Prevalence of interferon type I signature in CD14 monocytes of patients with Sjögren's syndrome and association with disease activity and *BAFF* gene expression. *Ann Rheum Dis* 2013;**72**:728–35.

80. Kimoto O, Sawada J, Shimoyama K, Suzuki D, Nakamura S, Hayashi H, et al. Activation of the interferon pathway in peripheral blood of patients with Sjögren's syndrome. *J Rheumatol* 2011;**38**:310–6.

81. Devauchelle-Pensec V, Cagnard N, Pers JO, Youinou P, Saraux A, Chiocchia G. Gene expression profile in the salivary glands of primary Sjögren's syndrome patients before and after treatment with rituximab. *Arthritis Rheum* 2010;**62**:2262–71.

82. Lavie F, Miceli-Richard C, Ittah M, Sellam J, Gottenberg JE, Mariette X. Increase of B cell-activating factor of the TNF family (BAFF) after rituximab treatment: insights into a new regulating system of BAFF production. *Ann Rheum Dis* 2007;**66**:700–3.

83. Naidoo N, Pawitan Y, Soong R, Cooper DN, Ku S-S. Human genetics and genomics a decade after the release of the draft sequence of the human genome. *Hum Genomics* 2011;**5**:577–622.

84. Giannopoulou EG, Elemento O, Ivashkiv LB. Use of RNA sequencing to evaluate rheumatic disease patients. *Arthritis Res Ther* 2015;**17**:167.

85. Scher JU, Bretz WA, Abramson SB. Periodontal disease and subgingival microbiota as contributors for rheumatoid arthritis pathogenesis: modifiable risk factors? *Curr Opin Rheumatol* 2014;**26**:424–9.

86. Scher JU, Ubeda C, Equinda M, Khanin R, Buischi Y, Viale A, et al. Periodontal disease and the oral microbiota in new-onset rheumatoid arthritis. *Arthritis Rheumatol* 2012;**64**:3083–94.

87. Scher JU, Sczesnak A, Longman RS, Segata N, Ubeda C, Bielski C, et al. Expansion of intestinal *Prevotella copri* correlates with enhanced susceptibility to arthritis. *Elife* 2013;**2**:e01202. http://dx.doi.org/10.7554/eLife.01202.

88. Zhang X, Zhang D, Jia H, Feng Q, Wang D, Liang D, et al. The oral and gut microbiomes are perturbed in rheumatoid arthritis and partly normalized after treatment. *Nat Med* 2015;**21**: 895–905.

89. Leung KC, Leung WK, McMillan AS. Supra-gingival microbiota in Sjögren's syndrome. *Clin Oral Investig* 2007;**11**:415–23.

90. Szymula A, Rosenthal J, Szczerba BM, Bagavant H, Fu SM, Deshmukh US. T cell epitope mimicry between Sjögren's syndrome antigen A (SSA)/Ro60 and oral, gut, skin and vaginal bacteria. *Clin Immunol* 2014;**152**:1–9.

91. Ryu OH, Atkinson JC, Hoehn GT, Illei GG, Hart TC. Identification of parotid salivary biomarkers in Sjögren's syndrome by surface-enhanced laser desorption/ionization time-of-flight mass spectrometry and two-dimensional difference gel electrophoresis. *Rheumatology* 2006;**45**:1077–86.

92. Baldini C, Giust L, Ciregia F, Valle YD, Giacomelli C, Donadio E, et al. Proteomic analysis of saliva: a unique tool to distinguish primary Sjögren's syndrome from secondary Sjögren's syndrome and other sicca syndromes. *Arthritis Res The* 2011;**13**:R194.

93. Delaleu N, Mydel P, Kwee I, Brun JG, Jonsson MV, Jonsson R. High fidelity between saliva proteomics and the biologic state of salivary glands defines biomarker signatures for primary Sjögren's syndrome. *Arthritis Rheumatol* 2015;**67**:1084–95.

94. Fitzpatrick MA, Young SP. Metabolomics: a novel window into inflammatory disease. *Swiss Med Wkly* 2013;**143**:w13743.

95. Gaber T, Haupl T, Sandig G, Tykwinska K, Fangradt M, Tschirschmann M, et al. Adaptation of human CD4+ T-cells to pathophysiological hypoxia: a transcriptome analysis. *J Rheumatol* 2009;**36**:2655–69.

96. Marchesi JR, Holmes E, Khan F, Kochhar S, Scanlon P, Shanahan F, et al. Rapid and non-invasive metabolomic characterization of inflammatory bowel disease. *J Proteome Res* 2007; **6**:546–51.

97. Kageyama G, Saegusa J, Irino Y, Tanaka S, Tsuda K, Takahashi S, et al. Metabolomics analysis of saliva from patients with primary Sjögren's syndrome. *Clin Exp Immunol* July 21, 2015. http://dx.doi.org/10.1111/cei.12683. [Epub ahead of print].

Chapter 9

# Autoantigens and Autoantibodies in the Pathogenesis of Sjögren's Syndrome

E. Tinazzi, G. Patuzzo, C. Lunardi
*University of Verona, Verona, Italy*

## 1. INTRODUCTION

It is well established that environmental factors in concert with an appropriate genetic background play a fundamental role in triggering Sjögren's syndrome (SS) leading to chronic inflammation of the target organs through different mechanisms, among which the molecular mimicry between infectious agents and autoantigens has been the most studied. An aberrant autoimmune response due to T- and B-lymphocyte hyperactivity and autoantibody production is known to be a crucial mechanism for the induction of autoimmune epitheliitis and the perpetuation of inflammation. In particular, histopathological damage ranges from mild to diffuse cell infiltrates characterized by a predominance of T and B cells. B-lymphocyte hyperactivity and the development of B-cell follicles containing germinal center–like structures represent a multistep process known as ectopic lymphoid neogenesis, which typically involves salivary glands and other SS target organs. As far as the T-cell compartment is concerned, different T-lymphocyte subpopulations participate in the development and maintenance of glandular inflammation. Indeed, T helper (Th) 1 lymphocytes and their soluble products, particularly interferons (IFNs), have long been considered to be the main players in the induction of chronic tissue damage, but the identification of Th17, Th22, T regulatory cells, and Th follicular cells has recently changed the view on the role played by the different T-cell subpopulations. Moreover, the interleukin (IL)-17-axis can favor B/T lymphocyte survival, protecting T cells from apoptosis and, as a consequence, potentiating aberrant autoimmune responses.[1,2]

B-cell hyperactivity and the production of autoantibodies against different autoantigens are typical features of SS. Nevertheless, these autoantibodies are

Sjögren's Syndrome. http://dx.doi.org/10.1016/B978-0-12-803604-4.00009-5

non–organ specific and their role in the pathogenesis of the disease is not clearly understood or defined (Table 9.1). However, immunoglobulins (Igs) such as rheumatoid factor (RF), antinuclear antigens (ANAs), antiextractable nuclear and cytoplasmic antigens, particularly anti-Ro/SSA and anti-La/SSB, which have all been included in the diagnostic criteria of the disease, and anti-α-fodrin, are present in 80% to 90% of patients.[3] Indeed, 10% to 20% of SS patients are considered seronegative and this condition seems to be associated with a potential delay in diagnosis, but also with a milder form of the disease, similar to what happens in other seronegative autoimmune disorders.[4,5] Besides the autoantibodies associated to SS described so far, recently the presence of novel autoantibodies has been investigated with the aim of identifying new autoantigens, which may be specific for the disease. Such novel autoantibodies may have different characteristics and functions: be present in a percentage of seronegative patients; play a role in the pathogenesis of the disease; have a prognostic role in case of a correlation with specific organ damage; be a marker of response to therapy and important.

Several players may participate in the development of the disease. Firstly, genetic background plays a fundamental role, including genes encoding molecules implicated in B-cell activation [such as B-cell activating factor (BAFF)], lymphotoxins α and β, and tumor necrosis factor (TNF), together with genes

**TABLE 9.1 Prevalence of Autoantibodies in SS Patients**

| Autoantibodies Against | Prevalence (%) |
| --- | --- |
| Nuclear antigens | 59–85 |
| Ro52/TRIM21 | 66.7 |
| Ro60/TROVE2 | 52.1 |
| La/SSB | 49 |
| U1RNP | 2 |
| Rheumatoid factor | 36–74 |
| Cryoglobulins | 9–15 |
| Centromere | 4–17 |
| Mitochondria | 1.7–27 |
| Smooth muscle | 30 |
| Cyclic citrullinated peptides | 3–10 |
| Calreticulin | 20 |
| Muscarinic 3 receptors | 11 |
| Carbonic anhydrase II | 12.5–20.8 |
| α-Fodrin | 50–90 |

involved in increased production of type I IFNs, known as IFN-signature, and with genes associated with specific human leukocyte antigens (HLAs), such as HLA-B8, HLA-Dw3, HLA-DR3, and DRw52. Secondly, infectious agents have been implicated in the pathogenesis of the disease including, Epstein–Barr virus (EBV), human T-cell virus type 1, cytomegalovirus, and hepatitis C virus, all characterized by selective tropism for epithelial and immune cells and by ability to induce neurohormonal disturbances which may interfere with sex hormone ratios affecting steroid-dependent cells such as epithelial and autoreactive cells, both involved in the pathogenesis of the disease.[6–8]

The interplay between genetic and environmental factors may facilitate an autoimmune response against self-antigens, leading to tissue infiltration by immune cells and tissue damage with exposure of novel autoantigens and to further autoantibody production.

In this chapter, we will analyze both identified and proposed autoantigens and autoantibodies with the aim of clarifying the possible link between these molecules and the pathogenic mechanisms of the disease.

## 2. PATHOGENESIS AND AUTOANTIGENS

The aberrant autoimmune response with T- and B-lymphocyte hyperactivity and autoantibody production has been described as the main mechanism for the induction of autoimmune damage typically related to the onset of SS. It has also been suggested that there is a cooperative role played by macrophages, natural killer (NK) cells, and dendritic cells (DCs), which have also been described in inflamed salivary glands.[9] Particularly, based on their ability to participate in peripheral tolerance, DCs play an important role in the maintenance of autoimmune aggression by both interfering with autoreactive T-cell functions and acting as a putative source of IFNγ. This cytokine plays an important role in immune regulatory processes and is strongly associated with SS, because high concentrations have been found in the biopsy of target organs, particularly at the salivary gland level.[10] Moreover, IFNγ is functionally linked to some of the established autoantigens of the disease, such as Ro/SSA and La/SS.

In this setting, the comprehension of the possible role played by self-antigens in the pathogenesis of the disease is crucial.

Indeed, various molecules have been reported as possible autoantigens. However, a causal connection has not been established for all the proposed molecules and in the majority of cases, we may only describe the presence of autoantibodies directed against such antigens as a mirror of the autoimmune aggression without any proof of pathogenic effect.

### 2.1 Ro/SSA and La/SSB

The Ro/La ribonucleoprotein (RNP) complexes are protein–RNA complexes formed by the association of the Ro52 kDa, Ro60 kDa, and La proteins with small cytoplasmic RNA.

In particular, Ro52 is an IFN-inducible protein belonging to the tripartite motif (TRIM) protein family,[11,12] acting as intracellular Fc-receptor, and is implicated in the regulation of cell proliferation and apoptosis.[13] Conversely, Ro60/TROVE2 protein is a ring-shaped RNA-binding protein participating in recognition and leading to degradation of misfolded defective RNAs.[14] Similar to Ro60/TROVE2, La/SSB protein appears to be involved in RNA metabolism and, in particular, in the regulation of micro RNA (miRNA) expression by protecting and stabilizing precursor miRNA from nuclease activity.[15–17]

Ro52 messenger RNA transcript may be spliced into a common or alternative form in relation to the presence or deletion of exon 4 in the process of transcription. The alternative form has been demonstrated in a variety of tissues, including the fetal heart and salivary glands,[18] but the significance of this alternative splicing is still unclear because the demonstration of the corresponding Ro52 isoform has never been identified at the protein level in vivo.

The Ro52 protein has an E3 ligase activity and plays a role in the ubiquitination of proteins, leading to the regulation of cellular levels and activity of specific proteins. In particular, several proteins have been suggested as substrate for Ro52-mediated ubiquitination, including several members of the IFN-regulatory factor (IRF) transcription factor family.[19] In a deficient Ro52 mouse model, it has been demonstrated that the lack of Ro52-mediated ubiquitination of IRF transcription factors lead to an aberrant expression of type I IFNs and proinflammatory cytokines, such as IL-6, IL-12/IL-23, and TNF-α, confirming a central role for Ro52 as negative regulators of IRFs and proinflammatory cytokines.[20] Of relevance, Ro52 resides in the cytoplasm of unstimulated cells and translocates into the nucleus upon INF stimulation after viral infection. It seems that upregulation and nuclear translocation of Ro52 might be a functional part of the negative feedback loop suppressing IFN-mediated immune activation.

Ro60, a component of Ro/La RNP complex, is involved in quality control of RNA. Several reports indicate a sequence homology between Ro60 and viral protein, such as Coxsackie virus 2B protein and EBV nuclear antigen 1, suggesting that Ro60 may be an antigen responsible for a molecular mimicry mechanism.[21] This hypothesis is in accordance with data which has reported Ro60 autoantibodies months before the appearance of Ro52 and La autoantibodies in systemic lupus erythematosus (SLE) patients, but unfortunately similar data are not available in SS.[22]

The phosphoprotein La/SSB is a member of the RNA-recognition motif protein family and is a part of the Ro/La RNP complex that associates with small cytoplasmic RNAs and viral RNAs. Several studies have reported that viral infections induce miRNA and La complexes able to induce TLR3-related secretion of type-1 IFN and of TNF.

In this setting, it may be hypothesized that at the time of viral infection of salivary gland epithelial cells, Ro52 is overexpressed as a defensive mechanism both to suppress viral replication and to protect cells from prolonged activation of the type-1 IFN system. Simultaneously, the viral pathogen may use La protein to escape from the immune response, leading to a La/SSB overexpression. Nevertheless, both Ro and La antigens contribute to the amplification of an exuberant immune response, leading to aggression toward target organs.

## 2.2 Calreticulin

Calreticulin is an endoplasmic reticulum resident protein of approximately 46 kDa molecular weight with multiple functions, including control of cellular adhesiveness, gene expression, calcium homeostasis regulation, and molecular chaperoning.[23] It acts as a multifunctional protein that behaves as a molecular chaperone and contributes to CD91-mediated antigen presentation. The major receptor of calreticulin is CD91. This receptor is involved in the cross-presentation of chaperoned peptides within classical antigen-presenting cells, leading to specific innate and adaptive immune responses, and it is also able to mediate a variety of cellular functions because it is expressed in other cell types, including hepatocytes, adipocytes, fibroblasts, neuronal cells, and epithelial cells of salivary glands. Of relevance, interaction of CD91 with calreticulin seems to be related to the clearance of apoptotic cells, a keystone in SS pathogenesis. It has been also demonstrated that calreticulin specifically binds to a linear chemically synthesized epitope of Ro60 and induces conformation-dependent recognition by autoantibodies obtained from human autoimmune patients' sera. Moreover, the complex calreticulin-Ro60 can be internalized by salivary glands epithelial cells by CD91. These cells can act as nonprofessional APCs and trigger specific cellular autoimmune response and autoantibody production, thus amplifying the autoimmune response against Ro60.[24]

In summary, calreticulin has been shown to be implicated in SS pathogenesis. It serves as molecular chaperone, has the ability to bind and induce processing of antigenic peptides, and colocalizes with Ro60 antigen in apoptotic blebs, leading to autoimmune response.

## 2.3 Muscarinic 3 Receptors

Five different subtypes of muscarine acetylcholine receptors (M1R–M5R) have been identified and, among all of them, muscarinic 3 receptor (M3R) is selectively expressed in exocrine glands and plays an important role in exocrine secretion.[25] Acetylcholine binds to and activates M3R on salivary gland cells, increasing intracellular $Ca^{2+}$ concentration and leading to an activation of apical $Cl^-$ channels and consequent up-stimulation of salivary secretion. Activation of M3R also induces trafficking of aquaporin-5 from the cytoplasm to the apical membrane, causing a rapid transport of water across the cell membrane.

M3R has four extracellular domains, known as the N-terminal region and three extracellular loops. The second extracellular loop plays an important role in intracellular signaling and is critical for receptor activation by agonists.[26] Moreover, the second extracellular domain of M3R seems to act as autoantigen both for T and B cells leading to an excess of INFγ secretion by autoreactive

T lymphocytes in glandular infiltrates and to autoantibody production. Indeed, M3R reactive T cells were detected in a variable percentage of SS patients and it has been demonstrated in animal models that M3R-reactive Th1 and Th17 cells are essential for the development of sialadenitis.[27] Similarly, detection of autoantibodies against the second loop of M3R is present in about 50% of SS patients and the same antibodies seem to be pathogenetic, because they are able to induce a variation in intracellular $Ca^{2+}$ influx.[28]

Taken together these data provide evidence for a pathogenic role of M3R and suggest the potential for both T- and B-cell targeted therapy in SS.

## 2.4 Carbonic Anhydrase II

Carbonic anhydrases form a family of enzymes classified as metalloproteases, because their active site contains a zinc ion and is able to catalyze the reversible hydration of carbon dioxide to generate a proton and a bicarbonate ion. Carbonic anhydrase II (CAII) is the only soluble form of the enzyme and regulates the acid–base homeostasis in erythrocytes and the aqueous chambers of the eyes and renal tubules. CAII can be shown in the cytosol of tubular renal cells of both proximal and distal tubules and also in the salivary gland epithelial cells of animal models. Moreover, in a mouse model, immunization of mice with CAII leads to a systemic exocrine gland inflammation and infiltration, similar to that observed in human SS.[29] There are no reports regarding the potential pathogenic role of CAII in inflammation of salivary gland epithelial cells and renal tubule cells, but only a strong association between anti-CAII antibodies and a high risk of renal tubular acidosis development.[30]

## 2.5 α-Fodrin

α-Fodrin is a 240 KDa protein forming a heterodimer with β-fodrin. It is a universally expressed membrane-associated cytoskeletal protein important for maintaining normal membrane structure and for supporting cell surface protein function, since it seems to be involved in exocytosis and secretion.[31] α-Fodrin is one of the important targets of caspases during the apoptotic process and its cleavage leads to membrane malfunction and cell shrinkage. α-Fodrin is cleaved in three different fragments, known as N-terminal 150 kDa, C-terminal 120 kDa, and 35 kDa, but only the first two fragments are able to induce a strong antibody response and, in particular, only the 120 kDa fragment has been proposed as an important organ-specific autoantigen in the pathogenesis of the disease. Particularly, in an animal model the 120 kDa fragments are present in a high concentration in epithelial cells from salivary glands. Moreover, in a mouse model the pathogenic role of α-fodrin as autoantigen is underlined by the use of mucosal administration of α-fodrin, which seems to lead to the induction of tolerance of the antigen, blocking the lymphocytic infiltration of salivary glands and reducing salivary dysfunction.[32]

## 2.6 Tear Lipocalin

Tear lipocalin is a protein belonging to the lipocalin family and the calycine super-family, which is a diverse set of proteins that function as extracellular binding proteins. Lipocalins are a family of low molecular weight proteins (18–40 kDa) with prevalent extracellular functions and in general are proteins with a common structure and possess multiple molecular recognition properties, including binding to either small hydrophobic molecules, macromolecular complexes, or soluble macromolecules through covalent and noncovalent bonds; moreover, they bind to specific cell surface receptors. In particular, tear lipocalin is highly expressed both in tears and saliva and it accounts for about 15% to 33% of the tear proteins and it is the major lipid binding protein in human tears.[33]

Together with other proteins of the lipocalin family, tear lipocalins have been termed immunocalins, owing to their role in immunity. The immunocalins behave as acute-phase proteins and play a role in the acute-phase response to infection and injury. Moreover, tear lipocalins may have protective immunoregulatory, antiinflammatory, and antimicrobial effects in the tears and ocular surface and, together with the other immunocalins, seem to act as part of the cytokine immune network and as key regulators of inflammatory cells, including NK cells, neutrophils, monocytes, macrophages, and B and T lymphocytes, and interfere with platelet aggregation and adherence of neutrophils and monocytes to vascular endothelium.[34]

## 3. AUTOANTIBODIES: THEIR ROLE IN THE PATHOGENESIS AND DIAGNOSIS

Multiple autoantibodies are reported to be associated with SS. However, their role in the pathogenesis or in the diagnosis and/or prognosis of the disease is still uncertain. In fact, the presence of autoantibodies in some cases has a pathogenic role, whereas in others it may be caused by polyclonal activation of the B-lymphocyte compartment, typically associated with the disease. Here we have reported data regarding the well-known autoantibodies commonly related to SS together with some data of new emerging or proposed autoantibodies.

### 3.1 Antinuclear Antibodies and Anti-Ro/SSA and Anti-La/SSB

Antinuclear antibodies are detectable in the large majority of SS patients, are predominantly associated with a glandular involvement, and are strongly associated to Ro/SSA and La/SSB expression. The presence of autoantibodies against Ro/SSA (Ro52 and Ro60) and La/SSB is considered one of the characteristic features of SS and represents the diagnostic tool for the disease even if they are found respectively in 50% to 70% and 30% to 60% of SS patients.[35,36]

Anti-Ro/SSA antibodies can be classified into two distinct types of autoantibodies that specifically react with two nonhomologous proteins, respectively the Ro52/TRIM21 and Ro60/TROVE2, characterized by different specificities.

Usually, clinical studies do not distinguish between anti-Ro52/TRIM21 and anti-Ro60/TROVE2 antibodies and although the same autoantibodies often coexist in a significant proportion of patients, they seem to be related to distinct clinical features.[4] In particular, as represented in Table 9.2, detection of these

**TABLE 9.2** Association Between Autoantibodies Expression and Clinical Features

| Autoantibodies Against | Clinical Association |
|---|---|
| Ro52/TRIM21 | • Younger age at diagnosis and longer disease duration<br>• Exocrine gland hypofunction as attested by functional tests |
| Ro60/TROVE2 | • Severe infiltration of salivary glands<br>• Salivary gland enlargement<br>• Extraglandular manifestations |
| La/SSB | • Hypergammaglobulinemia, cryoglobulinemia<br>• Neonatal lupus, congenital heart block |
| U1RNP | • Overlapping syndrome with MCTD |
| RF | • Younger age at diagnosis<br>• Extraglandular manifestations |
| Cryoglobulins | • Younger age at diagnosis<br>• Salivary gland enlargement<br>• Extraglandular manifestations<br>• MALT lymphoma<br>• Hypocomplementemia<br>• Hypergammaglobulinemia |
| Centromere | • Overlap with systemic sclerosis<br>• Milder disease<br>• Negative correlation with anti-Ro/SSA and anti-La/SSB antibodies |
| Mitochondria | • Primary biliary cirrhosis |
| Smooth muscle | • Autoimmune hepatitis |
| Cyclic citrullinated peptides | • Articular involvement, particularly erosive arthritis |
| Muscarinic receptor 3 | • Sicca syndrome |
| CAII | • Renal tubular acidosis |
| α-Fodrin | • Lymphocytic infiltration of salivary glands<br>• Sicca syndrome<br>• CNS involvement |

*CAII*, Carbonic anhydrase II; *CNS*, central nervous system; *MALT*, mucosa-associated lymphoid tissue; *MCTD*, mixed connective tissue disease; *RF*, rheumatoid factor.

autoantibodies in patients' sera has been correlated with longer disease duration before diagnosis, extensive lymphocytic infiltration of minor salivary glands, severe exocrine gland hypofunction, and recurrent parotid gland enlargement.

Of relevance, pregnancy in women with anti-Ro/SSA and anti-La/SSB may be complicated by the development of neonatal lupus syndrome in the fetus or neonate and the autoantibody title is strongly associated with increased risk for congenital heart block. It has been hypothesized that in this rare syndrome, maternal anti-Ro and anti-La IgG autoantibodies may pass through the placenta to fetal circulation, thereby directly causing tissue injury of the heart and skin.[37]

### 3.2 Rheumatoid Factor, Anticyclic Citrullinated Peptide Antibodies

Igs such as rheumatoid factor (RF), anticyclic citrullinated peptides (CCPs), and cryoglobulins are detectable with high prevalence in SS patient sera, with the former being present in 36% to 74%, the second in 3% to 10%, and the latter in 9% to 15%, respectively.[38] RF and anti-CPP autoantibodies are strongly associated with articular involvement and particularly with higher rates of erosive arthritis and with synovitis. RF, anti-CPPs, and cryoglobulins are associated with younger age at diagnosis and with higher incidence of parotid gland enlargement and extraglandular involvement, including evolution to lymphoma. Moreover, the presence of cryoglobulins correlates more specifically with RF positivity, anti-Ro/SSA and/or La/SSB antibodies, hypocomplementemia, and monoclonal gammopathy, which all lead to a high risk of evolution into lymphoma.[39]

### 3.3 Antibodies Against U1 Ribonucleoprotein

Antibodies directed against U1 ribonucleoprotein (U1RNP) are detectable in 25% to 47% of SLE patients and high titers of anti-U1RNP are a diagnostic feature of mixed connective tissue disorder. In SS, the presence of anti-U1RNP is variable but strongly associated with a low amount of salivary secretion.[40] The mechanism of hyposalivation caused by the presence of anti-U1RNP antibodies is still unknown, but it has been suggested that local antibody production may be correlated to infiltrating B cells in the salivary glands, leading to an autoimmune phenomenon and local loss of function.

### 3.4 Anticentromere Antibodies

Anticentromere antibodies (ACAs), which are typically associated to the limited form of systemic sclerosis, are detectable in a variable proportion (4–17%) of SS patients and they seem to be related to an overlap syndrome with milder manifestation compared with overlap syndrome in ACA-negative patients, but with a higher risk of developing non-Hodgkin lymphoma.[41] Furthermore, the presence of ACAs in SS seems to identify a distinct clinical subgroup characterized by a higher disease activity index but with a similar damage compared with ACA-negative subjects.[42] It is unclear whether the presence of ACA is an epiphenomenon similar to what happens in the course of systemic sclerosis or whether the same antibodies have a potential role in the pathogenesis of a particular subset of SS patients.

## 3.5 Antimitochondrial Antibodies

Antimitochondrial antibodies (AMAs) target the components of keto acid dehydrogenase complex and pyruvate dehydrogenase subunit, and are reported in 1.7% to 13% of SS patients, showing a strong association with liver involvement according to its role as diagnostic serological marker of primary biliary cirrhosis. The presence of these autoantibodies in SS patients leads to a comparable histopathologic profile of liver and salivary gland lesions described as "autoimmune epitheliitis," which apparently show no progression during the course of the disease.[42]

## 3.6 Anti–Smooth Muscle Antibodies

Another set of autoantibodies that can be found in SS patients are the anti–smooth muscle antibodies (ASMAs) with a prevalence of about 30%.[43] Usually, ASMAs along with ANA positivity are diagnostic for autoimmune hepatitis; however, their clinical value in SS is not clear and their suggested correlation with liver involvement is still controversial.[3,44,45] Again, prevalence of these autoantibodies is low and as a consequence their sensitivity in SS diagnosis is limited.

## 3.7 Antibodies Against Muscarinic Receptors Type 3

Antibodies against muscarinic receptors, such as anti-M3R, detected by functional methods or using synthetic peptides, have been described in SS sera. These antibodies are directed to M3 muscarinic acetylcholine receptor, a molecule that is highly expressed in exocrine glands such as salivary glands and lacrimal glands, and is involved in salivary and lacrimal production. Indeed some data from experimental animal models suggest that M3R is a molecule which is potentially involved in glandular dysfunction.[46] In particular, the most important evidence for the pathogenetic role of anti-M3R antibodies is obtained by passive transfer experiments. In this setting, transfer of IgG derived from SS patients to mice induces salivary glandular hypofunction as well as upregulation of M3R expression in bronchioles in the recipient mice.[47] Moreover, M3R has been suggested as a potential therapeutic target in SS, since a crucial role for M3R-reactive Th1 and Th17 cells has been demonstrated in the pathogenesis of autoimmune sialadenitis in experimental mouse models.[27]

Despite all these considerations, discrepancies in solid-based enzyme-linked immunosorbent assay (ELISA) and difficulties in detecting anti-M3R by conventional immunological techniques has failed to provide a consensus for the association of anti-M3R presence occurrence with clinical manifestations in SS.[48,49]

## 3.8 Autoantibodies Targeting Carbonic Anhydrase II

Autoantibodies targeting CAII are present in 12.5% to 20.8% of SS patients and seem to be associated with renal involvement, particularly with distal renal tubular acidosis.[5,30] These results suggest that distal renal tubular involvement may be at least partially caused by defective function of CAII, resulting from high plasma anti-CAII title.

## 3.9 Antibodies Against α-Fodrin

Antibodies against α-fodrin have been shown to be present in between 50% and 90% of untreated patients but their diagnostic value is strongly modified by any therapeutic approach which seems to quickly normalize antibody titer, causing loss of the potential diagnostic significance.[50,51]

Nevertheless, it is relevant to underline that diagnostic accuracy of anti–α-fodrin antibodies in diverse series of patients is different, leading to different sensitivity and specificity. Hu et al. for instance, analyzed 23 studies, including 7 Chinese and 16 English studies, reporting a pooled sensitivity and specificity of 39.3% and 83% respectively, showing moderate accuracy for SS diagnosis with relative low sensitivity.[51] Moreover, a specific subset of patients with a particular organ involvement in whom the detection of these autoantibodies might be important as a diagnostic and prognostic marker has not been identified yet.

## 4. NOVEL PROPOSED AUTOANTIGENS AND AUTOANTIBODIES

Because a key diagnostic criterion is the presence of ANA and Ro/SSA and/or La/SSB, which are still absent in a proportion of SS patients, attention has recently been focused on the development of diagnostic tests for immunodominant autoantigens potentially related to SS.

The screening of a random peptide library with IgG from the sera of SS patients identified an immunodominant peptide of tear lipocalin, against which are directed antibodies that can distinguish sera of SS patients, from sera of healthy donors, and individuals with other systemic autoimmune disorders by ELISA.[52] We recently tested the presence of antibodies in a large series of SS patients and a cohort of control subjects, including healthy donors and patients affected by other autoimmune diseases such as rheumatoid arthritis, SLE, and systemic sclerosis, showing a good sensitivity and specificity of the ELISA assay. In order to improve the sensitivity of the diagnostic test and to minimize the possible methodological difficulties related to the use of synthetic peptides, we have investigated the use of lipocalin peptide displayed as plant-made chimeric virus particles to be used in a diagnostic assay. A good specificity of antibodies against tear lipocalin has been found in order to discriminate SS patients from both healthy controls and patients with other autoimmune disease.[53]

Recently, studies with animal models of SS have identified new potential autoantigens, such as anti–salivary gland protein 1 (SP1), anti–carbonic anhydrase 6 (CA6), and anti–parotid secretory protein (PSP); however, autoantibodies against these proteins have been detected in SS patient sera as well as in sera of patients with idiopathic dry mouth and dry eyes. Suresh and colleagues investigated antibodies against SP1, CA6, and PSP in a large cohort of SS patients showing a correlation primarily with symptoms such as dry eyes and dry mouth, and not with the outcome of labial biopsies which provide a definitive SS diagnosis.[54,55]

Similarly, the analysis of miRNAs targeting the autoantigens Ro/SSA and La/SSB has suggested that miRNA expression levels could be used to diagnose SS, but a reproducible expression profile in the disease has not been confirmed. In this setting, the study of miRNAs does not demonstrate superiority as a predictor of disease over Ro/SSA and La/SSB themselves.[56]

The dosage of anti-poly(U)-binding-splicing factor (PUF60) by immunoblot, immunoprecipitation, and ELISA has also recently been proposed as a prominent new target of the autoimmune response both in SS and dermatomyositis. The analysis showed that the presence of anti-PUF60 antibodies correlates with higher prevalence of ANA positivity ($\geq$1:320), RF, and hypergammaglobulinemia, and is associated with the presence of anti-Ro/SSA and anti-La/SSB. Nevertheless, anti-PUF60 antibodies were detectable in 29.8% of SS patients and in a variable proportion of subjects affected by other autoimmune diseases, showing a low diagnostic sensitivity.[57]

Finally, Delaleu and colleagues have suggested saliva proteomics for the diagnosis of SS using an antibody-based multiplex assay including 187 proteomic biomarkers. The analysis showed a four-component biomarker signature consisting of clusterin, IL-5, fibroblast growth factor 4, and IL-4; and a six-biomarker signature of clusterin, IL-5, pregnancy-associated plasma protein A, C-reactive protein, apolipoprotein A-II, and IL-4, which correctly classified over 90% of SS patients and the majority of healthy control subjects. The application of proteomic analysis in routine clinical practice is hampered by high costs as well as by technical difficulties and needs validation and therefore it is a method still reserved for the identification of new potential biomarkers that need to be validated using methods which are more accessible in clinical practice.[58,59]

## 5. CONCLUSIONS

The etiology and many aspects of the pathogenesis of SS remain poorly understood. Nevertheless, the identification of novel autoantigen targets helps researchers to better understand the pathogenesis of the disease, although it is difficult to prove the effective role played in triggering and maintaining the autoimmune response. However, antibodies directed against such novel autoantigens may become a useful tool in the diagnostic process of the disease.

## REFERENCES

1. Boggio E, Clemente N, Mondino A, Cappellano G, Orilieri E, Gigliotti CL, et al. IL-17 protects T cells from apoptosis and contributes to development of ALPS-like phenotypes. *Blood* 2014;**123**:1178–86.

2. Alunno A, Carubbi F, Bartoloni E, Bistoni O, Caterbi S, Cipriani P, et al. Unmasking the pathogenic role of IL-17 axis in Sjögren's syndrome: a new era for therapeutic targeting? *Autoimm Rev* 2014;**13**:1167–73.

3. Nardi N, Brito-Zerón P, Ramos-Casals M, Aguiló S, Cervera R, Ingelmo M, et al. Circulating autoantibodies against nuclear and non-nuclear antigens in primary Sjögren's syndrome: prevalence and clinical significance in 335 patients. *Clin Rheumatol* 2006;**25**:341–6.

4. Ter Borg EJ, Risselada AP, Kelder JC. Relation of systemic autoantibodies to the number of extraglandular manifestations in primary Sjögren's syndrome: a retrospective analysis of 65 patients in the Netherlands. *Semin Arthr Rheum* 2011;**40**:547–51.

5. Kyriakidis NC, Kapsogeorgou EK, Tzioufas AG. A comprehensive review of autoantibodies in primary Sjögren's syndrome: clinical phenotypes and regulatory mechanism. *J Autoimmun* 2014;**51**:67–74.

6. Lucchesi D, Pitzalis C, Bombardieri M. EBV and other viruses as triggers of tertiary lymphoid structures in primary Sjögren's syndrome. *Expert Rev Clin Immunol* 2014;**10**:445–55.

7. Kivity S, Arango MT, Ehrenfeld M, Tehori O, Shoenfeld Y, Anaya JM, et al. Infection and autoimmunity in Sjögren's syndrome: a clinical study and comprehensive review. *J Autoimmun* 2014;**51**:17–22.

8. Nakamura H, Takahashi Y, Yamamoto-Fukuda T, Horai Y, Nakashima Y, Arima K, et al. Direct infection of primary salivary gland epithelial cells by human T lymphotropic virus type I in patients with Sjögren's syndrome. *Arthritis Rheum* 2015;**67**:1096–106.

9. Brito-Zerón P, Gheitasi H, Retamozo S, Bové A, Londoño M, Sánchez-Tapias JM, et al. How hepatitis C virus modifies the immunological profile of Sjögren syndrome: analysis of 783 patients. *Arthritis Res Ther* 2015;**17**:250.

10. Jonsson MV, Skarstein K. Follicular dendritic cells confirm lymphoid organization in the minor salivary glands of primary Sjögren's syndrome. *J Oral Pathol Med* 2008;**37**:515–21.

11. Hjelmervik TO, Petersen K, Jonassen I, Jonsson R, Bolstad AI. Gene expression profiling of minor salivary glands clearly distinguishes primary Sjögren's syndrome patients from healthy control subjects. *Arthritis Rheum* 2005;**52**:1534–44.

12. Rhodes DA, Ihrke G, Reinicke AT, Malcherek G, Towey M, Isenberg DA, et al. The 52,000 MW Ro/SS-A autoantigen in Sjögren's syndrome/systemic lupus erythematosus (Ro52) is an interferon-gamma inducible tripartite motif protein associated with membrane proximal structures. *Immunology* 2002;**106**:246–56.

13. Reymond A, Meroni G, Fantozzi A, Merla G, Cairo S, Luzi L, et al. The tripartite motif family identifies cell compartments. *EMBO J* 2001;**20**:2140–51.

14. Oke V, Wahren-Herlenius M. The immunobiology of Ro52 (TRIM21) in autoimmunity: a critical review. *J Autoimmun* 2012;**39**:77–82.

15. Hernan dez-Molina G, Leal-Alegre G, Michel-Peregrina M. The meaning of anti-Ro and anti-La antibodies in primary Sjögren's syndrome. *Autoimmun Rev* 2011;**10**:123–5.

16. Tzioufas AG, Wassmuth R, Dafni UG, Guialis A, Haga HJ, Isenberg DA, et al. Clinical, immunological and immunogenetic aspects of autoantibody production against Ro/SSA, La/SSB and their linear epitopes in primary Sjögren's syndrome (pSS): a European multicentre study. *Ann Rheum Dis* 2002;**61**:398–404.

17. Witte T. Diagnostic markers of Sjögren's syndrome. *Dev Ophthalmol* 2010;**45**:123–8.

18. Bolstad AI, Eiken HG, Rosenlund B, Alarcón-Riquelme ME, Jonsson R. Increased salivary gland tissue expression of Fas, Fas ligand, cytotoxic T-lymphocyte-associated antigen 4, and programmed cell death 1 in primary Sjögren's syndrome. *Arthritis Rheum* 2003;**48**:174–85.

19. Higgs R, Ní Gabhann J, Ben Larbi N, Breen EP, Fitzgerald KA, Jefferies CA. The E3 ubiquitin ligase Ro52 negatively regulates IFN-beta production post-pathogen recognition by polyubiquitin-mediated degradation of IRF3. *J Immunol* 2008;**181**:1780–6.

20. Espinosa A, Dardalhon V, Brauner S, Ambrosi A, Higgs R, Quintana FJ, et al. Loss of the lupus autoantigen Ro52/Trim21 induces tissue inflammation and systemic autoimmunity by disregulating the IL-23 Th17 pathway. *J Exp Med* 2009;**206**:1661–71.

21. McClain MT, Heinlen LD, Dennis GJ, Roebuck J, Harley JB, James JA. Early events in lupus humoral autoimmunity suggest initiation through molecular mimicry. *Nat Med* 2005;**11**:85–9.

22. Heinlen LD, McClain MT, Ritterhouse LL, Bruner BF, Edgerton CC, Keith MP, et al. 60 kD Ro and nRNP A frequently initiate human lupus autoimmunity. *PLoS One* 2010;**5**:e9599.

23. Staikou EV, Routsias JG, Makri AA, Terzoglou A, Sakarellos-Daitsiotis M, Sakarellos C, et al. Calreticulin binds preferentially with B cell linear epitopes of Ro60 kD autoantigen, enhancing recognition by anti-Ro60 kD autoantibodies. *Clin Exp Immunol* 2003;**134**:143–50.

24. Tatouli IP, Tzioufas AG. Pathogenetic aspects of humoral autoimmunity in Sjögren's syndrome. *Lupus* 2012;**21**:1151–4.

25. Dawson L, Tobin A, Smith P, Gordon T. Antimuscarinic antibodies in Sjögren's syndrome. *Arthritis Rheum* 2005;**52**:2984–95.

26. Scarselli M, Li B, Kim SK, Wess J. Multiple residues in the second extracellular loop are critical for M3 muscarinic acetylcholine receptor activation. *J Biol Chem* 2007;**282**:7385–96.

27. Sumida T, Tsuboi H, Iizuka M, Hirota T, Asashima H, Matsumoto I. The role of M3 muscarinic acetylcholine receptor reactive T cells in Sjögren's syndrome: a critical review. *J Autoimmun* 2014;**51**:44–50.

28. Tsuboi H, Nakamura Y, Iizuka M, Matsuo N, Matsumoto I, Sumida T. Generation and functional analysis of monoclonal antibodies against the second extracellular loop of human M3 muscarinic acetylcholine receptor. *Mod Rheumatol* 2012;**22**:264–71.

29. Nishimori I, Bratanova T, Toshkov I, Caffrey T, Mogaki M, Shibata Y, et al. Induction of experimental autoimmune sialoadenitis by immunization of PL/J mice with carbonic anhydrase II. *J Immunol* 1995;**154**:4865–73.

30. Takemoto F, Hoshino J, Sawa N, Tamura Y, Tagami T, Yokota M, et al. Autoantibodies against carbonic anhydrase II are increased in renal tubular acidosis associated with Sjögren's syndrome. *Am J Med* 2005;**118**:181–4.

31. Torsten W. Anti-fodrin antibodies in Sjögren's syndrome. *Ann N Y Acad Sci* 2005;**1051**:235–9.

32. He J, Zhao J, Li Z. Mucosal administration of alpha-fodrin inhibits experimental Sjögren's syndrome autoimmunity. *Arthritis Res Ther* 2008;**10**:R44.

33. Dartt DA. Tear lipocalin: structure and function. *Ocul Surf* 2011;**9**:126–38.

34. Gasymov OK, Abduragimov AR, Prasher P, Yusifov TN, Glasgow BJ. Tear lipocalin: evidence for a scavenging function to remove lipids from the human corneal surface. *Invest Ophthalmol Vis Sci* 2005;**46**:3589–96.

35. Vitali C, Bombardieri S, Jonsson R, Moutsopoulos HM, Alexander EL, Carsons SE, et al. Classification criteria for Sjögren's syndrome: a revised version of the European criteria proposed by the American-European Consensus Group. *Ann Rheum Dis* 2002;**61**:554–8.

36. Theander E, Jonsson R, Sjöström B, Brokstad K, Olsson P, Henriksson G. Autoantibodies profiling can predict primary Sjögren's syndrome years before diagnosis and identify those with early onset and severe disease course. *Arthritis Rheum* 2015;**67**:2427–36.

37. Buyon JP, Clancy RM. Neonatal lupus: basic research and clinical perspectives. *Rheum Dis Clin North Am* 2005;**31**:299–313.

38. Patel R, Shahane A. The epidemiology of Sjögren's syndrome. *Clin Epidemiol* 2014;**6**:247–55.

39. Baldini C, Pepe P, Quartuccio L, Priori R, Bartoloni E, Alunno A, et al. Primary Sjögren's syndrome as a multi-organ disease: impact of the serological profile on the clinical presentation of the disease in a large cohort of Italian patients. *Rheumatology* 2014;**53**:839–44.

40. Migliorini P, Baldini C, Rocchi V, Bombardieri S. Anti-Sm and anti-RNP antibodies. *Autoimmunity* 2005;**38**:47–54.

41. Baldini C, Mosca M, Della Rossa A, Pepe P, Notarstefano C, Ferro F, et al. Overlap of ACA-positive systemic sclerosis and Sjögren's syndrome: a distinct clinical entity with mild organ involvement but at high risk of lymphoma. *Clin Exp Rheumatol* 2013;**31**:272–80.

42. Lee KE, Kang JH, Lee JW, Wen L, Park DJ, Kim TJ, et al. Anti-centromere antibody-positive Sjögren's syndrome: a distinct clinical subgroup? *Int J Rheum Dis* 2015;**18**:776–82.

43. Bogdanps DP, Invernizzi P, Mackay IR, Vergani D. Autoimmune liver serology: current diagnostic and clinical challenges. *Word J Gastroenterol* 2008;**14**:3374–87.

44. Ramos-Casals M, Sánchez-Tapias JM, Parés A, Forns X, Brito-Zerón P, Nardi N, et al. Characterization and differentiation of autoimmune versus viral liver involvement in patients with Sjögren's syndrome. *J Rheumatol* 2006;**33**:1593–9.

45. Bournia VK, Vlachoyiannopoulos PG. Subgroups of Sjögren's syndrome patients according to serological profiles. *J Autoimmun* 2012;**39**:15–26.

46. Kim N, Shin Y, Choi S, Namkoong E, Kim M, Lee J, et al. Effect of antimuscarinic autoantibodies in primary Sjögren's syndrome. *J Dent Res* 2015;**94**:722–8.

47. Cavill D, Waterman SA, Gordon TP. Antibodies raised against the second extracellular loop of the human muscarinic M3 receptor mimic functional autoantibodies in Sjögren's syndrome. *Scand J Immunol* 2004;**59**:261–6.

48. Sumida T, Tsuboi H, Iizuka M, Asashima H, Matsumoto I. Anti-M3 muscarinic acetylcholine receptor antibodies in patients with Sjögren's syndrome. *Mod Rheumatol* 2013;**23**:841–5.

49. Preuss B, Tunaru S, Henes J, Offermanns S, Klein R. A novel luminescence-based method for the detection of functionally active antibodies to muscarinic acetylcholine receptors of the M3 type (mAchR3) in patient's sera. *Clin Exp Immunol* 2014;**177**:179–89.

50. Witte T. Anti-fodrin antibodies in Sjögren's syndrome: a review. *Ann N Y Acad Sci* 2005;**1051**:235–9.

51. Hu Q, Wang D, Chen W. The accuracy of the anti-α-fodrin antibody test for diagnosis of Sjögren's syndrome: a meta-analysis. *Clin Biochem* 2013;**46**:1372–6.

52. Navone R, Lunardi C, Gerli R, Tinazzi E, Peterlana D, Bason C, et al. Identification of tear lipocalin as a novel autoantigen target in Sjögren's syndrome. *J Autoimmun* 2005;**25**:229–34.

53. Tinazzi E, Merlin M, Bason C, Beri R, Zampieri R, Lico C, et al. Plant-made chimeric virus particles for Sjögren's syndrome diagnosis. *Front Plant Sci* 2015.

54. Shen L, Suresh L, Lindemann M, Xuan J, Kowal P, Malyavantham K, et al. Novel autoantibodies in Sjögren's syndrome. *Clin Immunol* 2012;**145**:251–5.

55. Suresh L, Malyavantham K, Shen L, Ambrus Jr JL. Investigation of novel autoantibodies in Sjögren's syndrome utilizing sera from Sjögren's international collaborative clinical alliance cohort. *BMC Ophthalmol* 2015;**15**:38.

56. Gourzi VC, Kapsogeorgou EK, Kyriakidis NC, Tzioufas AG. Study of microRNAs (miRNAs) that are predicted to target the autoantigen Ro/SSA and La/SSB in primary Sjögren's syndrome. *Clin Exp Immunol* 2015. http://dx.doi.org/10.1111/cei.12664.

57. Fiorentino DF, Presby M, Baer AN, Petri M, Rieger KE, Soloski M, et al. PUF60: a prominent new target of the autoimmune response in dermatomyositis and Sjögren's syndrome. *Ann Rheum Dis* 2015;**0**:1–7.

58. Delaleu N, Mydel P, Kwee I, Brun JG, Jonsson MV, Jonsson R. High fidelity between saliva proteomics and the biologic state of salivary glands defines biomarker signatures for primary Sjögren's syndrome. *Arthritis Rheumatol* 2015;**67**:1084–95.

59. Athanasios G, Tzioufas G, Kapsogeorgou EK. Saliva proteomics is a promising tool to study Sjögren's syndrome. *Nat Rev Rheumatol* 2015;**11**:202–3.

Chapter 10

# Sjögren's Syndrome and Environmental Factors

S. Colafrancesco, C. Perricone
*Sapienza University of Rome, Rome, Italy*

Y. Shoenfeld
*Chaim Sheba Medical Center, Tel-Hashomer, Israel; Tel Aviv University, Tel Aviv-Yafo, Israel*

## 1. INTRODUCTION

Sjögren's syndrome (SS) is a systemic, chronic, autoimmune, inflammatory condition involving the exocrine glands. First defined as "autoimmune epithelitis" by Moutsopoulos, SS is characterized by the presence of lymphocyte infiltrates in glandular tissue that might lead, over time, to a progressive glandular dysfunction.[1] The type I interferon (IFN) pathway is highly expressed and there is evidence of the so-called "IFN signature" in peripheral blood mononuclear cells and minor salivary gland biopsies coming from patients with SS. Expression of Toll-like receptors (TLRs) and major histocompatibility complex class I and II molecules by salivary gland epithelial cells is essential for autoantigen presentation and thus production of proinflammatory cytokines. B lymphocytes play a central role in the development of disease[2] and the production of B-cell activating factor (BAFF) by epithelial cells together with autoantigen presentation greatly contributes to the stimulation of the adaptive immune system and the potential development of lymphoma.

Both genetic[3] and environmental factors have been suggested to be responsible for SS development (Fig. 10.1).

## 2. SJÖGREN'S SYNDROME AND INFECTIONS

Among the environmental agents, infections seem to be the most important trigger of disease.[4] Several infections may mimic SS, including tuberculosis; leprosy; spirochetes; hepatitis A, B, or C; parvovirus B19; dengue fever; malaria; subacute bacterial endocarditis; and HIV.[5] In such conditions, viruses play a key role in activating the immune response; this is referred in particular to viruses expressing a specific tropism for salivary and lachrymal glandular tissue:

*Sjögren's Syndrome.* http://dx.doi.org/10.1016/B978-0-12-803604-4.00010-1

**157**

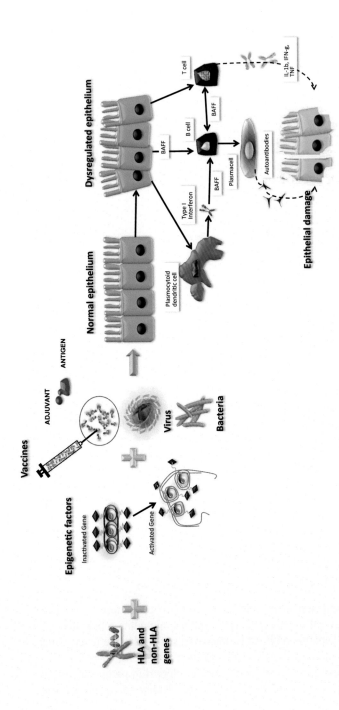

**FIGURE 10.1** Genetic, epigenetic, and environmental factors in the pathogenesis of SS. *BAFF*, B-cell activating factor; *HLA*, human leukocyte antigen; *IFN*, interferon; *IL*, interleukin; *TNF*, tumor necrosis factor.

cytomegalovirus, Epstein-Barr virus (EBV), and human herpes virus types 6, 7, and 8.[5–7] These viruses are able to induce an activation of the innate immune system via TLR pathways, which consequently stimulates the production of chemokines/cytokines such as type I IFN, whose expression is up-regulated in labial salivary glands, plasma, and peripheral blood cells of SS patients.[8] Over the last few years, an increasing body of evidence has confirmed the crucial role of type I IFNs in the multifactorial etiology of SS. The critical question that arises is what drives the production of a classical antiviral protein in the setting of autoimmunity.

It seems that one of the key targets of SS autoantibodies, Ro52, plays an essential role in the regulation of IFN production. Indeed, murine models with deficient expression of Ro52 overexpress type I IFN.[9] After type I IFN stimulation, Ro52, which is normally located in cytoplasm, migrates to the nucleus with subsequent increase of Ro52 transcription and negative regulation of IFN production.[9] To the same extent the phosphoprotein La seems to play a pleiotropic role. Actually, La is able to associate to small cytoplasmic RNAs as well as to viral RNA. Specifically, it interacts with the leader RNA sequence of respiratory syncytial virus, exercising a protective effect on the virus itself.[10] As result of such interaction, IFN activation is prevented and viral growth is favored. Moreover, cells infected by EBV are able to release a small RNA–La complex that seems to bind TLR3, inducing IFN I and tumor necrosis factor (TNF) production.[11]

In light of such considerations, we could hypothesize that after a viral infection, an increased expression of both Ro and La antigens is driven in salivary gland epithelial cells. On one hand, such overexpression might be the result of the prolonged IFN I activation and, on the other hand, of a viral strategy to escape from the immune response. In this context the inflammation pushes an increased cellular lysis and apoptosis, determining the external exposition of autoantigens and the production of autoantibodies.[12] In addition, a certain sequence homology between the protein Ro60 and the B2 protein of Coxsackie virus has been demonstrated to be able to activate CD4+ cells by molecular mimicry.[13] In patients with systemic lupus erythematosus, a molecular mimicry has been also discovered between Ro60 and the nuclear antigen 1 of EBV,[14] and for this reason it has been proposed as a mechanism responsible for the epitope spreading. Oral feeding with Ro60 proved to be able to prevent the epitope from spreading and the development of sicca symptoms in an experimental model of SS.[15]

## 3. SJÖGREN'S SYNDROME AND VACCINES

Even if rarely, development of SS has been observed after the administration of a vaccine.[16] In 2011, an expert committee of the European League Against Rheumatism addressed the role of vaccines in patients with rheumatic diseases including SS.[17] Despite the risk in patients with autoimmune diseases (ADs), including SS, several vaccines should be strongly considered (such as influenza, the 23-valent polysaccharidase pneumococcus, herpes zoster, and tetanus toxoid vaccinations), whereas others (such as *Bacillus* Calmette Guérin (BCG), hepatitis A and/or B, and human papilloma virus vaccines) should be avoided or at least considered only in select patients. Although the modern influenza vaccine seems to have a sufficient immunogenicity and a good safety profile in patients with ADs,[18] the A/California/7/2009/H1N1-like virus vaccine has demonstrated to lead to a significant increase in the mean levels of anti-Ro/SSA and anti-La/SSB antibodies in patients with primary SS for up to 1 year after vaccination.[19]

There are some studies dealing with the possible onset of SS after vaccine exposure (Table 10.1). Indeed, the administration of the hepatitis B vaccine has been associated with the development of clinical (dry mouth, dry eyes, arthralgia, fatigue) and laboratory (rheumatoid factor (RF), antinuclear antibodies (ANAs), and anti-Ro/SSA antibodies) features of SS.[23] In this specific case, lip biopsy also confirmed the presence of inflammatory cells infiltrates. However, also other vaccines have been suspected of causing SS, including the H1N1 vaccine. The case of a patient who developed a complete sicca syndrome 3 months after vaccine delivery has been reported. RF, ANA, and anti-Ro/SSA antibodies tested positive and a gland biopsy was compatible with SS.[26] In addition, a case of SS development after BCG immunotherapy exposure is described in the literature.[25] There are several possible links between SS and vaccines.[28]

Adjuvants may act by targeting the antigen-presenting cells via TLR, nonobese diabetes (NOD)-like receptors (NLRs), retinoic acid-inducible gene 1–like receptors, and C-type lectin receptors. The downstream signaling leads to the activation of transcription factors such as nuclear factor κB and interferon regulatory factor 3, finally inducing the production of cytokines and chemokines involved in priming, expansion, and polarization of the immune response. Aluminum, one of the most commonly used adjuvants, is able to trigger the activation of NLRP3 inflammasome signaling, leading to the production of proinflammatory cytokines (interleukin (IL) 1b, IL-18) via caspase 1 activation.[29] Although in this case, autoantibodies tested negative, histology of lip biopsy confirmed the presence of inflammatory infiltrates.

The role of an aluminum-based adjuvant (alum) in the induction of an SS-like disorder in the genetically susceptible female NZM2758 mouse strain that develops reduced salivary gland function and sialadenitis after injection with incomplete Freund adjuvants was recently investigated.[30] The alum-treated mice showed a persistent and significant reduction of salivary gland function, an increased submandibular salivary gland inflammation, and the production of ANA in comparison with the controls treated with phosphate-buffered saline.

## 4. SJÖGREN'S SYNDROME AND SILICONE

Not only the association between SS and vaccines, but also between silicone exposure and SS development, has been described. In 2003, the case of a male

**TABLE 10.1 Summary of Reported Cases of SS Possibly Associated With Silicone and Vaccines**

| Case Reports | Case | Adjuvants | Time | Signs and Symptoms | Autoantibodies | Histology | Genetic | Outcome |
|---|---|---|---|---|---|---|---|---|
| Sanchez-Roman et al.[20] | 6/50 Workers (3 pts, 6 SS) | Silicone | NS | Dry mouth<br>Dry eyes<br>Raynaud phenomenon | NS | NS | NS | NS |
| Puisieux et al.[21] | Silicotic coal miners (3 pts) | Silicone | NS | Dry mouth<br>Dry eyes<br>Raynaud phenomenon<br>Arthralgia<br>Purpura<br>Polyneuritis | 1 pt:<br>ANA<br>Anti-Ro/SSA<br>Anti-La/SSB<br>1 pt:<br>Cryoglobulinemia | ND | NS | NS |
| Orriols et al.[22] | Male, 28 years, sicca syndrome (dental technician) | Silicone | 5 years | Dry eyes<br>Interstitial pneumonia | Negative | Lymph Infiltrate Glandular sclerosis | NS | Lung transplant |
| Toussirot et al.[23] | Woman, 31 years | Hepatitis B vaccine | 1 month later | Arthralgia<br>Fatigue<br>Dry mouth<br>Dry eyes | RF<br>ANA<br>Anti-Ro/SSA | Positive | HLA-DRB1 P16/13 | CCS and HCQ with benefit |
| Astudillo et al.[24] | Male, 72 years, (dental technician) | Silicone | 3 months later | Dry mouth<br>Dry eyes<br>Arthralgia Raynaud phenomenon<br>Interstitial pneumonia | ANA<br>Anti-Ro/SSA | Positive | NS | HCQ with benefit |

*Continued*

**TABLE 10.1** Summary of Reported Cases of SS Possibly Associated With Silicone and Vaccines—cont'd

| Case Reports | Case | Adjuvants | Time | Signs and Symptoms | Autoantibodies | Histology | Genetic | Outcome |
|---|---|---|---|---|---|---|---|---|
| Narváez et al.[25] | Woman, 59 years | BCG immunotherapy | Several weeks later | Dry eyes<br>Dry mouth<br>Salivary gland enlargement | Negative | Positive | HLA B27<br>Negative | CCS with benefit |
| Toussirot et al.[26] | Woman, 30 years | H1N1 vaccine | 3 months later | Arthralgia<br>Dry mouth<br>Dry eye | RF<br>ANA<br>Anti-Ro/SSA | Positive | HLA DRB1*03, *15, DQB1*02, *06 | HCQ with benefit |
| Aykol et al.[27] | Woman, 34 years | Silicone | Soon later | Dry mouth<br>Dry eye<br>Raynaud phenomenon<br>Leukopenia | ANA<br>Anti-Ro/SSA<br>Anti-La/SSB | Positive | NS | HCQ with benefit |

*ANA*, Antinuclear antibody; *CCS*, corticosteroids; *HCQ*, hydroxychloroquine; *ND*, not determined; *NS*, not significant; *pt(s)*, patient(s); *RF*, rheumatoid factor; *SS*, Sjögren's syndrome.

dental technician who developed SS was diagnosed according to a positive serology and lip biopsy after silicone exposure was illustrated.[24] In a previous report, another case dealing with a dental technician who developed sicca syndrome after silicone exposure has been described.[22] More recently, Akyol and colleagues reported the case of a 34-year-old female patient who had a history of leukopenia, dry mouth, dry eyes, and cyanosis of her fingers that began soon after she underwent silicone breast implantation.[27] She was diagnosed with SS and successfully treated with hydroxychloroquine. Six cases of SS have been also described in coal miners and in workers from a factory producing scouring powder.[20] Puisieux et al.[21] reported on three cases of SS in silicotic coal miners. It is also important to underline how some cases of breast lymphomas, including non-Hodgkin lymphomas, have been reported in women with compromised silicone breast implants.[31] B-cell lymphoma development has been described as well in subjects with other kinds of implants.[32] These lymphomas can be primary breast lymphomas, the majority (~90%) of B-cell origin. The occurrence of anaplastic large cell lymphoma (ALCL), which accounts for 3% of newly diagnosed non-Hodgkin lymphoma cases, has been linked with breast implants for several years. Breast-implant–associated ALCL strongly expresses CD30, is more often negative for anaplastic lymphoma kinase, and is similar to primary cutaneous forms. The hypothesized mechanism for breast-implant–associated lymphoma has been addressed in a recently published review.[33] It has been suggested that silicone-triggered chronic inflammation, leading to a polyclonal B-cell activation with local production of cytokines, can result in full-blown SS. The B-cell oligoclonal and monoclonal expansion in infiltrated glands can in turn result in the development of a lymphoid malignancy. Although the transition from a chronic inflammatory condition to malignant lymphoma is a poorly understood multistep process, there is increasing evidence that chronic antigenic stimulation by an exoantigen or autoantigens plays an essential role in the development of SS-associated lymphoproliferation.[34]

## 5. SJÖGREN'S SYNDROME AND ASIA SYNDROME

The term "Autoimmune/inflammatory syndrome induced by adjuvants (ASIA)" was coined in 2011[35] to illustrate an "umbrella" of clinical conditions such as siliconosis, Gulf War syndrome, macrophage myofasciitis syndrome, sick building syndrome, and postvaccination phenomena sharing similar signs or symptoms.[36] The presence of shared symptoms suggests the existence of a common denominator able to trigger the development of such conditions. This common denominator has been subsequently identified in the adjuvant. The adjuvant is defined as "any substance that acts to accelerate, prolong, or enhance antigen specific immune response."[37] The adjuvant has the property to boost the immune response without having any specific antigenic effect itself. Taking advantage of this characteristic, vaccines usually contain adjuvants in their composition. The clinical conditions included in ASIA syndrome represent immune-mediated diseases that usually appear after a chronic stimulation of the immune system by agents with adjuvant characteristics. The development of such conditions implies the existence of a predisposing genetic background on which different external or endogenous environmental agents act as triggers. These environmental factors belong to a group of agents, namely "exposomes."[38] The evidence of a predisposing genetic background gives not only an explanation for the rarity of ASIA syndrome but also clarifies why physicians should be aware of the existence of such possible complications after vaccine exposure in specific individuals.[39] ASIA syndrome comprises a wide spectrum of symptoms including myalgia, myositis, arthralgia, neurological manifestations, fever, dry mouth, cognitive alterations,[40] and also the presence of chronic fatigue syndrome.[41] Major and minor criteria, including the previously mentioned symptoms, as well as auto-antibodies or antibodies directed at the suspected adjuvant or specific human leukocyte antigen (HLA) (ie, HLA DRB1, HLA DQB1), have been suggested in order to perform diagnosis of ASIA syndrome.[35] Interestingly, most of the clinical features included in such criteria are commonly observed in patients with SS, including dry mouth and/or dry eyes, myalgia and/or muscle weakness, and arthralgia and/or arthritis. Fatigue is also another key feature that is usually present in both conditions.

The most common agents acting as adjuvants are represented by silicone, aluminum, pristane, and infectious components. In addition, other oil substances, sometimes illegally injected for cosmetic purposes, may have an immune adjuvant effect and are reported as possible inducers of ASIA syndrome.[42] Concerning the mechanism of action, one of the main systems by which adjuvants induce an immune response is represented by molecular mimicry. Molecular mimicry refers to the concept that an immune response, initially directed against bacterial or viral antigens, can target host molecules that share sequence homology or structural similarities with microbial epitopes.[37] Also, other different mechanisms of actions have been described, such as the polyclonal activation of B cells,[43] the bystander activation (which enhances cytokine production and induces the expansion of autoreactive T cells),[44] and the epitope spreading, by which invading antigens accelerate the local activation of antigen-presenting cells and the overprocessing of antigens.[45]

Aluminum embodies one of the main adjuvants used in vaccine formulations and is possibly responsible for ASIA syndrome development. The mechanisms by which aluminum compounds function as adjuvants is explained by the evidence that aluminum salts induce activation of dendritic cells and complement components and increase the level of chemokine secretion in the injection site.[46] Similar to aluminum, the exposure to silicone has been said to boost the immune response. Silicone is considered an inert material and, for this reason, it has been incorporated in different medical products and devices such as breast implants. After the rupture of a breast prosthesis, local cutaneous inflammation, regional lymphadenopathy, and silicone granuloma have been reported and a remission of these conditions after implant removal has been described as well.[47] It seems that silicone implants trigger a specific antigen-driven local immune response through activated T helper (Th) 1/Th17 cells.[48] Moreover, patients with severe immune-mediated reactions to implanted silicone devices were found to have increased immunoglobulin G in the surrounding tissue and higher levels of antisilicone antibodies.[49] These findings suggest a possible adjuvant action of silicone.

Thus given these premises, the shared features between SS and ASIA are evident. Despite the evidence of a number of SS cases after the exposure to vaccines as well as to silicone, it is fundamental to remind that until recently, evidence strongly supports the idea that the benefit of vaccines largely overwhelms the eventual risks of developing an autoimmune condition. Concerning silicone, larger cohorts are awaited to better define the true existence of such association.

## 6. SJÖGREN'S SYNDROME, HORMONAL FACTORS, AND VITAMIN D

Advanced age of onset, together with the female preponderance, points toward a hormonal etiology of SS. To elucidate the synergistic contribution of genetic factors and hormones in the development of the disease, Czerwinski et al.[50] have investigated the NOD.B10.H2b mouse model of SS. It was reported that a decrease in the concentration of sex hormones after ovariectomy (OVX) in these genetically predisposed mice resulted in lacrimal gland lymphocytic infiltration, consisting of T cells and B cells, followed by epithelial cell death.[51] Moreover, the treatment with physiological doses of dihydrotestosterone or 17b-estradiol at the time of OVX prevented these changes. In a more recent study, the same authors found that OVX caused a significant increase in the expression and levels of the cytokines IL-1b, TNF-α, and IL-4 in the lacrimal glands of the NOD.B10.H2b mice. OVX in the NOD.B10.H2b mice also caused an increase in the levels of anti-Ro/SSA autoantibodies in the serum only. Thus a decrease in the concentrations of ovarian hormones in the genetically predisposed mice seems to accelerate the onset of SS by up-regulating various proinflammatory cytokines at different times and promoting the formation of anti-Ro/SSA serum autoantibodies, creating an environment favorable for the initiation of the disease.[50] Other studies from animal models revealed that whereas estrogenic receptor (both α and β) deficiency protects against the development of SS, the aromatase knock-out mouse develops a lymphoproliferative disease resembling SS, also characterized by B-cell infiltration of the kidneys and the spleen.[52] Low levels of dehydroepiandrosterone have been also detected at SS salivary gland tissues, compared with controls to an extent that dehydroepiandrosterone was considered as a potential therapeutic strategy.[53]

Recently, low levels of vitamin D have been associated with several autoimmune conditions, including SS.[7] The levels of vitamin D and their association with manifestations of SS were studied in a large international multicenter cohort[54] suggesting an association with neuropathy and lymphoma. In this view, there is some evidence from case-control studies that low dietary intake of vitamin D is associated with an increased risk for non-Hodgkin lymphoma in the normal population, probably because of the antiproliferative effect on lymphoma cell lines of vitamin D. This evidence may suggest a role for vitamin D supplementation in the therapeutic approach to SS.

## 7. SJÖGREN'S SYNDROME, STRESS, AND ENVIRONMENTAL POLLUTION

It was recently shown that before disease onset, patients with SS experience high psychological stress after major negative life events without developing satisfactory adaptive coping strategies to confront their stressful life changes. Thus it was suggested that lack of social support may contribute to the relative risk of disease development.[55] Also, patients with nonapneic sleep disorder have been associated with a higher risk for developing ADs.[56]

The relationship between SS and pollution has been addressed in different studies. Epidemiological analyses have associated air particulate matter (PM) inhalation with a decline in lung function and increased morbidity and mortality caused by cardiorespiratory diseases, particularly in susceptible populations. A mouse model of SS (NOD mice) which develops SS was exposed to intranasal instillation either with saline (control) or residual oil fly ash solution (1 mg/kg body weight) and compared with BALB/c mice. It was shown that whereas BALB/c mice showed normal histoarchitecture, NOD mice showed lymphocytic peribronchial infiltrates. The lesions in NOD mice were more severe than those in BALB/c mice. Indeed, cellular infiltration in the alveoli and a greater decrease in the alveolar space was observed.[57] Since this experimental evidence, other studies have been performed on human cohorts. In a recent study from Calgary (Alberta, Canada) it was found that the odds of acquiring an AD are increased with fine particulate levels (PM 2.5), but the results were inconclusive for nitrogen dioxide. Unfortunately it was not possible to differentiate whether the higher risk was for SS or for the other autoimmune conditions considered in the study.[58]

In another study that aimed at evidencing any difference between occupational exposure to organic solvents and the risk of developing SS, it was found that a number of substances could contribute to the pathogenesis of the disease.[59] Despite no difference observed in cases and controls for smoking habits, socioeconomic levels, and socioprofessional categories, significantly increased odds rations (ORs) were observed for dichloromethane, perchlorethylene, chlorinated solvents, benzene, toluene, white spirit, and aromatic solvents. Exposure to any types of solvent was also associated with an increased OR (OR 2.76, 95% confidence interval 1.70–4.47).

# 8. CONCLUSIONS

There is broad evidence that certain microbial agents and substances, by stimulating the immune system, may provoke the full-blown acquisition of an AD such as SS. Clarifying these common mechanisms and addressing the key pathological pathways will endeavor to manage patients with SS and to find innovative treatment strategies.

## REFERENCES

1. Moutsopoulos HM. Sjögren's syndrome: autoimmune epitheliitis. *Clin Immunol Immunopathol* 1994;**72**:162–5.
2. Cornec D, Devauchelle-Pensec V, Tobon GJ, Pers JO, Jousse-Joulin S, Saraux A. B cells in Sjögren's syndrome: from pathophysiology to diagnosis and treatment. *J Autoimmun* 2012;**39**:161–7.
3. Ice JA, Li H, Adrianto I, Lin PC, Kelly JA, Montgomery CG, et al. Genetics of Sjögren's syndrome in the genome-wide association era. *J Autoimmun* 2012;**39**:57–63.
4. Kivity S, Arango MT, Ehrenfeld M, Tehori O, Shoenfeld Y, Anaya JM, et al. Infection and autoimmunity in Sjögren's syndrome: a clinical study and comprehensive review. *J Autoimmun* 2014;**51**:17–22.
5. Igoe A, Scofield RH. Autoimmunity and infection in Sjögren's syndrome. *Curr Opin Rheumatol* 2013;**25**:480–7.
6. Sipsas NV, Gamaletsou MN, Moutsopoulos HM. Is Sjögren's syndrome a retroviral disease? *Arthritis Res Ther* 2011;**13**:212.
7. Tincani A, Andreoli L, Cavazzana I, Doria A, Favero M, Fenini MG, et al. Novel aspects of Sjögren's syndrome in 2012. *BMC Med* 2013;**11**:93.
8. Brkic Z, Versnel MA. Type I IFN signature in primary Sjögren's syndrome patients. *Expert Rev Clin Immunol* 2014;**10**:457–67.
9. Ronnblom L, Eloranta ML, Alm GV. The type I interferon system in systemic lupus erythematosus. *Arthritis Rheum* 2006;**54**:408–20.
10. Bitko V, Musiyenko A, Bayfield MA, Maraia RJ, Barik S. Cellular La protein shields non-segmented negative-strand RNA viral leader RNA from RIG-I and enhances virus growth by diverse mechanisms. *J Virol* 2008;**82**:7977–87.
11. Iwakiri D, Zhou L, Samanta M, Matsumoto M, Ebihara T, Seya T, et al. Epstein-Barr virus (EBV)-encoded small RNA is released from EBV-infected cells and activates signaling from Toll-like receptor 3. *J Exp Med* 2009;**206**:2091–9.
12. Stetson DB. Connections between antiviral defense and autoimmunity. *Curr Opin Immunol* 2009;**21**:244–50.
13. Stathopoulou EA, Routsias JG, Stea EA, Moutsopoulos HM, Tzioufas AG. Cross-reaction between antibodies to the major epitope of Ro60 kD autoantigen and a homologous peptide of Coxsackie virus 2B protein. *Clin Exp Immunol* 2005;**141**:148–54.
14. McClain MT, Heinlen LD, Dennis GJ, Roebuck J, Harley JB, James JA. Early events in lupus humoral autoimmunity suggest initiation through molecular mimicry. *Nat Med* 2005;**11**:85–9.
15. Jonsson R, Vogelsang P, Volchenkov R, Espinosa A, Wahren-Herlenius M, Appel S. The complexity of Sjögren's syndrome: novel aspects on pathogenesis. *Immunol Lett* 2011;**141**:1–9.
16. Colafrancesco S, Perricone C, Priori R, Valesini G, Shoenfeld Y. Sjögren's syndrome: another facet of the autoimmune/inflammatory syndrome induced by adjuvants (ASIA). *J Autoimmun* 2014;**51**:10–6.

17. van Assen S, Agmon-Levin N, Elkayam O, Cervera R, Doran MF, Dougados M, et al. EULAR recommendations for vaccination in adult patients with autoimmune inflammatory rheumatic diseases. *Ann Rheum Dis* 2011;**70**:414–22.

18. Milanovic M, Stojanovich L, Djokovic A, Kontic M, Gvozdenovic E. Influenza vaccination in autoimmune rheumatic disease patients. *Tohoku J Exp Med* 2013;**229**:29–34.

19. Pasoto SG, Ribeiro AC, Viana VS, Leon EP, Bueno C, Neto ML, et al. Short- and long-term effects of pandemic unadjuvanted influenza A(H1N1)pdm09 vaccine on clinical manifestations and autoantibody profile in primary Sjögren's syndrome. *Vaccine* 2013;**31**:1793–8.

20. Sanchez-Roman J, Wichmann I, Salaberri J, Varela JM, Nunez-Roldan A. Multiple clinical and biological autoimmune manifestations in 50 workers after occupational exposure to silica. *Ann Rheum Dis* 1993;**52**:534–8.

21. Puisieux F, Hachulla E, Brouillard M, Hatron PY, Devulder B. Silicosis and primary Gougerot-Sjogren syndrome. *Rev Med Interne* 1994;**15**:575–9.

22. Orriols R, Ferrer J, Tura JM, Xaus C, Coloma R. Sicca syndrome and silicoproteinosis in a dental technician. *Eur Respir J* 1997;**10**:731–4.

23. Toussirot E, Lohse A, Wendling D, Mougin C. Sjögren's syndrome occurring after hepatitis B vaccination. *Arthritis Rheum* 2000;**43**:2139–40.

24. Astudillo L, Sailler L, Ecoiffier M, Giron J, Couret B, Arlet-Suau E. Exposure to silica and primary Sjögren's syndrome in a dental technician. *Rheumatology* 2003;**42**:1268–9.

25. Narvaez J, Castro-Bohorquez FJ, Vilaseca-Momplet J. Sjögren's-like syndrome following intravesical *Bacillus* Calmette-Guerin immunotherapy. *Am J Med* 2003;**115**:418–20.

26. Toussirot E, Bossert M, Herbein G, Saas P. Comments on the article by Tabache F. et al. "Acute polyarthritis after influenza A H1N1 immunization", Joint Bone Spine, 2011, doi:10.1016/j. jbs.2011.02.007: primary Sjögren's syndrome occurring after influenza A H1N1 vaccine administration. *Joint Bone Spine* 2012;**79**:107.

27. Akyol L, Önem S, Özgen M, Sayarlıoğlu M. Sjögren's syndrome after silicone breast implantation. *Eur J Rheumatol* 2015.

28. Soriano A, Afeltra A, Shoenfeld Y. Immunization with vaccines and Sjögren's syndrome. *Expert Rev Clin Immunol* 2014;**10**:429–35.

29. Eisenbarth SC, Colegio OR, O'Connor W, Sutterwala F, Flavell RA. Crucial role for the NALP3 inflammasome in the immunostimulatory properties of aluminium adjuvants. *Nature* 2008;**453**:1122–6.

30. Bagavant H, Nandula SR, Kaplonek P, Rybakowska PD, Deshmukh US. Alum, an aluminum-based adjuvant, induces Sjögren's syndrome-like disorder in mice. *Clin Exp Rheumatol* 2014;**32**:251–5.

31. Nichter LS, Mueller MA, Burns RG, Stallman JM. First report of nodal marginal zone B-cell lymphoma associated with breast implants. *Plast Reconstr Surg* 2012;**129**:576e–8e.

32. Kellogg BC, Hiro ME, Payne WG. Implant-associated anaplastic large cell lymphoma: beyond breast prostheses. *Ann Plast Surg* 2014;**73**:461–4.

33. Bizjak M, Selmi C, Praprotnik S, Bruck O, Perricone C, Ehrenfeld M, et al. Silicone implants and lymphoma: the role of inflammation. *J Autoimmun* 2015;**65**:64–73.

34. Ramos-Casals M, De Vita S, Tzioufas AG. Hepatitis C virus, Sjögren's syndrome and B-cell lymphoma: linking infection, autoimmunity and cancer. *Autoimmun Rev* 2005;**4**:8–15.

35. Shoenfeld Y, Agmon-Levin N. 'ASIA': autoimmune/inflammatory syndrome induced by adjuvants. *J Autoimmun* 2011;**36**:4–8.

36. Agmon-Levin N, Hughes GR, Shoenfeld Y. The spectrum of ASIA: 'autoimmune (auto-inflammatory) syndrome induced by adjuvants'. *Lupus* 2012;**21**:118–20.

37. Israeli E, Agmon-Levin N, Blank M, Shoenfeld Y. Adjuvants and autoimmunity. *Lupus* 2009;**18**:1217–25.

38. Bogdanos DP, Smyk DS, Invernizzi P, Rigopoulou EI, Blank M, Pouria S, et al. Infectome: a platform to trace infectious triggers of autoimmunity. *Autoimmun Rev* 2013;**12**:726–40.

39. Toubi E. ASIA-autoimmune syndromes induced by adjuvants: rare, but worth considering. *Isr Med Assoc J* 2012;**14**:121–4.

40. Perricone C, Colafrancesco S, Mazor RD, Soriano A, Agmon-Levin N, Shoenfeld Y. Autoimmune/inflammatory syndrome induced by adjuvants (ASIA) 2013: unveiling the pathogenic, clinical and diagnostic aspects. *J Autoimmun* 2013;**47**:1–16.

41. Rosenblum H, Shoenfeld Y, Amital H. The common immunogenic etiology of chronic fatigue syndrome: from infections to vaccines via adjuvants to the ASIA syndrome. *Infect Dis Clin North Am* 2011;**25**:851–63.

42. Vera-Lastra O, Medina G, Cruz-Dominguez Mdel P, Ramirez P, Gayosso-Rivera JA, Anduaga-Dominguez H, et al. Human adjuvant disease induced by foreign substances: a new model of ASIA (Shoenfeld's syndrome). *Lupus* 2012;**21**:128–35.

43. Barzilai O, Ram M, Shoenfeld Y. Viral infection can induce the production of autoantibodies. *Curr Opin Rheumatol* 2007;**19**:636–43.

44. Murali-Krishna K, Altman JD, Suresh M, Sourdive DJ, Zajac AJ, Miller JD, et al. Counting antigen-specific CD8 T cells: a reevaluation of bystander activation during viral infection. *Immunity* 1998;**8**:177–87.

45. Lehmann PV, Forsthuber T, Miller A, Sercarz EE. Spreading of T-cell autoimmunity to cryptic determinants of an autoantigen. *Nature* 1992;**358**:155–7.

46. HogenEsch H. Mechanisms of stimulation of the immune response by aluminum adjuvants. *Vaccine* 2002;**20**(Suppl. 3):S34–9.

47. Caldeira M, Ferreira AC. Siliconosis: autoimmune/inflammatory syndrome induced by adjuvants (ASIA). *Isr Med Assoc J* 2012;**14**:137–8.

48. Wolfram D, Rabensteiner E, Grundtman C, Bock G, Mayerl C, Parson W, et al. T regulatory cells and TH17 cells in peri-silicone implant capsular fibrosis. *Plast Reconstr Surg* 2012;**129**:327e–37e.

49. Goldblum RM, Pelley RP, O'Donell AA, Pyron D, Heggers JP. Antibodies to silicone elastomers and reactions to ventriculoperitoneal shunts. *Lancet* 1992;**340**:510–3.

50. Czerwinski S, Mostafa S, Rowan VS, Azzarolo AM. Time course of cytokine upregulation in the lacrimal gland and presence of autoantibodies in a predisposed mouse model of Sjögren's syndrome: the influence of sex hormones and genetic background. *Exp Eye Res* 2014;**128**: 15–22.

51. Mostafa S, Seamon V, Azzarolo AM. Influence of sex hormones and genetic predisposition in Sjögren's syndrome: a new clue to the immunopathogenesis of dry eye disease. *Exp Eye Res* 2012;**96**:88–97.

52. Iwasa A, Arakaki R, Honma N, Ushio A, Yamada A, Kondo T, et al. Aromatase controls Sjögren syndrome-like lesions through monocyte chemotactic protein-1 in target organ and adipose tissue-associated macrophages. *Am J Pathol* 2015;**185**:151–61.

53. Hartkamp A, Geenen R, Godaert GL, Bootsma H, Kruize AA, Bijlsma JW, et al. Effect of dehydroepiandrosterone administration on fatigue, well-being, and functioning in women with primary Sjögren syndrome: a randomised controlled trial. *Ann Rheum Dis* 2008;**67**:91–7.

54. Agmon-Levin N, Kivity S, Tzioufas AG, Lopez Hoyos M, Rozman B, Efes I, et al. Low levels of vitamin-D are associated with neuropathy and lymphoma among patients with Sjögren's syndrome. *J Autoimmun* 2012;**39**:234–9.

55. Karaiskos D, Mavragani CP, Makaroni S, Zinzaras E, Voulgarelis M, Rabavilas A, et al. Stress, coping strategies and social support in patients with primary Sjögren's syndrome prior to disease onset: a retrospective case-control study. *Ann Rheum Dis* 2009;**68**:40–6.

56. Hsiao YH, Chen YT, Tseng CM, Wu LA, Lin WC, Su VY, et al. Sleep disorders and increased risk of autoimmune diseases in individuals without sleep apnea. *Sleep* 2015;**38**:581–6.

57. Ferraro S, Orona N, Villalon L, Saldiva PH, Tasat DR, Berra A. Air particulate matter exacerbates lung response on Sjögren's syndrome animals. *Exp Toxicol Pathol* 2015;**67**:125–31.

58. Bernatsky S, Smargiassi A, Johnson M, Kaplan GG, Barnabe C, Svenson L, et al. Fine particulate air pollution, nitrogen dioxide, and systemic autoimmune rheumatic disease in Calgary, Alberta. *Environ Res* 2015;**140**:474–8.

59. Chaigne B, Lasfargues G, Marie I, Huttenberger B, Lavigne C, Marchand-Adam S, et al. Primary Sjögren's syndrome and occupational risk factors: a case-control study. *J Autoimmun* 2015;**60**:80–5.

Chapter 11

# Histology of Sjögren's Syndrome

**F. Barone**
*University of Birmingham, Birmingham, United Kingdom*

**S. Colafrancesco**
*Sapienza University of Rome, Rome, Italy*

**J. Campos**
*University of Birmingham, Birmingham, United Kingdom*

## 1. INTRODUCTION

The formation of periductal lymphocytic infiltrates within the inflamed salivary glands represents the histological hallmark of primary Sjögren's syndrome (pSS). Lymphomonocytic aggregates can spread within the tissue, affecting salivary gland morphology and function. On a discrete percentage of patients (~25%),[1] it is possible to observe the formation of organized germinal center (GC)-like structure, detection of which has been correlated to lymphoma development.[1,2] Salivary gland histopathology is considered the gold standard for pSS diagnosis and is highly recommended in early phase clinical trials as a disease biomarker.[3] This chapter reviews the histological features of normal and diseased salivary glands in the context of pSS and provides the reader with a tool to understand pSS histopathology and differential diagnosis, and to identify in the tissue key elements that characterize pSS pathogenesis.

## 2. SALIVARY GLAND ANATOMY

Major salivary glands include the paired parotid, submandibular, and sublingual glands.[4] The parotid glands are wedge-shaped, located in front of the ear and the posterior surface of the mandible. These are the largest salivary glands and are covered by fascia and parotid capsule. Each parotid gland weighs between 15 and 30 g and is divided by the facial nerve into a superficial and a deep lobe; the latter lies within the parapharyngeal space.[5,6] The parotid glands are in close association with some branches of the facial nerve (cranial nerve [CN] VII).[6]

Sjögren's Syndrome. http://dx.doi.org/10.1016/B978-0-12-803604-4.00011-3

The submandibular glands are about half the size of the parotid glands and weigh between 7 and 16 g. They are located in the submandibular triangle, which has a superior margin formed by the inferior edge of the mandible and inferior margins designed by the anterior and posterior bellies of the digastric muscle. Most of the submandibular gland lies posterolateral to the mylohyoid muscle.[4,6]

The sublingual glands are the smallest of the major salivary glands, about one-fifth the size of the submandibular gland and weighing between 2 and 4 g. They lie as a flat structure in a submucosal plane within the anterior floor of the mouth, superior to the mylohyoid muscle and deep to the sublingual folds opposite the lingual frenulum.[7] There is no true fascial capsule surrounding the glands, which are instead covered by oral mucosa. Several ducts from the superior portion of the sublingual gland either secrete directly into the floor of the mouth, or empty into the Bartholin duct that then continues into the Wharton duct.[4,6]

About 600 to 1000 minor salivary glands line the oral cavity and oropharynx in the submucosa between muscle fibers.[8] The greatest number of these glands, ranging in size from 1 to 5 mm, is in the lips, tongue, buccal mucosa, and palate, although they can also be found along the tonsils, supraglottis, and paranasal sinuses. Each gland has a single duct which secretes, directly into the oral cavity, saliva which can be either serous, mucous, or mixed.[4]

## 3. HISTOLOGY OF NORMAL SALIVARY GLANDS

Salivary glands are classified as exocrine glands, which secrete saliva through a duct system from a secretory structure called the *salivary acinus*.[4] There are three main types of acini: serous, mucous, and mixed. Serous acini are roughly spherical and release via exocytosis a watery protein secretion. The acinar cells are pyramidal, with basally located nuclei surrounded by dense cytoplasm and secretory granules that are most abundant in the apex. Mucinous acini store a viscous glycoprotein (mucin) within secretory granules that become hydrated when released to form mucus. Mucinous acinar cells are commonly simple columnar cells with flattened, basally situated nuclei and water-soluble granules that make the intracellular cytoplasm appear clear. Mixed or seromucous acini contain components of both types, but one type of secretory unit may dominate.[4] Between the epithelial cells and basal lamina of the acinus, flat myoepithelial cells form a lattice work and possess cytoplasmic filaments on their basal side to aid in contraction, and thus forced secretion, of the acini. Spindle-shaped myoepithelial cells are also observed around the intercalated ducts.[4,6]

Salivary glands exhibit three types of ducts. The acini first secrete through small canaliculi into intercalated ducts, which are comprised of an irregular myoepithelial cell layer with narrow lumen. These in turn empty into striated ducts within the glandular lobe. Striated ducts are lined by columnar cells with basal striations caused by membrane invagination and mitochondria.[4,6] Lastly, excretory ducts, lined by cuboidal epithelium, which turns into stratified squamous epithelium toward the terminal end of the duct, deliver the secrete into the mouth for the large salivary glands, namely the Bartholin duct, the Wharton duct, and the Steins duct.[4]

The minor salivary glands are found throughout the oral cavity, with the greatest density in the buccal and labial mucosa, the posterior hard palate, and the tongue base. The majority of these glands are either mucinous or seromucinous, which secrete highly glycosylated mucins, antimicrobial proteins, and immunoglobulins.[8] The minor salivary gland duct system is simpler than that of the major salivary glands, where the intercalated ducts are longer and the intralobular ducts lack basal striations.[4,8]

## 4. SALIVARY GLAND BIOPSY

Salivary gland histological examination is usually undertaken in order to perform differential diagnosis of pSS, lymphoma associated to SS, or other conditions such as sarcoidosis or amyloidosis. Biopsy can be used to confirm a pSS clinical diagnosis, at any time during the disease course to stage the disease and provide the patient with a prognostic tool,[2] or to monitor disease changes upon therapeutic intervention or during clinical trials.[3]

Salivary glands are easily accessible either via the buccal mucosa or through the skin. Because of the invasiveness of the procedure and the need for general anesthesia, there are no study reports on the use of submandibular glands as a possible biopsy site. Only few reports deal with the use of sublingual and palate glands, the latest with reported complications.[9]

The biopsy of the parotid gland is used in few specialized centers.[10] It has the potential to provide larger and well-preserved tissue for histological examination and is characterized by better organized lymphocytic aggregates and larger and more frequent areas of lymphoepithelial proliferation, as compared with minor salivary glands.[11-14] Parotid gland biopsy is usually obtained by a 1–2-cm skin incision below the earlobe that gives access to the parotid tail.[15] If executed by expert hands, major complications may be easily avoided; nonetheless, occasionally the surgery may be followed by serious complications including salivary fistula, temporary change in sensation in the preauricular area, and, rarely, sialocele and facial nerve damage.[15] Given its invasiveness, parotid biopsies are not really suited to perform repeated tests over a time.

Because of its easy accessibility and low-risk profile, minor salivary gland biopsy is the most used technique to obtain salivary gland tissue. Biopsy of the minor salivary glands presents a number of advantages, such as the easy accessibility via the buccal mucosa (thus avoiding skin incisions), the use of simple local anesthesia, and the access to a large number of salivary glands without the risk of damage to histological structures.[16] Possible complications are more commonly minor and transient. They may include transient or persistent hypesthesia of the lower lip, arterial bleeding, vasovagal collapse, and burning sensation of the mouth while drinking hot beverages.[17-19]

Studies have compared the utility of labial versus parotid biopsy.[20,21] When the two techniques were compared, it was concluded that using as criteria the presence of focus score ≥1 or the presence of smaller lymphocytic infiltrates in combination with the presence of benign lymphoepithelial sialadenitis (LESA), the sensitivity and specificity of the two procedures was comparable.[10] For labial biopsy, a sensitivity and specificity of 60% to 82% and 91% to 94%, respectively, has been reported but false positive and false negative results may occur as a result of sampling.[22]

The distribution of the inflammatory infiltrates in pSS can be extremely heterogeneous, thereby requiring an adequate number of good quality salivary glands to be analyzed in order to satisfy the requirement for the histological diagnosis. For this reason, the introduction of a multilevel analysis of minor salivary gland samples in order to increase the glandular area as well as the number of foci has been proposed.[23]

## 5. HISTOLOGICAL FINDINGS IN SALIVARY GLANDS FROM SJÖGREN'S SYNDROME PATIENTS

The formation of small lymphocytic foci around the intralobular and interlobular ducts represents the pathognomonic histological lesion in pSS.[24–26] CD4+ T cells and dendritic cells mainly inhabit early aggregates. Progressive B-cell infiltration is often observed during the disease course and is reflected in the negative correlation between the T/B cell ratio and the degree of salivary gland inflammation.[26,27]

Loss of tissue architecture, atrophic involution of the acini, hyperplasia of the lining cells of the intraglandular ducts, and accumulation of hyaline material are some of the common histological features if the gland is extensively infiltrated.[25,28]

Within the glands, several components of the immune response have been detected. Higher number of T regulatory cells have been found in patients with pSS as compared with patients with secondary Sjögren's syndrome (SS) or connective tissue disease patients without SS.[29] Sarigul et al. also described a higher percentage of FoxP3-expressing CD4+ T cells in the salivary glands of pSS patients, even though similar numbers were found in peripheral blood from pSS and rheumatoid arthritis patients and healthy controls.[30] The rate of T regulatory cell detection appears to correlate with lesion severity.[30] A consistent number of plasma cells has also been detected at the periphery of the largest aggregates in the glands; however, the detection of high number of plasma cells is still considered an exclusion criteria for pSS diagnosis. The possibility to evaluate the ratio between immunoglobulin (Ig) M/IgA and IgG plasma cells as part of the diagnostic process in pSS is cause of debate in the oral medicine/rheumatology community.[3,25] Plasmacytoid dendritic cells, the main source of interferon (IFN) α,[31] have also been identified as CD123 + BDCA-2+ cells in all analyzed pSS salivary gland biopsies by Gottenberg et al.[32] Circulatory plasmacytoid dendritic cells have been shown to be more activated in pSS patients with a higher expression of CD40.[33]

In approximately 20–25% of SS patients, the salivary gland aggregates are organized into segregated T- and B-cell areas, and are characterized by the formation of follicular dendritic cell (FDC) networks within areas of active B-cell proliferation defined as GC-like structures.[34] These structures and their functional role in disease development/progression will be discussed in the following section.

Infiltrating lymphocytes in the ducts can give rise to the formation of LESA (previously named myoepithelial lesions [MESA]). These areas of lymphocytic infiltration (mainly B cells) can lead to atrophy of the columnar ductal epithelium and proliferation of the basal epithelial cells.[11] Hyperplasia of epithelium may be observed and the lumens may be not completely visible, thus reducing the ducts to irregularly shaped islands of polygonal and spindled cells. B cells represent the predominant infiltrating cell type, often acquiring monocytoid features or centrocyte-like morphology commonly accompanied by immunoblasts, plasmacytoid lymphocytes, and plasma cell differentiation.[35] In up to 50% of cases, clonal intraepithelial B-cell infiltration is present[11] and in some cases it is possible to observe, either by in situ hybridization or immunohistochemistry, κ or λ light chain excess production in the infiltrating cells.[36] It is still controversial whether such finding in the absence of proliferating/expanding B-cell clones represents an early sign of extranodal marginal zone B-cell lymphoma transition.[35]

## 6. DIFFERENTIAL DIAGNOSIS

Salivary glands are not the exclusive target of SS and differential diagnosis is required to exclude other possible undergoing inflammatory processes.[37]

Several viruses may be responsible for an exocrine gland lymphocytic infiltration, which is in some cases indistinguishable from SS. Hepatitis C virus (HCV) and HIV represent the most common viruses able to affect salivary glands and because of their similarities with pSS have been included in the exclusion criteria for PSS diagnosis.[38] The first histological evidence in patients with chronic HCV liver disease of focal lymphocytic sialadenitis resembling SS was provided in 1992.[39] There is a specific tropism of HCV for exocrine gland epithelial cells[40,41] and a chronic focal SS-like sialadenitis can be observed in up to 50% of HCV-infected patients.[42] HCV sialadenitis is histologically indistinguishable from SS. Indeed, over the course of HCV infection, analogous immunohistochemical characteristics as well as a Chisholm–Mason classification grade between 3 and 4 have been described.[43] In murine models of HCV, a pericapillary distribution of the lymphocytic aggregates has been described, and, although milder, a localization in the lachrymal glands has been observed too.[40] Accordingly, in humans, HCV-related lymphocytic infiltrates are mainly located in the pericapillary area and a lack of real glandular tissue damage has been observed.[44] However, the infiltrate extension and the focus scores appear to be milder in HCV as compared with pSS.[45] Finally, whereas in PSS the infiltrating lymphocytes are mainly composed of CD4+ cells; a mixed population of CD4+ and CD8+ cells is found in HCV sialadenitis with evidence of few prevalent CD8+ cells areas. In line with such evidence, the CD4/CD8 ratio is reduced in HCV patients compared with patients who have SS.[46] This finding has been further confirmed by Caldeira et al. who demonstrated a prevalence of CD3+ cells in diffused and focal infiltrates of the salivary glands with a ratio CD3+/CD20+ of 1.17 and a slight prevalence of CD8+ cells.[47]

A much higher predominance of CD8+ infiltrating cells may be observed in sialadenitis induced by HIV infection. Indeed, HIV infection may lead to the development of an SS-like clinical picture. A diffuse infiltrative lymphocytosis syndrome (DILS) has been described in 3–50% of salivary glands coming from these patients.[48] In the West African population the prevalence of DILS appears to be higher, with evidence of ductal atypia in up to 96% of patients, and more than one lymphocytic focus in up to 48%.[49] In 1958, Bernier et al. coined the term *lymphoepithelial cystic lesions* to describe the peculiar lesions of this condition.[50] These are composed by a mix of lymphoepithelial and cystic lesions developing as a result of striated duct compression by hyperplastic lymphoid tissue.[51] Lymphoepithelial cystic lesions are estimated to occur in about 10% of HIV cases, usually in advanced stages.[35] In the early stage of disease, the cysts are usually not present and features more similar to SS may be identified, such as follicular lymphoid hyperplasia and atrophic glands.[52] Histiocytes and plasma cells can be found in the cyst walls together with multinucleated giant cells.[53] Even if rarely, lymphoepithelial cystic lesions may take place also in other conditions, including SS or sarcoidosis. In these cases a markedly decreased interfollicular CD4/CD8 T-cell ratio might help to distinguish HIV-associated lymphoepithelial cystic lesions from HIV-negative cases.[54]

One of the principal disorders mimicking SS is sarcoidosis. In this case, the lip biopsy is the main method to detect the condition.[55] Sarcoidosis is a distinct entity from SS but it has been described in 1–2% of SS patients.[56] Sarcoidosis can affect both lacrimal and salivary glands in 3% and 6% of cases, respectively.[57] Parotid glands are often involved, although submandibular localizations have been described.[58] Sarcoidosis-associated sialadenitis is commonly characterized by the presence of noncaseating granulomas.[56] However, granulomas may be not always present and the presence of scattered lymphoplasmacytic infiltrates and multinucleated cells makes it difficult to perform a differential diagnosis.[55] For this reason if there is clinical doubt, the detection of mild lymphocytic infiltrates (grades I or II according to Chisholm–Mason score) should be interpreted with caution. The presence of multinucleate giant cells, pathognomonic of the sarcoidosis[55] associated to prevalent CD8+ cells infiltrates[59] might support the diagnosis.

The IgG4-related sclerosing diseases represent an important differential diagnosis for SS. IgG4-related disease is a systemic condition characterized by extensive IgG4-positive plasma cells and T-lymphocyte infiltration of various organs. The involvement of salivary glands usually leads to a characteristic sclerosing sialadenitis previously known as of "Kuttner tumor."[60] The IgG4-related sclerosing disease is distinguished by the evidence of a prominent cellular interlobular fibrosis composed of fibroblasts, lymphocytes, and plasma cells associated to a florid follicular hyperplasia.[61] It is characterized by a marked lymphoplasmacytic inflammation with evidence of infiltrating IgG4-positive plasma cells, lymphoid follicles, sclerosis, acinar atrophy, obliterative phlebitis, and the absence of prominent lymphoepithelial lesions.[61] This condition has a predilection for the submandibular gland, although parotid gland involvement has been described, too.[62]

# 7. GERMINAL CENTERS AS PREDICTORS OF LYMPHOMA DEVELOPMENT

The GC is represented by an area of intense, confined, and organized B-cell proliferation. Histologically, GCs are identifiable in the hematoxylin-eosin (H&E) stained histological section as areas of lighter staining within densely aggregated lymphoid follicles (Fig. 11.1). The lighter staining is caused by lymphoblasts (characterized by large light cytoplasm) and the dendrites of the FDCs that displace the dense and darker B cells (B cells have a small cytoplasm; in the H&E the predominant feature of these cells is the nuclear material that binds the darker hematoxylin staining). GCs are mainly composed of B lymphocytes but also macrophages, dendritic cells (DC)s, specialized FDCs, and T lymphocytes. DCs play a key role in ectopic GC formation and drive their maintenance

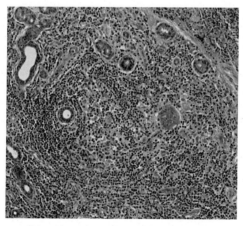

**FIGURE 11.1**    Hematoxylin-eosin (H&E) staining of salivary gland biopsy with an evident germinal center (GC)–like structure.

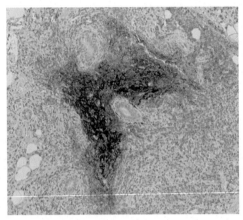

**FIGURE 11.2**   Immunohistochemical staining for CD21 in a labial salivary gland sample showing a large follicular dendritic cell network.

by supporting the antigen presentation and producing key cytokines for B-cell maturation and proliferation.[63] Structurally, GCs are formed by a dark zone that is inhabited by highly proliferating centroblasts and a light zone populated by FDCs and centrocytes. Whereas the dark zone represents the area where the B-cell clones undergo expansion; the light zone is the site of antigen presentation and affinity maturation of the B-cell compartment.

Within the major salivary glands, this segregation in dark and light zone compartments is more often detected; this distinction might be more difficult in the smaller minor salivary glands. Nonetheless, within the minor gland, areas of lighter staining in the B-cell area can be clearly visible; this is consistently associated with the presence of positive staining for CD21 long isoform at the sequential section, thus confirming the presence of FDC networks (Fig. 11.2). In this area, it is possible to detect expression of activation-induced cytidine deaminase (AID), the enzyme that, regulating the process of somatic hypermutation and class switch recombination, is instrumental for the whole process of B-cell affinity maturation.[12,13] Although conflicting results dealing with AID level of expression inside GCs have been reported,[13,64] there is a general agreement on the presence of local proliferation and chronic antigenic stimulation in the salivary glands.[65]

In secondary lymphoid organ GC, the process of antigen selection is tightly regulated; it is believed that in ectopic GC the chronic antigen stimulation may contribute to the aberrant mutation pattern.[66,67] Indeed, the chronic antigenic stimulation together with the local ectopic expression of B- and T-cell survival factors are likely to provide the ideal microenvironment for the development of hyperactive clones.[68] Salivary gland lymphoid organization and GC formation is accompanied by the ectopic production of the lymphoid chemokines CXCL13, CCL21, and CXCL12[12,13] that localize within the aggregates in discrete areas, resembling the lymphoid organization observed in secondary lymphoid organs. Lymphoid chemokines are required for the movement and positioning of the B- (and T-) cell compartment within the diverse areas of the GC and the follicle in general. Disruption of the chemokine gradient results in aberrant GC reaction.[69–72] Accordingly, local expression of lymphoid chemokines has been shown to correlate with the degree of organization of the foci[12,13] and with systemic autoantibody production and clinical manifestation of the disease.[73,74]

During the disease course, the detection of GCs in the salivary gland biopsy has been associated to more aggressive development both serologically and clinically.[75] The presence of histologically detectable GCs ($25.1 \pm 5.0\%$ standard deviation) in pSS patients has been found to correlate with a higher focus score (1.25 points higher).[75] Specifically, positive rheumatoid factor (RF) or anti-Ro/SSA and anti-La/SSB antibodies is much higher in patients with GCs than in patients without, suggesting a possible contribution of these structures in their local production.[75] Although the occurrence of GCs appears to be strictly correlated with a more aggressive disease, a number of studies demonstrate similar laboratory features between patients with GCs in salivary glands and patients with only a high lymphocyte focus score. Specifically, in terms of autoantibody production and inflammatory modulating cytokine release, no significant differences have been observed between SS patients with positive or negative GCs.[76,77]

A recent work has also described how active Epstein–Barr virus (EBV) in SS salivary glands seems to be associated with the development of ectopic lymphoid structures.[78] According to this study, latent EBV infection appears associated with ectopic GC and EBV seems to be able to transform latently infected B cells in proliferating blasts and convert them into long-lived memory B cells. Such a finding suggests the contribution of this infection to the activation of GC B cells and plasma cell differentiation in pSS.[78]

Although the potential association between GC formation within the glands and development of lymphoma has been suggested for long time,[13,34] evidence of the correlation between the two is a more recent achievement.[2] Theander et al. have reported the strong negative correlation (99% negative predictive value) between the absence of GC detection and development of B-cell lymphoma[2]; nonetheless, the positive predictive value of GC for lymphoma development is low (14%).[2] In a different study by Johnsen SJ et al.,[79] although patients with lymphoma were more likely to have a positive minor salivary gland biopsy and a higher focus score, no significant difference in GC prevalence was detected between patients developing lymphoma or not. This clearly suggests that in the process of lymphomagenesis, the formation of ectopic GC is a requirement, but is not alone responsible for the malignancy development. The work from Theander advocates for the report of GC detection in the biopsy report alongside the classical focus score, thus providing both patients and clinicians with a stratification tool to identify patients that will require more frequent monitoring. In the Theander study, the identification of the GC structures was performed on H&E

stained samples, a procedure that required an expert histopathologist's review of the sections. Further work is required to validate whether alternative methods of GC detection, ie, staining for FDC networks or bcl2/bcl6 will add value and specificity to this report. Validation of these methods for GC detection is undergoing.

## 8. LYMPHOMA HISTOPATHOLOGY

Within the inflammatory aggregates in the salivary gland of patients with pSS, B-cell lymphoma might arise. Classically salivary gland lymphomas are non-Hodgkin malignancies of the mucosa-associated lymphoid tissue (MALT) type and form predominantly in the major salivary glands (parotid). Fixed or recurrent parotid swelling will raise the clinical suspicion and the patient will undergo further investigations, including fine-needle biopsy or core biopsy of the glands.[80] MALT lymphomas have the tendency to occupy the large majority of the gland, disrupting the glandular anatomy and its function. MALT lymphomas are histologically characterized by different areas; the reactive area characterized by the presence of large follicles with IgD+ naive B cells and a sizable T zone[1] that represent the expansion of the pSS inflammatory component. The malignant areas, inhabited by marginal zone–like lymphocytes (centrocytes), small lymphocytes, immunoblasts, and centroblast-like cells represent the expansion of the neoplastic clones that can infiltrate the reactive follicles, assuming the characteristic distribution observed in the marginal zone of the spleen and Peyer patches or might occupy the interfollicular area.[81] Areas of LESA are often associated with the expansion of the malignant clones.[1] The neoplastic cells are generally small to medium-sized with moderately abundant clear or pale eosinophilic cytoplasm. Tumor cells express CD20, IgM, and the antiapoptotic factor bcl-2; although they are generally negative for IgD, CD5, and CD10. In some cases, the malignant clones can undergo plasma cell differentiation or transformation in to diffuse large B-cell lymphoma (DLBC). In this latter case, malignant B cells are larger cells (usually 5 times larger than normal lymphocytes) and resemble immunoblasts or centroblasts. DLBC malignancies loose the characteristic distribution of the MALT lymphoma in marginal zone–like structures and completely subvert the reactive lymphocytic aggregates as well as the glandular structure.

## 9. THE VALUE OF HISTOPATHOLOGICAL ASSESSMENT DURING CLINICAL TRIALS

The necessity to provide reliable and objective biomarkers to stratify patients or measure efficacy in early phases and proof of principle trials has raised the opportunity to use salivary gland histology analysis as a biological outcome measure in pSS. Although a general consensus on the items to consider and measure has not been achieved,[3] several studies have already used this tool to monitor biological effects in the tissue.

The classical tool to use to measure the extent of the salivary gland infiltrate is the focus score. It is defined as "focus" of an aggregate of 50 or more lymphocytes per 4 mm$^2$. According to the Chisholm and Mason[24] grading system, there are five possible levels of severity of inflammatory infiltrate: 0 = absence of infiltrates; 1 = slight infiltrate; 2 = moderate infiltrate or less than one focus; 3 = one focus; and 4 = more than one focus. Later, Greenspan et al.[25] developed the "focus score" that is commonly used to diagnose and also reassess disease activity after treatment. They used the definition of focus provided by Chisholm and Mason to elaborate a grading scale aimed at quantifying the number of foci. Specifically, the focus score is calculated by dividing the number of foci for the total glandular area and then multiplying for 4 mm$^2$. Although focus score provides a useful tool to assess disease activity, it still has some limitations. The focus score does not provide information on the size of infiltrates, nor does it report qualitative aspects such as the cellular composition (CD3+, CD20+, CD21+) or the organization of the aggregates in organized structures. Finally, the presence of GCs is not reported in the focus score, because the foci are only enumerated. The lack of critical information such as the organization or the extent of the inflammatory aggregates turns the focus score into an incomplete prognostic instrument and limited tool for the analysis of the salivary glands during clinical trials.[3]

Therefore it is not surprising that different studies have used different measurements to evaluate the histological response post therapy.

Pijpe et al. evaluated the efficacy of rituximab (RTX) (4 weekly infusions of 375 mg/m$^2$) after 12 weeks of treatment in eight patients with early pSS (disease duration not longer than 4 years, B-cell hyperactivity [IgG > 15 g/L] and positive RF, and anti-Ro/SSA and anti-La/SSB antibodies).[82] A significant improvement of subjective symptoms and increased salivary secretion was observed in all patients. Biopsies were taken before and 12 weeks post treatment in five of these patients and different parameters were considered in order to analyze the spreading and organization of the infiltrate: focus score, B-/T-cell ratio, disappearance of the GC-like structures, and the reduction of the infiltrating lymphocytes in the ducts.[83] Actively proliferating parenchyma and the evaluation of parenchyma/fat representation in the biopsies was also quantified. The data showed a reduction in lymphocyte infiltrates (specifically of B cells) in all patients with a decrease of the B-/T-cell ratio. In four of the five patients presenting GC in the first biopsy, a reduction in incidence was observed, and in three cases the GC completely disappeared. The amount and extent of lymphoepithelial lesions decreased in three patients and disappeared in two patients. Cellular proliferation of acinar parenchyma was reduced in all patients after therapy. The amount of acinar parenchyma did not change or was slightly decreased, whereas the amount of fat after treatment did not change or was increased.[83]

Carubbi et al.[84] also reported changes in salivary gland lesions in 19 patients with early pSS (maximum 2 years from the onset of first symptoms and a

European League Against Rheumatism Sjögren's Syndrome Disease Activity Index ≥6) treated with RTX compared with 22 patients treated with classical disease-modifying antirheumatic drugs after 120 weeks of therapy.[84] Patients received 1000-mg infusions of RTX 2 weeks apart (at day 1 and at day 15), and this course was repeated every 24 weeks for a total amount of six courses of therapy for each patient. Histological evaluation included a measurement of the focus score (89.4% of patients presented a focus score below 1 by the end of the study) alongside data on B-/T-cell areas and consequent formation of GC-like structures, the incidence of which was found to be significantly reduced (from 52.6% to 5.2% in the second biopsy).[84]

In the abatacept study performed in 2013, histology was used to integrate the clinical data from 11 patients treated with eight doses of CTLA-4Ig (weeks 0, 2, 4, 8, 12, 16, 20, and 24) (500 mg below 60 kg body weight or 750 mg above 60 kg body weight per infusion). In this case a reduction of the focus score was not observed, but a significant reduction in the number of the inflammatory foci, with a detailed report of the T-cell infiltration, was described.[85]

## 10. CONCLUSIONS

The histological interpretation of salivary gland biopsies provides a key clinical and research tool. Novel data highlighting the prognostic value of certain histological lesions make the salivary gland histopathology a potential stratification tool and a critical biomarker in the context of clinical trials. Research projects are in place to provide consensus on the use of histology and more flexible and complete criteria for biopsy analysis.

## REFERENCES

1. Barone F, Bombardieri M, Rosado MM, Morgan PR, Challacombe SJ, De Vita S, et al. CXCL13, CCL21, and CXCL12 expression in salivary glands of patients with Sjögren's syndrome and MALT lymphoma: association with reactive and malignant areas of lymphoid organization. *J Immunol* 2008;**180**:5130–40.
2. Theander E, Vasaitis L, Baecklund E, Nordmark G, Warfvinge G, Liedholm R, et al. Lymphoid organisation in labial salivary gland biopsies is a possible predictor for the development of malignant lymphoma in primary Sjögren's syndrome. *Ann Rheum Dis* 2011;**70**:1363–8.
3. Fisher BA, Brown RM, Bowman SJ, Barone F. A review of salivary gland histopathology in primary Sjögren's syndrome with a focus on its potential as a clinical trials biomarker. *Ann Rheum Dis* 2015;**74**(9):1645–50.
4. Holsinger F, Bui D. Salivary gland disorders – anatomy, function, and evaluation of the salivary glands. In: Eugene NM, Ferris RL, editors. Berlin Heidelberg: Springer; 2007.
5. Grant J. *An atlas of anatomy.* 6th ed. Baltimore: Williams & Wilkins; 1972.
6. Dawes C, O'Mullane D, Edgar M. *Saliva and oral health.* 4th ed. Stephen Hancocks Ltd; 2012. p. 154.
7. Hollinshead W. Anatomy for surgeons. 3rd ed. *The head and neck,* vol. I. Philadelphia: J.B. Lippincott Company; 1982.

8. Hand AR, Pathmanathan D, Field RB. Morphological features of the minor salivary glands. *Arch Oral Biol* 1999;**44**:S3–10.

9. Eisenbud L, Platt N, Stern M, D'Angelo W, Sumner P. Palatal biopsy as a diagnostic aid in the study of connective tissue diseases. *Oral Surg Oral Med Oral Pathol* 1973;**35**:642–8.

10. Pijpe J, Kalk WW, van der Wal JE, Vissink A, Kluin PM, Roodenburg JL, et al. Parotid gland biopsy compared with labial biopsy in the diagnosis of patients with primary Sjögren's syndrome. *Rheumatology* 2007;**46**:335–41.

11. Carbone A, Gloghini A, Ferlito A. Pathological features of lymphoid proliferations of the salivary glands: lymphoepithelial sialadenitis versus low-grade B-cell lymphoma of the malt type. *Ann Otol Rhinol Laryngol* 2000;**109**:1170–5.

12. Barone F, Bombardieri M, Manzo A, Blades MC, Morgan PR, Challacombe SJ, et al. Association of CXCL13 and CCL21 expression with the progressive organization of lymphoid-like structures in Sjögren's syndrome. *Arthritis Rheum* 2005;**52**:1773–84.

13. Bombardieri M, Barone F, Humby F, Kelly S, McGurk M, Morgan P, et al. Activation-induced cytidine deaminase expression in follicular dendritic cell networks and interfollicular large B cells supports functionality of ectopic lymphoid neogenesis in autoimmune sialoadenitis and MALT lymphoma in Sjögren's syndrome. *J Immunol* 2007;**179**:4929–38.

14. Jordan RC, Speight PM. Lymphoma in Sjögren's syndrome: from histopathology to molecular pathology. *Oral Surg Oral Med Oral Pathol Oral Radiol Endod* 1996;**81**:308–20.

15. Colella G, Cannavale R, Vicidomini A, Itro A. Salivary gland biopsy: a comprehensive review of techniques and related complications. *Rheumatology* 2010;**49**:2117–21.

16. Alsaad K, Lee TC, McCartan B. An anatomical study of the cutaneous branches of the mental nerve. *Int J Oral Maxillofac Surg* 2003;**32**:325–33.

17. Friedman JA, Miller EB, Huszar M. A simple technique for minor salivary gland biopsy appropriate for use by rheumatologists in an outpatient setting. *Clin Rheumatol* 2002;**21**:349–50.

18. Caporali R, Bonacci E, Epis O, Morbini P, Montecucco C. Comment on: parotid gland biopsy compared with labial biopsy in the diagnosis of patients with primary Sjögren's syndrome. *Rheumatology* 2007;**46**:1625. author reply 1625–1626.

19. Daniels TE. Labial salivary gland biopsy in Sjögren's syndrome: assessment as a diagnostic criterion in 362 suspected cases. *Arthritis Rheum* 1984;**27**:147–56.

20. Marx RE, Hartman KS, Rethman KV. A prospective study comparing incisional labial to incisional parotid biopsies in the detection and confirmation of sarcoidosis, Sjögren's disease, sialosis and lymphoma. *J Rheumatol* 1988;**15**:621–9.

21. Wise CM, Agudelo CA, Semble EL, Stump TE, Woodruff RD. Comparison of parotid and minor salivary gland biopsy specimens in the diagnosis of Sjögren's syndrome. *Arthritis Rheum* 1988;**31**:662–6.

22. Vitali C, Monti P, Giuggioli C, Tavoni A, Neri R, Genovesi-Ebert F, et al. Parotid sialography and lip biopsy in the evaluation of oral component in Sjögren's syndrome. *Clin Exp Rheumatol* 1989;**7**:131–5.

23. Morbini P, Manzo A, Caporali R, Epis O, Villa C, Tinelli C, et al. Multilevel examination of minor salivary gland biopsy for Sjögren's syndrome significantly improves diagnostic performance of AECG classification criteria. *Arthritis Res Ther* 2005;**7**:R343–8.

24. Chisholm DM, Mason DK. Labial salivary gland biopsy in Sjögren's disease. *J Clin Pathol* 1968;**21**:656–60.

25. Greenspan JS, Daniels TE, Talal N, Sylvester RA. The histopathology of Sjögren's syndrome in labial salivary gland biopsies. *Oral Surg Oral Med Oral Pathol* 1974;**37**:217–29.

26. Christodoulou MI, Kapsogeorgou EK, Moutsopoulos HM. Characteristics of the minor salivary gland infiltrates in Sjögren's syndrome. *J Autoimmun* 2010;**34**:400–7.

27. Christodoulou MI, Kapsogeorgou EK, Moutsopoulos NM, Moutsopoulos HM. Foxp3+ T-regulatory cells in Sjögren's syndrome: correlation with the grade of the autoimmune lesion and certain adverse prognostic factors. *Am J Pathol* 2008;**173**:1389–96.

28. Gonzalez S, Aguilera S, Alliende C, Urzua U, Quest AF, Herrera L, et al. Alterations in type I hemidesmosome components suggestive of epigenetic control in the salivary glands of patients with Sjögren's syndrome. *Arthritis Rheum* 2011;**63**:1106–15.

29. Furuzawa-Carballeda J, Sanchez-Guerrero J, Betanzos JL, Enriquez AB, Avila-Casado C, Llorente L, et al. Differential cytokine expression and regulatory cells in patients with primary and secondary Sjögren's syndrome. *Scand J Immunol* 2014;**80**:432–40.

30. Sarigul M, Yazisiz V, Bassorgun CI, Ulker M, Avci AB, Erbasan F, et al. The numbers of Foxp3+ Treg cells are positively correlated with higher grade of infiltration at the salivary glands in primary Sjögren's syndrome. *Lupus* 2010;**19**:138–45.

31. Fitzgerald-Bocarsly P, Dai J, Singh S. Plasmacytoid dendritic cells and type I IFN: 50 years of convergent history. *Cytokine Growth Factor Rev* 2008;**19**:3–19.

32. Gottenberg JE, Cagnard N, Lucchesi C, Letourneur F, Mistou S, Lazure T, et al. Activation of IFN pathways and plasmacytoid dendritic cell recruitment in target organs of primary Sjögren's syndrome. *Proc Natl Acad Sci USA* 2006;**103**:2770–5.

33. Wildenberg ME, van Helden-Meeuwsen CG, van de Merwe JP, Drexhage HA, Versnel MA. Systemic increase in type I interferon activity in Sjögren's syndrome: a putative role for plasmacytoid dendritic cells. *Eur J Immunol* 2008;**38**:2024–33.

34. Salomonsson S, Jonsson MV, Skarstein K, Brokstad KA, Hjelmstrom P, Wahren-Herlenius M, et al. Cellular basis of ectopic germinal center formation and autoantibody production in the target organ of patients with Sjögren's syndrome. *Arthritis Rheum* 2003;**48**:3187–201.

35. Greaves WO, Wang SA. Selected topics on lymphoid lesions in the head and neck regions. *Head Neck Pathol* 2011;**5**:41–50.

36. Harris NL. Lymphoid proliferations of the salivary glands. *Am J Clin Pathol* 1999;**111**:S94–103.

37. Ramos-Casals M, Solans R, Rosas J, Camps MT, Gil A, Del Pino-Montes J, et al. Primary Sjögren syndrome in Spain: clinical and immunologic expression in 1010 patients. *Medicine* 2008;**87**:210–9.

38. Vitali C. Immunopathologic differences of Sjögren's syndrome versus sicca syndrome in HCV and HIV infection. *Arthritis Res Ther* 2011;**13**:233.

39. Haddad J, Deny P, Munz-Gotheil C, Ambrosini JC, Trinchet JC, Pateron D, et al. Lymphocytic sialadenitis of Sjögren's syndrome associated with chronic hepatitis C virus liver disease. *Lancet* 1992;**339**:321–3.

40. Koike K, Moriya K, Ishibashi K, Yotsuyanagi H, Shintani Y, Fujie H, et al. Sialadenitis histologically resembling Sjögren syndrome in mice transgenic for hepatitis C virus envelope genes. *Proc Natl Acad Sci USA* 1997;**94**:233–6.

41. Arrieta JJ, Rodriguez-Inigo E, Ortiz-Movilla N, Bartolome J, Pardo M, Manzarbeitia F, et al. In situ detection of hepatitis C virus RNA in salivary glands. *Am J Pathol* 2001;**158**:259–64.

42. Loustaud-Ratti V, Riche A, Liozon E, Labrousse F, Soria P, Rogez S, et al. Prevalence and characteristics of Sjögren's syndrome or Sicca syndrome in chronic hepatitis C virus infection: a prospective study. *J Rheumatol* 2001;**28**:2245–51.

43. Ramos-Casals M, la Civita L, de Vita S, Solans R, Luppi M, Medina F, et al. Characterization of B cell lymphoma in patients with Sjögren's syndrome and hepatitis C virus infection. *Arthritis Rheum* 2007;**57**:161–70.

44. Carrozzo M. Oral diseases associated with hepatitis C virus infection. Part 1. Sialadenitis and salivary glands lymphoma. *Oral Dis* 2008;**14**:123–30.

45. Pirisi M, Scott C, Fabris C, Ferraccioli G, Soardo G, Ricci R, et al. Mild sialoadenitis: a common finding in patients with hepatitis C virus infection. *Scand J Gastroenterol* 1994;**29**:940–2.

46. Freni MA, Artuso D, Gerken G, Spanti C, Marafioti T, Alessi N, et al. Focal lymphocytic aggregates in chronic hepatitis C: occurrence, immunohistochemical characterization, and relation to markers of autoimmunity. *Hepatology* 1995;**22**:389–94.

47. Caldeira PC, Oliveira e Silva KR, Vidigal PV, Grossmann SM, do Carmo MA. Inflammatory cells in minor salivary glands of patients with chronic hepatitis C: immunophenotype, pattern of distribution, and comparison with liver samples. *Hum Immunol* 2014;**75**:422–7.

48. Kordossis T, Paikos S, Aroni K, Kitsanta P, Dimitrakopoulos A, Kavouklis E, et al. Prevalence of Sjögren's-like syndrome in a cohort of HIV-1-positive patients: descriptive pathology and immunopathology. *Br J Rheumatol* 1998;**37**:691–5.

49. McArthur CP, Subtil-DeOliveira A, Palmer D, Fiorella RM, Gustafson S, Tira D, et al. Characteristics of salivary diffuse infiltrative lymphocytosis syndrome in West Africa. *Arch Pathol Lab Med* 2000;**124**:1773–9.

50. Bernier JL, Bhaskar SN. Lymphoepithelial lesions of salivary glands; histogenesis and classification based on 186 cases. *Cancer* 1958;**11**:1156–79.

51. Maiorano E, Favia G, Viale G. Lymphoepithelial cysts of salivary glands: an immunohistochemical study of HIV-related and HIV-unrelated lesions. *Hum Pathol* 1998;**29**:260–5.

52. Ihrler S, Steger W, Riederer A, Zietz C, Vogl I, Lohrs U. HIV-associated cysts of the parotid glands: an histomorphologic and magnetic resonance tomography study of formal pathogenesis. *Laryngorhinootologie* 1996;**75**:671–6.

53. Elliott JN, Oertel YC. Lymphoepithelial cysts of the salivary glands: histologic and cytologic features. *Am J Clin Pathol* 1990;**93**:39–43.

54. Kreisel FH, Frater JL, Hassan A, El-Mofty SK. Cystic lymphoid hyperplasia of the parotid gland in HIV-positive and HIV-negative patients: quantitative immunopathology. *Oral Surg Oral Med Oral Pathol Oral Radiol Endod* 2010;**109**:567–74.

55. Giotaki H, Constantopoulos SH, Papadimitriou CS, Moutsopoulos HM. Labial minor salivary gland biopsy: a highly discriminatory diagnostic method between sarcoidosis and Sjögren's syndrome. *Respiration* 1986;**50**:102–7.

56. Ramos-Casals M, Brito-Zeron P, Garcia-Carrasco M, Font J. Sarcoidosis or Sjögren syndrome? Clues to defining mimicry or coexistence in 59 cases. *Medicine* 2004;**83**:85–95.

57. James DG, Sharma OP. Overlap syndromes with sarcoidosis. *Sarcoidosis* 1985;**2**:116–21.

58. Vourexakis Z, Dulguerov P, Bouayed S, Burkhardt K, Landis BN. Sarcoidosis of the submandibular gland: a systematic review. *Am J Otolaryngol* 2010;**31**:424–8.

59. Gal I, Kovacs J, Zeher M. Case series: coexistence of Sjögren's syndrome and sarcoidosis. *J Rheumatol* 2000;**27**:2507–10.

60. Chan JK. Kuttner tumor (chronic sclerosing sialadenitis) of the submandibular gland: an under-recognized entity. *Adv Anat Pathol* 1998;**5**:239–51.

61. Geyer JT, Ferry JA, Harris NL, Stone JH, Zukerberg LR, Lauwers GY, et al. Chronic sclerosing sialadenitis (Kuttner tumor) is an IgG4-associated disease. *Am J Surg Pathol* 2010;**34**:202–10.

62. Rasanen O, Jokinen K, Dammert K. Sclerosing inflammation of the submandibular salivary gland (Kuttner's tumor). *Duodecim* 1972;**88**:646–51.

63. Aguzzi A, Kranich J, Krautler NJ. Follicular dendritic cells: origin, phenotype, and function in health and disease. *Trends Immunol* 2014;**35**:105–13.

64. Le Pottier L, Devauchelle V, Fautrel A, Daridon C, Saraux A, Youinou P, et al. Ectopic germinal centers are rare in Sjögren's syndrome salivary glands and do not exclude autoreactive B cells. *J Immunol* 2009;**182**:3540–7.

65. Tzioufas AG, Kapsogeorgou EK, Moutsopoulos HM. Pathogenesis of Sjögren's syndrome: what we know and what we should learn. *J Autoimmun* 2012;**39**:4–8.

66. Berg AR, Weisenburger DD, Linder J, Armitage JO. Lymphoplasmacytic lymphoma: report of a case with three monoclonal proteins derived from a single neoplastic clone. *Cancer* 1986;**57**:1794–7.

67. Vinuesa CG, Sanz I, Cook MC. Dysregulation of germinal centres in autoimmune disease. *Nat Rev Immunol* 2009;**9**:845–57.

68. Pitzalis C, Jones GW, Bombardieri M, Jones SA. Ectopic lymphoid-like structures in infection, cancer, and autoimmunity. *Nat Rev Immunol* 2014;**14**:447–62.

69. Ansel KM, Ngo VN, Hyman PL, Luther SA, Forster R, Sedgwick JD, et al. A chemokine-driven positive feedback loop organizes lymphoid follicles. *Nature* 2000;**406**:309–14.

70. Luther SA, Tang HL, Hyman PL, Farr AG, Cyster JG. Coexpression of the chemokines ELC and SLC by T zone stromal cells and deletion of the *ELC* gene in the plt/plt mouse. *Proc Natl Acad Sci USA* 2000;**97**:12694–9.

71. Luther SA, Bidgol A, Hargreaves DC, Schmidt A, Xu Y, Paniyadi J, et al. Differing activities of homeostatic chemokines CCL19, CCL21, and CXCL12 in lymphocyte and dendritic cell recruitment and lymphoid neogenesis. *J Immunol* 2002;**169**:424–33.

72. Mebius RE. Organogenesis of lymphoid tissues. *Nat Rev Immunol* 2003;**3**:292–303.

73. Kramer JM, Klimatcheva E, Rothstein TL. CXCL13 is elevated in Sjögren's syndrome in mice and humans and is implicated in disease pathogenesis. *J Leukoc Biol* 2013;**94**:1079–89.

74. Salomonsson S, Larsson P, Tengner P, Mellquist E, Hjelmstrom P, Wahren-Herlenius M. Expression of the B cell-attracting chemokine CXCL13 in the target organ and autoantibody production in ectopic lymphoid tissue in the chronic inflammatory disease Sjögren's syndrome. *Scand J Immunol* 2002;**55**:336–42.

75. Risselada AP, Looije MF, Kruize AA, Bijlsma JW, van Roon JA. The role of ectopic germinal centers in the immunopathology of primary Sjögren's syndrome: a systematic review. *Sem Arthritis Rheum* 2013;**42**:368–76.

76. Szodoray P, Alex P, Jonsson MV, Knowlton N, Dozmorov I, Nakken B, et al. Distinct profiles of Sjögren's syndrome patients with ectopic salivary gland germinal centers revealed by serum cytokines and BAFF. *Clin Immunol* 2005;**117**:168–76.

77. Jonsson MV, Salomonsson S, Oijordsbakken G, Skarstein K. Elevated serum levels of soluble E-cadherin in patients with primary Sjögren's syndrome. *Scand J Immunol* 2005;**62**:552–9.

78. Croia C, Astorri E, Murray-Brown W, Willis A, Brokstad KA, Sutcliffe N, et al. Implication of Epstein-Barr virus infection in disease-specific autoreactive B cell activation in ectopic lymphoid structures of Sjögren's syndrome. *Arthritis Rheumatol* 2014;**66**:2545–57.

79. Johnsen SJ, Berget E, Jonsson MV, Helgeland L, Omdal R, Jonsson R. Evaluation of germinal center-like structures and B cell clonality in patients with primary Sjögren syndrome with and without lymphoma. *J Rheumatol* 2014;**41**:2214–22.

80. Nocturne G, Mariette X. Sjögren Syndrome-associated lymphomas: an update on pathogenesis and management. *Br J Haematol* 2015;**168**:317–27.

81. Isaacson PG, Wotherspoon AC, Diss T, Pan LX. Follicular colonization in B-cell lymphoma of mucosa-associated lymphoid tissue. *Am J Surg Pathol* 1991;**15**:819–28.

82. Pijpe J, van Imhoff GW, Vissink A, van der Wal JE, Kluin PM, Spijkervet FK, et al. Changes in salivary gland immunohistology and function after rituximab monotherapy in a patient with Sjögren's syndrome and associated MALT lymphoma. *Ann Rheum Dis* 2005;**64**:958–60.

83. Pijpe J, Meijer JM, Bootsma H, van der Wal JE, Spijkervet FK, Kallenberg CG, et al. Clinical and histologic evidence of salivary gland restoration supports the efficacy of rituximab treatment in Sjögren's syndrome. *Arthritis Rheum* 2009;**60**:3251–6.

84. Carubbi F, Cipriani P, Marrelli A, Benedetto P, Ruscitti P, Berardicurti O, et al. Efficacy and safety of rituximab treatment in early primary Sjögren's syndrome: a prospective, multi-center, follow-up study. *Arthritis Res Ther* 2013;**15**:R172.

85. Adler S, Korner M, Forger F, Huscher D, Caversaccio MD, Villiger PM. Evaluation of histologic, serologic, and clinical changes in response to abatacept treatment of primary Sjögren's syndrome: a pilot study. *Arthritis Care Res* 2013;**65**:1862–8.

Chapter 12

# Glandular Epithelium: Innocent Bystander or Leading Actor?

**E.K. Kapsogeorgou, A.G. Tzioufas**
*National University of Athens, Athens, Greece*

## 1. INTRODUCTION

Sjögren's syndrome (SS) is an autoimmune disease with heterogeneous clinical pictures, which extend from benign local exocrinopathy that affects primarily the salivary and lachrymal glands to systemic disorder, and in approximately 5% of patients evolves to B-cell malignancies.[1] Furthermore, SS can be expressed as an isolated clinical entity or coexpressed with virtually every other systemic autoimmune rheumatic disorder. Most of these features are present at diagnosis and do not change during follow-up treatment,[2] suggesting that SS is a slowly progressive disease. Studies have identified clinical, laboratory, and histopathologic features, which predict the patients that are at high risk to develop lymphoproliferative disorder. Thus purpura, cryoglobulinemia, leukopenia, C3 and C4 hypocomplementemia, as well as persistent salivary gland enlargement, have been recognized as adverse prognostic indicators.[2-6] Most importantly, in the majority of SS patients who are at high risk of lymphoma development, palpable purpura, cryoglobulinemia, and C4 hypocomplementemia are present at the time of diagnosis and thus can be used as predicting factors of adverse outcome.[2-6] All these features along with the fact that the histopathologic lesions in minor salivary glands (MSGs) are easily accessible render SS as an ideal model for the study of autoimmunity and associated malignancy.

The extensive study of MSG autoimmune lesions revealed that, in accordance with the clinical picture of the disease, the severity and the composition of the histopathologic lesions vary among SS patients and do not significantly change over time.[7-10] In fact, T cells predominate in mild lesions and B cells in severe, whereas macrophages increase with lesion severity and high incidence has been linked to lymphoma development.[7,11] Most importantly, the severity and the composition of inflammatory lesions is fully blown at diagnosis and does not significantly change thereafter, with the exception of development of lymphoma in predisposed patients, suggesting that distinct

Sjögren's Syndrome. http://dx.doi.org/10.1016/B978-0-12-803604-4.00012-5

**189**

pathogenetic pathways and immune responses operate in SS patients with variable degree of infiltration.[10] Furthermore, the association between the intense salivary gland inflammation and the occurrence of extraglandular systemic manifestations such as Raynaud phenomenon, vasculitis, lymph node/spleen enlargement, and leukopenia,[9] as well as of various histopathological parameters such as formation of ectopic germinal centers, infiltration by certain types of immune cells, and production of cytokines (eg, B-cell activating factor [BAFF], interleukin [IL]18, etc.) with lymphoma development,[7–13] suggest that the local immune responses in SS are linked to the systemic manifestations of the disorder.

The mechanisms mediating the development and perpetuation of lymphocytic infiltrates, their severity, and the predominance of certain types of immune responses (T- or B-cell driven), as well as the way these could affect the outcome of the disease, have not been fully understood. Emerging data during the past two decades indicate that epithelial cells, which are the major targets of autoimmune responses, are not innocent bystanders but active, key regulators of SS autoimmune responses.[1] Herein we summarize the factors that have been implicated in epithelial cell dysfunction, as well as the findings supporting the significant role of glandular epithelium in the development and regulation of autoimmune responses.

## 2. DYSFUNCTION OF GLANDULAR EPITHELIA IN SJÖGREN'S SYNDROME: "INNOCENT BYSTANDERS"?

Historically, glandular epithelia in SS were considered to be innocent bystanders experiencing the injurious effects of chronic inflammation and its byproducts, such as function-modulating cytokines and cytotoxic and apoptotic signals that lead to epithelial dysfunction and/or destruction with ultimate result the salivary gland hypofunction. Nevertheless, the severity of salivary gland dysfunction in SS does not necessarily correlate with the degree of lymphocytic infiltration and epithelial loss and destruction,[14] suggesting that the SS secretory functional impairment is not completely dependent on inflammatory processes. On the contrary, oral dryness in SS seems to be a complex phenomenon possibly owing to the reduction and/or inhibition of water transport machinery, as well as an altered quality of the saliva produced by epithelia. Autoimmune responses seem to affect both epithelial secretory function by modulating the underlying pathways and epithelial survival by promoting apoptotic cell death.

### 2.1 Altered Epithelial Secretory Function in Sjögren's Syndrome

The secretion process in salivary glands is controlled by sympathetic and parasympathetic nerve fibers, whereas the differential stimulation of epithelial cholinergic and adrenergic receptors determines the quantity and quality of secreted saliva.[15] Thus acetylcholine stimulation of cholinergic receptors results in saliva rich in water and electrolytes, but low in proteins and glycoproteins, whereas adrenergic stimulation results in exocytosis of protein and glycoproteins with a low water and electrolyte content. Hypothesizing that lymphocytic infiltration could affect glandular innervation, initial observations suggested that vasoactive intestinal peptide–containing nerve fibers are reduced in areas of strong inflammation at the MSG lesions of SS patients; however, later studies showed that innervation and consequent nerve stimulation are not altered in SS patients.[16,17] Data from mouse models suggested that cytokine-mediated reduced release of neurotransmitters may participate in the salivary hypofunction of SS.[18–24] Furthermore, the development of autoimmune responses against the muscarinic type 3 acetylcholine receptor (M3R) has been implicated in reduced salivary function of SS patients. M3R plays a critical role in the parasympathetic control of salivation.[25,26] Autoantibodies against M3R have been described in SS patients and have been shown to reduce fluid secretion by acinar cells via intracellular trafficking of the water transport protein aquaporin-5 (AQP5) in epithelial cells, whereas cellular immune responses against M3R have been associated to epithelial cell destruction; hence immune responses are directly linked with epithelial cell dysfunction in affected salivary glands.[27–30] AQP5-disturbed expression may also participate in the secretory dysfunction of epithelial cells in SS; even though reports are controversial.[31,32] Altered distribution of AQP5 in the acini of salivary glands of SS patients has been described. Instead of normal apical membrane distribution, AQP5 was found to localize in the basal membranes of acini in the inflamed MSG tissues of SS patients, whereas tumor necrosis factor (TNF) α, which is abundant in MSG lesions of SS patients, has been implicated in the altered AQP5 expression.[32–35]

Secretion abnormalities in SS patients do not only involve the quantity of fluid secretion, but also the quality of saliva and particularly mucin production. Mucins are complex O-linked glycoproteins with high content of anionic oligosaccharides acting as hydrophilic polymers that bind water on the epithelial surface and thereby preserve mucosa humidity.[36] Altered expression and trafficking of mucins have been associated with SS.[37] Increased levels, as well as accumulation of mucin 1 (MUC1) in acini cytoplasm, have been described in the MSGs of SS patients and have been linked to proinflammatory cytokine expression.[38] Similar to MUC1, MUC7 was found to accumulate in the cytoplasm of acini in SS patients, and along with MUC5B, was also released via exocytosis in the extracellular matrix.[39,40] Furthermore, mucins (MUC5B) seem to be hypoglycosylated in SS. In particular, MUC5B hyposulfation has been associated with reduced Gal3-O-sulfotransferase activity, which in turn has been inversely correlated with lymphocyte infiltration and glandular levels of proinflammatory cytokines, suggesting that inflammation might inhibit its activity in SS.[41,42]

## 2.2 Apoptotic Cell Death of Epithelial Cells in Sjögren's Syndrome

Apoptosis plays a significant role in the pathogenesis of all autoimmune disorders, including SS, by representing a major pathway whereby intracellular antigens are presented to the immune system in an immunogenic fashion. Several studies have demonstrated increased rates of apoptotic cell death in glandular epithelia at the MSG autoimmune lesions of SS patients.[43-46] During early apoptosis, nuclear Ro52/TRIM21, Ro60/TROVE2, and La/SSB autoantigens, which are the major target of SS humoral autoimmune responses, redistribute to the cytoplasm, whereas in later phases, they move to the surface of apoptotic blebs and bodies.[47] The subsequent engagement and processing of the autoantibody containing apoptotic particles by antigen presenting cells (APCs), which in turn are presented to T cells, most likely represent the major triggering for the initiation of SS autoimmune responses.[48] The significance of epithelial apoptosis in the pathogenesis of SS has been recently shown in an experimental mouse model. In particular, silencing of IκB-ζ expression in lacrimal epithelial cells led to increased epithelial apoptosis within the lacrimal glands and the development of an SS-like inflammatory lesion associated with high titers of serum anti-Ro/SSA and anti-La/SSB antibodies. The significant pathogenetic role of epithelial apoptotic cell death in this model was further verified by the reverse of the phenotype by apoptosis blockade using caspase inhibitors.[49] The etiopathogenical causes of epithelial apoptosis in the MSG lesions of SS are not known. Most likely, multiple factors are implicated. Cytotoxic cells and other T cells, as well as B cells, have been reported to provide proapoptotic signals to epithelial cells through either the secretion of enzymes and cytokines or direct interaction of death receptors, particularly the Fas/FasL pathway.[50-52] Special attention has been given to the role of Fas-mediated apoptosis of epithelial cells in SS. Although in MSG tissues, glandular epithelia express high levels of Fas molecules, and this expression is associated with elevated epithelial apoptosis, in vitro studies using long-term cultured salivary gland epithelial cells (SGECs) from SS patients revealed that epithelia are resistant to Fas-mediated apoptosis and a second signal provided either by CD40 ligation or cytokines, such as interferon (IFN) γ, is needed to sensitize and drive them to apoptotic cell death.[44,46,52-54] In addition, cytokines that are abundant in the MSG autoimmune lesions, such as IFNγ and TNF-α, have been described as promoting directly or indirectly (by the upregulation of other proapoptotic molecules) the apoptotic cell death of glandular epithelia.[52,55-59] On the other hand, autoantibodies against Ro/SSA and La/SSB autoantigens have been also shown to induce caspace-3 mediated epithelial apoptosis.[60] Furthermore, stimulation of the innate Toll-like receptor (TLR) 3 has been shown to result in epithelial apoptosis, partially mediated by anoikis.[61,62] Finally, estrogen deprivation and endoplasmic stress has been implicated in SGEC apoptosis.[63,64] All these data suggest that the salivary gland microenvironment regulates the survival or death of glandular epithelial cells.

## 3. THE CLINICAL EXPRESSION OF "AUTOIMMUNE EPITHELIITIS"

The aforementioned data support the notion that glandular epithelial cell function and survival in SS patients are dictated by tissue microenvironment, suggesting that epithelial cells are innocent bystanders suffering from the influence of autoimmune responses. However, the clinical picture of the disease suggests that this is not the case. The vast majority of patients (90–100%) experience dry eyes and dry mouth as a result of dysfunction and/or destruction of exocrine glands. Systemic manifestations are common in SS patients and can be categorized as parenchymal organ involvement (lung, kidneys, interstitial nephritis) or lesions related to hyperproduction of immune complexes and/or vasculitic involvement (purpura, peripheral neuropathy, glomerulonephritis).[1] Both SS-related exocrinopathy and parenchymal organ involvement are associated with the development of lymphocytic infiltrates around or invading epithelial structures, suggesting that the disease is in fact an autoimmune epitheliitis.[65] This was further strengthened by subsequent histopathological and in vitro studies, as described in the following section.

## 4. EPITHELIUM AS THE LEADING ACTOR OF AUTOIMMUNE RESPONSES

A plethora of studies during the past 20 years analyzing epithelial cells both in situ in MSG tissues and in vitro by using long-term cultured non-neoplastic SGECs from SS patients and controls proved that epithelia are not innocent bystanders, but the orchestrators of local autoimmune responses in the MSG lesions of SS patients.[1,65,66] Extensive in situ immunohistopathological analyses revealed that SGECs are able to mediate the development, maintenance, and progression of the local autoimmune inflammatory responses. However, the break-through in the study of the epithelial properties in SS came with the development of an in vitro system for the long-term culture of non-neoplastic SGEC lines from SS patients and control individuals with sicca that were established from one lobule of MSG obtained during diagnostic biopsy.[67] This facilitated the study of SGECs in an environment devoid of the effect of other cell types and tissue microenvironmental factors, thus permitting the evaluation of the constitutive epithelial phenotype and function, as well as the influence of intrinsic or exogenous factors on them, and strengthen their immunoregulatory role in the development and perpetuation of autoimmune lesions in SS.[67]

## 4.1 Epithelial Cells Are Suitably Equipped to Mediate the Development and Perpetuation of SS Autoimmune Responses

The study of SGECs in situ and in long-term cultures revealed that the epithelial cells of SS patients express a plethora of immune-competent molecules implicated in innate and acquired immune responses. The later involves molecules implicated in lymphoid cell recruitment, homing, activation, differentiation, and proliferation, as well as the expansion and organization of lymphoid infiltrates.[1,66] In this context, SGECs have been shown to express functional major histocompatibility complex (MHC) class I and class II molecules, B7 and CD40 costimulatory molecules, adhesion molecules, Fas and Fas ligand apoptosis–related molecules, proinflammatory cytokines, and cytokines involved in lymphoid cell differentiation, as well as a plethora of T cell–attracting and germinal-center–forming chemokines (summarized in Table 12.1).[66]

The expression of B7.2 costimulatory molecules by SGECs deserves particular attention, because these proteins are typically expressed by classical APCs and are critical for the regulation of naive T-cell activation. SGECs express all three known splice variants of B7.2, including a novel ligand-independent cell surface variant with regulatory function.[68] In fact, the expression pattern of B7.2 molecules by SGECs simulates that of monocytes,[68] which are one of the major types of classical APCs. Furthermore, the full-length B7.2 protein that is expressed by SGECs displays unique binding properties, denoted by the functional interaction with the stimulating CD28-receptor and reduced binding to the negative regulator of immune response cytotoxic T-lymphocyte antigen 4 (CTLA4).[69] These properties are most likely related to the elevated glycosylation status of B7.2 molecules in SGECs,[68,69] because treatment with N-glycosidases resulted in regaining of CTLA4 binding by epithelial B7.2 molecules (our unpublished data).

SGECs have also the capacity to sense innate immunity signals through the expression of several TLR and CD91 molecules.[70,71] TLR signaling in SGECs results in the upregulation of MHC-I, CD54/ICAM-1, CD40, and CD95/Fas protein expression, thus linking innate and adaptive immune responses.[71] Among the several innate receptors that are expressed by SGEC, TLR3 is of particular importance. SGECs express constitutively significantly high surface levels of TLR3 molecules. Signaling through TLR3 induces apoptosis of SGECs,[61] whereas it has been recently shown that it also upregulates the expression of Ro/SSA and La/SSB autoantigens in SGECs, suggesting that it might be implicated in autoantigen presentation.[72] The major role of TLR3 in SS pathogenesis is further supported by experimental mouse models where TLR3 signaling results in significant salivary gland hypofunction accompanied by the upregulation of various type I IFN-responsive genes, chemokines, early recruitment of dendritic and natural killer cells, and later of B cells at the submandibular glands.[73,74]

Finally, SGECs seem able to mediate the exposure and presentation of intracellular proteins to the immune system (see Table 12.1). Two pathways have been implicated in this procedure: (1) the elevated in situ apoptotic death of SGECs and the release of autoantigen-containing apoptotic blebs, as mentioned previously,[46,47,52,66,75] and (2) the release of exosomes loaded with Ro/SSA, La/SSB, and Sm autoantigens.[76] Exosomes are small endosomal vesicles

**TABLE 12.1 Expression of Immune-Competent Molecules by SGECs, Indicating Their Capacity to Regulate Local SS Autoimmune Responses**

| Immune-Related Processes/Responses | Expression of Immune-Modulatory Molecules by SGECs | |
|---|---|---|
| Innate immunity | Toll-like receptors | TLR1, TLR2, TLR3, TLR4, TLR7, TLR9 |
| | | CD91 |
| Immune cell homing | Adhesion | ICAM-1/CD54, VCAM/CD106, E-selectin |
| T-cell activation | Antigen presentation | MHC class I (HLA-ABC) |
| | | MHC class II (HLA-DR, HLA-DP, HLA-DQ) |
| | Costimulatory | B7-1 (CD80), B7-2 (CD86) |
| | | PD-L1 |
| | | CD40 |
| B-cell survival, maturation and differentiation | | BAFF |
| | | CD40 |
| Macrophage/dendritic cell differentiation | | GM-CSF |
| Granulocytes | | G-CSF |
| Expansion/perpetuation/ organization of infiltrates | Cytokines | IL-1, IL-6, IL-8, TNFα, IFNs, IL-18 (pro- active), BAFF, adiponectin, GM-CSF, G-CSF |
| | T-cell attracting/ germinal-center– forming chemokines | CCL3/MIP-1α, CCL4/MIP-1β, IL-8, CCL5/RANTES, CCL20/LARC,STCP-1/MDC, CXCL-9/Mig, CXCL-10/IP-10, CXCL12/SDF-1, CXCL13/BCA-1, CXCR3, CCL17/TARC, CCL19/ELC CCL21/SLC/TCA |
| Exposure of intracellular | Apoptotic cell death | Fas, FasL |
| Autoantigens | Exosome secretion | |

*BAFF*, B-cell activating factor; *FasL*, Fas ligand; *G-CSF*, Granulocyte colony-stimulating factor; *GM-CSF*, granulocyte-macrophage colony-stimulating factor; *HLA*, human leukocyte antigen; *IFN*, interferon; *IL*, interleukin; *MHC*, major histocompatibility complex; *SGEC*, salivary gland epithelial cell; *TLR*, Toll-like receptor; *TNF*, tumor necrosis factor.

(30–100 nm) that, among a plethora of physiological roles, have been shown to mediate the transfer of antigens to APCs, a property with significant applications in vaccine development and cancer treatment.[77]

## 4.2 Epithelial Cells Are Able to Mediate the Activation and Differentiation of Immune Cells

In the histopathological lesions at the MSG tissues of SS patients, infiltrating mononuclear cells (particularly T and B lymphocytes and dendritic cells) are often found to invade ducts or to be in close proximity with ductal epithelial cells, suggesting that glandular epithelia communicate and interact with immune cells. Indeed, in vitro studies involving coculture of non-neoplastic SGECs with immune cells provided evidence that epithelial cells are able to fruitfully interact with immune cells. Thus SGECs have been found able to mediate the activation of CD4+ T cells,[69] whereas recently it has been shown that SGECs are also able to promote the differentiation of naive CD4+ T cells to follicular helper T (Tfh) cells through IL-6 and inducible costimulator-ligand expression.[78] In fact, SGEC-differentiated Tfh cells have been proved able to enhance B lymphocyte survival, thus indirectly implicating SGECs with B-cell survival and differentiation as well. Furthermore, the epithelial expression of functional BAFF[79,80] suggests that SGECs may also be directly involved in the altered B-cell differentiation[12,81] and the formation of ectopic germinal-center–like structures that characterize the disorder.[82] Indeed, in accordance with the findings in MSGs, coculture of SGECs with peripheral blood B cells was found to promote a switch of B-cell differentiation to the Bm5p and Bm2 phenotype with concomitant decrease of the Bm1 subpopulation, as well as to augment a transitional type 2-like phenotype of B cells.[83] The expression of granulocyte-macrophage colony-stimulating factor (GM-CSF) by SGECs (our unpublished data) indicates that they are probably capable of participating in the differentiation of macrophages and dendritic cells, a point that remains to be elucidated. All these findings support the active role of SGECs in the regulation of lymphocytic infiltrates in the MSG tissues of SS patients. Considering the role of epithelial cells in the accumulation, activation, and differentiation of immune cells, it would be tempting to hypothesize that epithelial cells also determine the type of immune cell predominance and the degree of infiltration in MSG inflammatory lesions. Indeed, our unpublished data from gene expression and microRNA arrays indicate that long-term cultured SGECs from patients with mild, intermediate, and severe MSG infiltration display a distinct constitutive expression pattern that distinguishes SGECs from the three SS subgroups, as well as from controls with sicca. Sophisticated bioinformatic analysis is needed to reveal differentially expressed pathways and their significance for the regulation of autoimmune lesion size and composition. In addition, further in-depth studies are needed to illuminate complex interactions between SGECs and immune cells and reveal underlying key regulatory pathways, with the ultimate goal being therapeutic intervention.

## 4.3 Epithelial Cells of Sjögren's Syndrome Patients Are Intrinsically Activated

The comparative assessment of long-term cultured SGECs derived from SS patients and controls complaining of sicca revealed significantly higher constitutive expression of the majority of the immunoactive molecules studied in SS-SGEC lines, which was stable after several months of culture.[66] The elevated expression of immunoregulatory molecules by long-term cultured SGECs from SS patients, along with in situ evidence indicating the expression of the protooncogene c-myc[84] and the aberrant redistribution of Ro/SSA and La/SSB autoantigens in the cytoplasm[47,85] of the epithelia of SS patients, suggest that intrinsic activation processes operate in the epithelial cells of SS patients.[66] The offending factor(s) of the epithelial activation are not known. Epigenetic changes or latent viral infections, which have long been suspected to participate in SS pathogenesis, may be causally implicated in the epithelial activation of SS patients. The IFN signature[86–89] in the MSG lesions of SS patients and the high expression and responsiveness to TLR3 by SGECs further support the implication of viral infection in SS pathogenesis. Indeed, infection by certain viruses, such as hepatitis C virus or HIV, is associated with chronic sialadenitis that mimics SS without presenting humoral responses against Ro/SSA and La/SSB autoantigens and sex preference.[90,91] In this setting, several viruses, such as cytomegalovirus, Epstein-Barr virus, retroviral elements, human herpes virus type 6, human T lymphotropic virus type I, human herpes virus type 8, and, lately, Coxsackie viral sequences, have been described as harboring the salivary gland tissues of SS patients.[59,92–100] The lack of elevated cytolysis suggests that persistent, nonlytic, viral infection of epithelial cells may occur. The persisting residence of viral genetic material within the epithelial cell may alter its biological properties and initiate an aberrant immune response; however, highly sophisticated techniques are needed to evaluate the existence of forensic sequences in SGECs.

## 5. SUMMARY

Epithelial cells in SS are not innocent bystanders that pathetically experience the influence of inflammatory factors, but key players that drive and regulate local autoimmune responses by actively mediating the accumulation, activation, and differentiation of immune cells. On the other hand, immune cells and inflammatory microenvironment further activate epithelial cells or regulate their survival, thus creating a vicious cycle of epithelial/immune cell responses that perpetuates SS autoimmune responses (Fig. 12.1). The delineation of the interactions of SGECs with immune cells and the underlying pathways, as well as of the offending factors of epithelial activation, is of great significance for the understanding of disease pathogenesis and the development of effective therapeutic interventions.

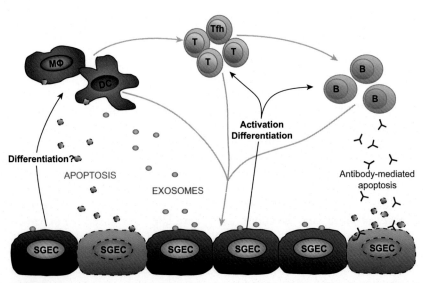

**FIGURE 12.1** Glandular epithelial cells are leading actors in the development and maintenance of SS autoimmune responses. Salivary gland epithelial cells (*SGECs*) are suitably equipped to mediate the recruitment activation and/or differentiation of T and B lymphocytes, macrophages (*MΦs*), and dendritic cells (*DCs*), as well as the organization of infiltrates in the minor salivary glands (MSGs) of SS patients through the production of cytokines/chemokines. In more detail, SGECs, through interaction of surface receptors and/or soluble factors, advance the activation of CD4+ T cells, as well as their differentiation to T follicular helper (*Tfh*) cells, which are essential for B-cell survival and differentiation. Also, SGECs directly promote the differentiation of B cells, whereas the secretion of granulocyte-macrophage colony-stimulating factor suggests that they may be able to drive the activation/differentiation of MΦs and DCs as well. Furthermore, SGECs release autoantigen-loaded vesicles, such as exosomes or apoptotic bodies, that are captured by MΦs and DCs, which in turn are presented in T cells. Activated T cells subsequently activate and differentiate B cells, with final result being the production of autoantibodies. These autoantibodies are able to induce apoptotic cell death in SGECs, resulting in perpetuation of tissue damage and subsequent autoimmune responses. Finally, activated immunocytes through cell-to-cell interactions and/or cytokine and chemokine secretion further activate epithelial cells or induce their apoptotic death, thus amplifying autoimmune responses and creating a vicious cycle of inflammation. *Black arrows* represent activation signals provided by SGECs to immune cells, whereas *gray arrows* indicate the activation/differentiation/death signals from immune cells to SGECs.

## ABBREVIATIONS

**MSG** Minor salivary gland
**SGEC** Salivary gland epithelial cells

## REFERENCES

1. Tzioufas AG, Kapsogeorgou EK, Moutsopoulos HM. Pathogenesis of Sjögren's syndrome: what we know and what we should learn. *J Autoimmun* 2012;**39**:4–8.
2. Skopouli FN, Dafni U, Ioannidis JP, Moutsopoulos HM. Clinical evolution, and morbidity and mortality of primary Sjögren's syndrome. *Semin Arthritis Rheum* 2000;**29**: 296–304.

3. Ioannidis JP, Vassiliou VA, Moutsopoulos HM. Long-term risk of mortality and lymphoproliferative disease and predictive classification of primary Sjögren's syndrome. *Arthritis Rheum* 2002;**46**:741–7.

4. Ramos-Casals M, Brito-Zeron P, Yague J, Akasbi M, Bautista R, Ruano M, et al. Hypocomplementaemia as an immunological marker of morbidity and mortality in patients with primary Sjögren's syndrome. *Rheumatology* 2005;**44**:89–94.

5. Sutcliffe N, Inanc M, Speight P, Isenberg D. Predictors of lymphoma development in primary Sjögren's syndrome. *Semin Arthritis Rheum* 1998;**28**:80–7.

6. Voulgarelis M, Dafni UG, Isenberg DA, Moutsopoulos HM. Malignant lymphoma in primary Sjögren's syndrome: a multicenter, retrospective, clinical study by the European Concerted Action on Sjögren's syndrome. *Arthritis Rheum* 1999;**42**:1765–72.

7. Christodoulou MI, Kapsogeorgou EK, Moutsopoulos HM. Characteristics of the minor salivary gland infiltrates in Sjögren's syndrome. *J Autoimmun* 2010;**34**:400–7.

8. Christodoulou MI, Kapsogeorgou EK, Moutsopoulos NM, Moutsopoulos HM. Foxp3+ T-regulatory cells in Sjögren's syndrome: correlation with the grade of the autoimmune lesion and certain adverse prognostic factors. *Am J Pathol* 2008;**173**:1389–96.

9. Gerli R, Muscat C, Giansanti M, Danieli MG, Sciuto M, Gabrielli A, et al. Quantitative assessment of salivary gland inflammatory infiltration in primary Sjögren's syndrome: its relationship to different demographic, clinical and serological features of the disorder. *Br J Rheumatol* 1997;**36**:969–75.

10. Kapsogeorgou EK, Christodoulou MI, Panagiotakos DB, Paikos S, Tassidou A, Tzioufas AG, et al. Minor salivary gland inflammatory lesions in Sjögren syndrome: do they evolve? *J Rheumatol* 2013;**40**:1566–71.

11. Manoussakis MN, Boiu S, Korkolopoulou P, Kapsogeorgou EK, Kavantzas N, Ziakas P, et al. Rates of infiltration by macrophages and dendritic cells and expression of interleukin-18 and interleukin-12 in the chronic inflammatory lesions of Sjögren's syndrome: correlation with certain features of immune hyperactivity and factors associated with high risk of lymphoma development. *Arthritis Rheum* 2007;**56**:3977–88.

12. Groom J, Kalled SL, Cutler AH, Olson C, Woodcock SA, Schneider P, et al. Association of BAFF/BLyS overexpression and altered B cell differentiation with Sjögren's syndrome. *J Clin Invest* 2002;**109**:59–68.

13. Salomonsson S, Jonsson MV, Skarstein K, Brokstad KA, Hjelmstrom P, Wahren-Herlenius M, et al. Cellular basis of ectopic germinal center formation and autoantibody production in the target organ of patients with Sjögren's syndrome. *Arthritis Rheum* 2003;**48**:3187–201.

14. Dawson LJ, Fox PC, Smith PM. Sjögren's syndrome: the non-apoptotic model of glandular hypofunction. *Rheumatology* 2006;**45**:792–8.

15. Aps JK, Martens LC. Review: the physiology of saliva and transfer of drugs into saliva. *Forensic Sci Int* 2005;**150**:119–31.

16. Konttinen YT, Hukkanen M, Kemppinen P, Segerberg M, Sorsa T, Malmstrom M, et al. Peptide-containing nerves in labial salivary glands in Sjögren's syndrome. *Arthritis Rheum* 1992;**35**:815–20.

17. Pedersen AM, Dissing S, Fahrenkrug J, Hannibal J, Reibel J, Nauntofte B. Innervation pattern and Ca2+ signalling in labial salivary glands of healthy individuals and patients with primary Sjögren's syndrome (pSS). *J Oral Pathol Med* 2000;**29**:97–109.

18. Zoukhri D, Kublin CL. Impaired neurotransmitter release from lacrimal and salivary gland nerves of a murine model of Sjögren's syndrome. *Invest Ophthalmol Vis Sci* 2001;**42**:925–32.

19. Roescher N, Tak PP, Illei GG. Cytokines in Sjögren's syndrome. *Oral Dis* 2009;**15**:519–26.

20. Hurst S, Collins SM. Interleukin-1 beta modulation of norepinephrine release from rat myenteric nerves. *Am J Physiol* 1993;**264**:G30–5.

21. Hurst SM, Collins SM. Mechanism underlying tumor necrosis factor-alpha suppression of norepinephrine release from rat myenteric plexus. *Am J Physiol* 1994;**266**:G1123–9.

22. Zoukhri D, Kublin CL. Impaired neurotransmission in lacrimal and salivary glands of a murine model of Sjögren's syndrome. *Adv Exp Med Biol* 2002;**506**:1023–8.

23. Kublin CL, Hodges RR, Zoukhri D. Proinflammatory cytokine inhibition of lacrimal gland secretion. *Adv Exp Med Biol* 2002;**506**:783–7.

24. Dawson LJ, Christmas SE, Smith PM. An investigation of interactions between the immune system and stimulus-secretion coupling in mouse submandibular acinar cells: a possible mechanism to account for reduced salivary flow rates associated with the onset of Sjögren's syndrome. *Rheumatology* 2000;**39**:1226–33.

25. Nakamura T, Matsui M, Uchida K, Futatsugi A, Kusakawa S, Matsumoto N, et al. M(3) muscarinic acetylcholine receptor plays a critical role in parasympathetic control of salivation in mice. *J Physiol* 2004;**558**:561–75.

26. Beroukas D, Goodfellow R, Hiscock J, Jonsson R, Gordon TP, Waterman SA. Up-regulation of M3-muscarinic receptors in labial salivary gland acini in primary Sjögren's syndrome. *Lab Invest* 2002;**82**:203–10.

27. Lee BH, Gauna AE, Perez G, Park YJ, Pauley KM, Kawai T, et al. Autoantibodies against muscarinic type 3 receptor in Sjögren's syndrome inhibit aquaporin 5 trafficking. *PLoS One* 2013;**8**:e53113.

28. Sumida T, Tsuboi H, Iizuka M, Asashima H, Matsumoto I. Anti-M3 muscarinic acetylcholine receptor antibodies in patients with Sjögren's syndrome. *Mod Rheumatol* 2013;**23**:841–5.

29. Iizuka M, Wakamatsu E, Tsuboi H, Nakamura Y, Hayashi T, Matsui M, et al. Pathogenic role of immune response to M3 muscarinic acetylcholine receptor in Sjögren's syndrome-like sialoadenitis. *J Autoimmun* 2010;**35**:383–9.

30. Dawson LJ, Stanbury J, Venn N, Hasdimir B, Rogers SN, Smith PM. Antimuscarinic antibodies in primary Sjögren's syndrome reversibly inhibit the mechanism of fluid secretion by human submandibular salivary acinar cells. *Arthritis Rheum* 2006;**54**:1165–73.

31. Beroukas D, Hiscock J, Jonsson R, Waterman SA, Gordon TP. Subcellular distribution of aquaporin 5 in salivary glands in primary Sjögren's syndrome. *Lancet* 2001;**358**:1875–6.

32. Steinfeld S, Cogan E, King LS, Agre P, Kiss R, Delporte C. Abnormal distribution of aquaporin-5 water channel protein in salivary glands from Sjögren's syndrome patients. *Lab Invest* 2001;**81**:143–8.

33. Tsubota K, Hirai S, King LS, Agre P, Ishida N. Defective cellular trafficking of lacrimal gland aquaporin-5 in Sjögren's syndrome. *Lancet* 2001;**357**:688–9.

34. Yamamura Y, Motegi K, Kani K, Takano H, Momota Y, Aota K, et al. TNF-alpha inhibits aquaporin 5 expression in human salivary gland acinar cells via suppression of histone H4 acetylation. *J Cell Mol Med* 2012;**16**:1766–75.

35. Steinfeld SD, Appelboom T, Delporte C. Treatment with infliximab restores normal aquaporin 5 distribution in minor salivary glands of patients with Sjögren's syndrome. *Arthritis Rheum* 2002;**46**:2249–51.

36. Wu AM, Csako G, Herp A. Structure, biosynthesis, and function of salivary mucins. *Mol Cell Biochem* 1994;**137**:39–55.

37. Castro I, Sepulveda D, Cortes J, Quest AF, Barrera MJ, Bahamondes V, et al. Oral dryness in Sjögren's syndrome patients: not just a question of water. *Autoimmun Rev* 2012;**12**:567–74.

38. Sung HH, Castro I, Gonzalez S, Aguilera S, Smorodinsky NI, Quest A, et al. MUC1/SEC and MUC1/Y overexpression is associated with inflammation in Sjögren's syndrome. *Oral Dis* 2015;**21**.

39. Bahamondes V, Albornoz A, Aguilera S, Alliende C, Molina C, Castro I, et al. Changes in Rab3D expression and distribution in the acini of Sjögren's syndrome patients are associated with loss of cell polarity and secretory dysfunction. *Arthritis Rheum* 2011;**63**:3126–35.

40. Barrera MJ, Sanchez M, Aguilera S, Alliende C, Bahamondes V, Molina C, et al. Aberrant localization of fusion receptors involved in regulated exocytosis in salivary glands of Sjögren's syndrome patients is linked to ectopic mucin secretion. *J Autoimmun* 2012;**39**:83–92.

41. Alliende C, Kwon YJ, Brito M, Molina C, Aguilera S, Perez P, et al. Reduced sulfation of MUC5b is linked to xerostomia in patients with Sjögren syndrome. *Ann Rheum Dis* 2008;**67**:1480–7.

42. Castro I, Aguilera S, Brockhausen I, Alliende C, Quest AF, Molina C, et al. Decreased salivary sulphotransferase activity correlated with inflammation and autoimmunity parameters in Sjögren's syndrome patients. *Rheumatology* 2012;**51**:482–90.

43. Jimenez F, Aiba-Masago S, Al Hashimi I, Vela-Roch N, Fernandes G, Yeh CK, et al. Activated caspase 3 and cleaved poly(ADP-ribose)polymerase in salivary epithelium suggest a pathogenetic mechanism for Sjögren's syndrome. *Rheumatology* 2002;**41**:338–42.

44. Kong L, Ogawa N, Nakabayashi T, Liu GT, D'Souza E, McGuff HS, et al. Fas and Fas ligand expression in the salivary glands of patients with primary Sjögren's syndrome. *Arthritis Rheum* 1997;**40**:87–97.

45. Manganelli P, Quaini F, Andreoli AM, Lagrasta C, Pilato FP, Zuccarelli A, et al. Quantitative analysis of apoptosis and bcl-2 in Sjögren's syndrome. *J Rheumatol* 1997;**24**:1552–7.

46. Polihronis M, Tapinos NI, Theocharis SE, Economou A, Kittas C, Moutsopoulos HM. Modes of epithelial cell death and repair in Sjögren's syndrome (SS). *Clin Exp Immunol* 1998;**114**:485–90.

47. Ohlsson M, Jonsson R, Brokstad KA. Subcellular redistribution and surface exposure of the Ro52, Ro60 and La48 autoantigens during apoptosis in human ductal epithelial cells: a possible mechanism in the pathogenesis of Sjögren's syndrome. *Scand J Immunol* 2002;**56**:456–69.

48. Rosen A, Casciola-Rosen L, Ahearn J. Novel packages of viral and self-antigens are generated during apoptosis. *J Exp Med* 1995;**181**:1557–61.

49. Okuma A, Hoshino K, Ohba T, Fukushi S, Aiba S, Akira S, et al. Enhanced apoptosis by disruption of the STAT3-IkappaB-zeta signaling pathway in epithelial cells induces Sjögren's syndrome-like autoimmune disease. *Immunity* 2013;**38**:450–60.

50. Varin MM, Guerrier T, Devauchelle-Pensec V, Jamin C, Youinou P, Pers JO. In Sjögren's syndrome, B lymphocytes induce epithelial cells of salivary glands into apoptosis through protein kinase C delta activation. *Autoimmun Rev* 2012;**11**:252–8.

51. Xanthou G, Tapinos NI, Polihronis M, Nezis IP, Margaritis LH, Moutsopoulos HM. CD4 cytotoxic and dendritic cells in the immunopathologic lesion of Sjögren's syndrome. *Clin Exp Immunol* 1999;**118**:154–63.

52. Abu-Helu RF, Dimitriou ID, Kapsogeorgou EK, Moutsopoulos HM, Manoussakis MN. Induction of salivary gland epithelial cell injury in Sjögren's syndrome: in vitro assessment of T cell-derived cytokines and Fas protein expression. *J Autoimmun* 2001;**17**:141–53.

53. Ping L, Ogawa N, Sugai S. Novel role of CD40 in Fas-dependent apoptosis of cultured salivary epithelial cells from patients with Sjögren's syndrome. *Arthritis Rheum* 2005;**52**:573–81.

54. Bolstad AI, Eiken HG, Rosenlund B, Alarcon-Riquelme ME, Jonsson R. Increased salivary gland tissue expression of Fas, Fas ligand, cytotoxic T lymphocyte-associated antigen 4, and programmed cell death 1 in primary Sjögren's syndrome. *Arthritis Rheum* 2003;**48**:174–85.

55. Matsumura R, Umemiya K, Goto T, Nakazawa T, Ochiai K, Kagami M, et al. Interferon gamma and tumor necrosis factor alpha induce Fas expression and anti-Fas mediated apoptosis in a salivary ductal cell line. *Clin Exp Rheumatol* 2000;**18**:311–8.

56. Cha S, Brayer J, Gao J, Brown V, Killedar S, Yasunari U, et al. A dual role for interferon-gamma in the pathogenesis of Sjögren's syndrome-like autoimmune exocrinopathy in the nonobese diabetic mouse. *Scand J Immunol* 2004;**60**:552–65.

57. Wang Y, Shnyra A, Africa C, Warholic C, McArthur C. Activation of the extrinsic apoptotic pathway by TNF-alpha in human salivary gland (HSG) cells in vitro, suggests a role for the TNF receptor (TNF-R) and intercellular adhesion molecule-1 (ICAM-1) in Sjögren's syndrome-associated autoimmune sialadenitis. *Arch Oral Biol* 2009;**54**: 986–96.

58. Sisto M, D'Amore M, Caprio S, Mitolo V, Scagliusi P, Lisi S. Tumor necrosis factor inhibitors block apoptosis of human epithelial cells of the salivary glands. *Ann N Y Acad Sci* 2009;**1171**:407–14.

59. Kulkarni K, Selesniemi K, Brown TL. Interferon-gamma sensitizes the human salivary gland cell line, HSG, to tumor necrosis factor-alpha induced activation of dual apoptotic pathways. *Apoptosis* 2006;**11**:2205–15.

60. Sisto M, Lisi S, Lofrumento D, D'Amore M, Scagliusi P, Mitolo V. Autoantibodies from Sjögren's syndrome trigger apoptosis in salivary gland cell line. *Ann N Y Acad Sci* 2007;**1108**:418–25.

61. Manoussakis MN, Spachidou MP, Maratheftis CI. Salivary epithelial cells from Sjögren's syndrome patients are highly sensitive to anoikis induced by TLR-3 ligation. *J Autoimmun* 2010;**35**:212–8.

62. Horai Y, Nakamura H, Nakashima Y, Hayashi T, Kawakami A. Analysis of the downstream mediators of toll-like receptor 3-induced apoptosis in labial salivary glands in patients with Sjögren's syndrome. *Mod Rheumatol* 2015;**26**:1–6.

63. Katsiougiannis S, Tenta R, Skopouli FN. Endoplasmic reticulum stress causes autophagy and apoptosis leading to cellular redistribution of the autoantigens Ro/SSA and La/SSB in salivary gland epithelial cells. *Clin Exp Immunol* 2015;**62**:414–9.

64. Ishimaru N, Arakaki R, Watanabe M, Kobayashi M, Miyazaki K, Hayashi Y. Development of autoimmune exocrinopathy resembling Sjögren's syndrome in estrogen-deficient mice of healthy background. *Am J Pathol* 2003;**163**:1481–90.

65. Moutsopoulos HM. Sjögren's syndrome: autoimmune epitheliitis. *Clin Immunol Immunopathol* 1994;**72**:162–5.

66. Manoussakis MN, Kapsogeorgou EK. The role of intrinsic epithelial activation in the pathogenesis of Sjögren's syndrome. *J Autoimmun* 2010;**35**:219–24.

67. Dimitriou ID, Kapsogeorgou EK, Abu-Helu RF, Moutsopoulos HM, Manoussakis MN. Establishment of a convenient system for the long-term culture and study of non-neoplastic human salivary gland epithelial cells. *Eur J Oral Sci* 2002;**110**:21–30.

68. Kapsogeorgou EK, Moutsopoulos HM, Manoussakis MN. A novel B7-2 (CD86) splice variant with a putative negative regulatory role. *J Immunol* 2008;**180**:3815–23.

69. Kapsogeorgou EK, Moutsopoulos HM, Manoussakis MN. Functional expression of a costimulatory B7.2 (CD86) protein on human salivary gland epithelial cells that interacts with the CD28 receptor, but has reduced binding to CTLA4. *J Immunol* 2001;**166**:3107–13.

70. Bourazopoulou E, Kapsogeorgou EK, Routsias JG, Manoussakis MN, Moutsopoulos HM, Tzioufas AG. Functional expression of the alpha 2-macroglobulin receptor CD91 in salivary gland epithelial cells. *J Autoimmun* 2009;**33**:141–6.

71. Spachidou MP, Bourazopoulou E, Maratheftis CI, Kapsogeorgou EK, Moutsopoulos HM, Tzioufas AG, et al. Expression of functional Toll-like receptors by salivary gland epithelial cells: increased mRNA expression in cells derived from patients with primary Sjögren's syndrome. *Clin Exp Immunol* 2007;**147**:497–503.

72. Kyriakidis NC, Kapsogeorgou EK, Gourzi VC, Konsta OD, Baltatzis GE, Tzioufas AG. Toll-like receptor 3 stimulation promotes Ro52/TRIM21 synthesis and nuclear redistribution in salivary gland epithelial cells, partially via type I interferon pathway. *Clin Exp Immunol* 2014;**178**:548–60.

73. Nandula SR, Dey P, Corbin KL, Nunemaker CS, Bagavant H, Deshmukh US. Salivary gland hypofunction induced by activation of innate immunity is dependent on type I interferon signaling. *J Oral Pathol Med* 2013;**42**:66–72.

74. Nandula SR, Scindia YM, Dey P, Bagavant H, Deshmukh US. Activation of innate immunity accelerates sialoadenitis in a mouse model for Sjögren's syndrome–like disease. *Oral Dis* 2011;**17**:801–7.

75. Cohen JJ, Duke RC, Fadok VA, Sellins KS. Apoptosis and programmed cell death in immunity. *Annu Rev Immunol* 1992;**10**:267–93.

76. Kapsogeorgou EK, Abu-Helu RF, Moutsopoulos HM, Manoussakis MN. Salivary gland epithelial cell exosomes: a source of autoantigenic ribonucleoproteins. *Arthritis Rheum* 2005;**52**:1517–21.

77. Thery C, Zitvogel L, Amigorena S. Exosomes: composition, biogenesis and function. *Nat Rev Immunol* 2002;**2**:569–79.

78. Gong YZ, Nititham J, Taylor K, Miceli-Richard C, Sordet C, Wachsmann D, et al. Differentiation of follicular helper T cells by salivary gland epithelial cells in primary Sjögren's syndrome. *J Autoimmun* 2014;**51**:57–66.

79. Daridon C, Devauchelle V, Hutin P, Le Berre R, Martins-Carvalho C, Bendaoud B, et al. Aberrant expression of BAFF by B lymphocytes infiltrating the salivary glands of patients with primary Sjögren's syndrome. *Arthritis Rheum* 2007;**56**:1134–44.

80. Ittah M, Miceli-Richard C, Eric Gottenberg J, Lavie F, Lazure T, Ba N, et al. B cell-activating factor of the tumor necrosis factor family (BAFF) is expressed under stimulation by interferon in salivary gland epithelial cells in primary Sjögren's syndrome. *Arthritis Res Ther* 2006;**8**:R51.

81. Hansen A, Daridon C, Dorner T. What do we know about memory B cells in primary Sjögren's syndrome? *Autoimmun Rev* 2010;**9**:600–3.

82. Jonsson MV, Szodoray P, Jellestad S, Jonsson R, Skarstein K. Association between circulating levels of the novel TNF family members APRIL and BAFF and lymphoid organization in primary Sjögren's syndrome. *J Clin Immunol* 2005;**25**:189–201.

83. Morva A, Kapsogeorgou EK, Konsta OD, Moutsopoulos HM, Tzioufas AG. Salivary gland epithelial cells (SGECs) promote the differentiation of B cells. In: *12th International Symposium on Sjögren's Syndrome, Kyoto, Japan*; 2013.

84. Skopouli FN, Kousvelari EE, Mertz P, Jaffe ES, Fox PC, Moutsopoulos HM. c-myc mRNA expression in minor salivary glands of patients with Sjögren's syndrome. *J Rheumatol* 1992;**19**:693–9.

85. Yannopoulos DI, Roncin S, Lamour A, Pennec YL, Moutsopoulos HM, Youinou P. Conjunctival epithelial cells from patients with Sjögren's syndrome inappropriately express major histocompatibility complex molecules, La(SSB) antigen, and heat-shock proteins. *J Clin Immunol* 1992;**12**:259–65.

86. Hjelmervik TO, Petersen K, Jonassen I, Jonsson R, Bolstad AI. Gene expression profiling of minor salivary glands clearly distinguishes primary Sjögren's syndrome patients from healthy control subjects. *Arthritis Rheum* 2005;**52**:1534–44.

87. Gottenberg JE, Cagnard N, Lucchesi C, Letourneur F, Mistou S, Lazure T, et al. Activation of IFN pathways and plasmacytoid dendritic cell recruitment in target organs of primary Sjögren's syndrome. *Proc Natl Acad Sci USA* 2006;**103**:2770–5.

88. Hall JC, Casciola-Rosen L, Berger AE, Kapsogeorgou EK, Cheadle C, Tzioufas AG, et al. Precise probes of type II interferon activity define the origin of interferon signatures in target tissues in rheumatic diseases. *Proc Natl Acad Sci USA* 2012;**109**:17609–14.
89. Gliozzi M, Greenwell-Wild T, Jin W, Moutsopoulos NM, Kapsogeorgou E, Moutsopoulos HM, et al. A link between interferon and augmented plasmin generation in exocrine gland damage in Sjögren's syndrome. *J Autoimmun* 2013;**40**:122–33.
90. Kordossis T, Paikos S, Aroni K, Kitsanta P, Dimitrakopoulos A, Kavouklis E, et al. Prevalence of Sjögren's-like syndrome in a cohort of HIV-1-positive patients: descriptive pathology and immunopathology. *Br J Rheumatol* 1998;**37**:691–5.
91. Mariette X, Zerbib M, Jaccard A, Schenmetzler C, Danon F, Clauvel JP. Hepatitis C virus and Sjögren's syndrome. *Arthritis Rheum* 1993;**36**:280–1.
92. Brookes SM, Pandolfino YA, Mitchell TJ, Venables PJ, Shattles WG, Clark DA, et al. The immune response to and expression of cross-reactive retroviral gag sequences in autoimmune disease. *Br J Rheumatol* 1992;**31**:735–42.
93. Couty JP, Ranger-Rogez S, Vidal E, Rogez JP, Denis F. Study of HHV-8 in primary Sjögren's syndrome. *Clin Exp Rheumatol* 1997;**15**:333–4.
94. Fox RI, Pearson G, Vaughan JH. Detection of Epstein-Barr virus-associated antigens and DNA in salivary gland biopsies from patients with Sjögren's syndrome. *J Immunol* 1986;**137**:3162–8.
95. Saito I, Nishimura S, Kudo I, Fox RI, Moro I. Detection of Epstein-Barr virus and human herpes virus type 6 in saliva from patients with lymphoproliferative diseases by the polymerase chain reaction. *Arch Oral Biol* 1991;**36**:779–84.
96. Shattles WG, Brookes SM, Venables PJ, Clark DA, Maini RN. Expression of antigen reactive with a monoclonal antibody to HTLV-1 P19 in salivary glands in Sjögren's syndrome. *Clin Exp Immunol* 1992;**89**:46–51.
97. Shillitoe EJ, Daniels TE, Whitcher JP, Vibeke Strand C, Talal N, Greenspan JS. Antibody to cytomegalovirus in patients with Sjögren's syndrome: as determined by an enzyme-linked immunosorbent assay. *Arthritis Rheum* 1982;**25**:260–5.
98. Talal N, Dauphinee MJ, Dang H, Alexander SS, Hart DJ, Garry RF. Detection of serum antibodies to retroviral proteins in patients with primary Sjögren's syndrome (autoimmune exocrinopathy). *Arthritis Rheum* 1990;**33**:774–81.
99. Triantafyllopoulou A, Tapinos N, Moutsopoulos HM. Evidence for coxsackievirus infection in primary Sjögren's syndrome. *Arthritis Rheum* 2004;**50**:2897–902.
100. Venables PJ, Ross MG, Charles PJ, Melsom RD, Griffiths PD, Maini RN. A seroepidemiological study of cytomegalovirus and Epstein-Barr virus in rheumatoid arthritis and sicca syndrome. *Ann Rheum Dis* 1985;**44**:742–6.

Chapter 13

# T Cells in the Pathogenesis of Sjögren's Syndrome: More Than Just Th1 and Th2

A. Alunno, E. Bartoloni, R. Gerli
*University of Perugia, Perugia, Italy*

## 1. INTRODUCTION

In the last few decades, T lymphocytes have been widely investigated in the pathogenic scenario of autoimmune diseases. To date, a consistent body of evidence points out the key role of this arm of the immune system in the induction and perpetuation of primary Sjögren's syndrome (SS). The first milestone in this field is the study by Fox et al. who reported in 1983 that the vast majority of infiltrating cells in minor salivary glands (MSGs) of SS patients were T lymphocytes.[1] In fact, these lymphocytes were activated CD4+ cells polarized toward a T helper (Th) 1 phenotype.[2] On this basis, and according to the so-called "Th1/Th2 paradigm," which emerged in the 1990s, SS was classified as a Th1-driven autoimmune disease.[3] In recent years, however, this paradigm was challenged by the discovery of an increasing number of different T-lymphocyte subsets. Therefore several studies attempted to characterize the involvement of regulatory T (Treg) cells, Th17, and other T-cell subpopulations in the induction and perpetuation of chronic autoimmune sialadenitis (Fig 13.1).

Herein we summarize the recent insights on the T-lymphocyte pathogenic role in SS.

## 2. REGULATORY T CELLS IN SJÖGREN'S SYNDROME

Treg cells represent a specialized T-lymphocyte subset able to orchestrate physiological immune responses against pathogens and to interfere with aberrant immune responses against self-antigens, thereby preventing autoimmunity.[4] In 1995, the group of Sakaguchi and colleagues identified a

Sjögren's Syndrome. http://dx.doi.org/10.1016/B978-0-12-803604-4.00013-7

205

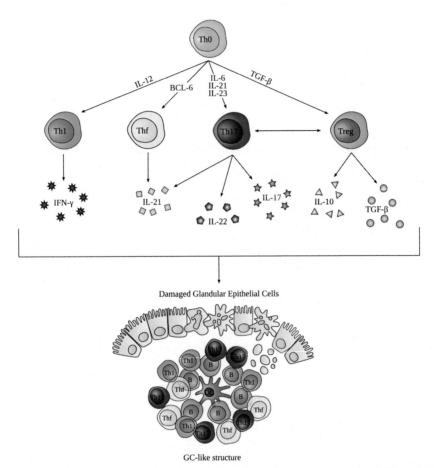

**FIGURE 13.1** T-cell subpopulations and their products in the pathogenesis of Sjögren's syndrome. *BCL*, B-cell lymphoma; *GC*, germinal center; *IFN*, interferon; *IL*, interleukin; *TGF*, transforming growth factor; *Th*, T helper; *Tfh*, follicular T helper; *Treg*, regulatory T cell.

CD4+ T-cell population expressing high surface levels of the interleukin (IL) 2 receptor α-chains (CD25) that was able to prevent systemic autoimmunity in thymectomized mice.[5] Subsequent studies in humans revealed that these cells, named *regulatory* because of their capability to "regulate" autoreactive immune responses, were consistently present in the peripheral blood (PB) of healthy subjects.[6] In the light of the most recent studies, CD4+ Treg cells can be divided into: (1) thymus-derived Treg cells that develop in the thymus in early phases of life and whose phenotype and function remain stable overtime; (2) peripherally derived Treg cells, including Tr1 and Th3, that arise from the extrathymic conversion of effector T cells in the presence of a specific cytokine microenvironment and that are highly flexible and prompt to expand under appropriate signals.[7,8] Although a variety of molecules have been identified in addition to CD25 on Treg cell surface, the forkhead box protein P3 (FoxP3) transcriptional factor remains to date the most specific Treg marker that is also required to confer a regulatory function.[9,10] The upregulation of FoxP3 in naive T cells, namely the polarization toward a Treg phenotype, is mainly driven by transforming growth factor (TGF)-β.

The capability of Treg cells to hamper autoimmune responses by selective deletion of autoreactive lymphocytes via either cell–cell contact or the release of soluble mediators, including IL-10 and TGF-β, represented the rationale to investigate their possible numerical or functional abnormalities in systemic and organ-specific autoimmune disorders. A consistent number of studies have been performed in the last 10 years in SS, often yielding conflicting results.[11–20] Indeed, it should be taken into account that recent studies put forward the hypothesis that high surface expression of CD25 is not mandatory to identify Treg cells, because FoxP3+ suppressive T lymphocytes lacking CD25 have been identified in the PB of normal subjects and patients with systemic lupus erythematosus or SS.[20–22]

On this basis, although the aforementioned studies provided conflicting results concerning the proportion of circulating Treg cells in the PB of SS patients, there is general agreement regarding the consistent expression of FoxP3, independently of that of CD25, within the mononuclear cell infiltrate of SS-MSGs.[12,15,17,20] Of interest, some authors identified a direct association between FoxP3 glandular expression and the severity of the local inflammatory infiltrate.[15,17] This observation is similar to that reported in rheumatoid synovial tissue[23,24] and allows the speculation that Treg cells are actually present in the inflammatory infiltrate, but their suppressive activity may be affected by the local microenvironment. This hypothesis is further supported by in vitro studies revealing that SS circulating Treg cells display a normal suppressive function.[11,12,16,20]

In conclusion, although it is difficult to verify the function of Treg cells in vivo and therefore to draw definitive conclusions, it is reasonable to postulate their involvement in disease pathogenesis (Table 13.1).

## 3. IL-17–PRODUCING T CELLS IN SJÖGREN'S SYNDROME

IL-17 is a family of cytokines which includes six members, from A to F, although the currently used term *IL-17* usually refers to IL-17A.[25] IL-17, identified in 1993 in rodents and in 1995 in humans,[26,27] is a multifaceted cytokine. In fact, since IL-17 receptor is present on the surface of many immune and nonimmune cells, IL-17 is involved in a plethora of physiological processes, including immune defense against infections. Gram-positive and gram-negative bacteria as well as fungi elicit IL-17–mediated immune

**TABLE 13.1 Currently Available Data Concerning Regulatory T Cells and IL-17 Axis in Sjögren's Syndrome**

| Source | Regulatory T Cells | Th17 Cells/IL-17 |
|---|---|---|
| Salivary glands | • FoxP3 expression is associated to the severity of glandular inflammation<br>• Inverse relationship between glandular and circulating FoxP3+ cells<br>• Lower FoxP3+ cells correlate with adverse predictors for lymphoma development<br>• CD25low/-GITR+ T cells are present in mononuclear cell infiltrate | • High expression of IL-17 and IL-17 receptor<br>• High expression of IL-6, IL-21, IL-22, IL-23<br>• CD4+, CD8+, mast cells, and DN T cells produce IL-17<br>• IL-17 is associated with the severity of glandular damage<br>• DN T cells are associated with GCs |
| Saliva/tears | NA | • Increased levels of IL-17 in saliva<br>• Increased levels of IL-17 in tears<br>• No association between salivary IL-17 and glandular damage |
| Serum | NA | • Increased levels of IL-17<br>• Increased levels of IL-6, IL-21, and IL-23<br>• IL-17 prevalence is dependent on disease duration<br>• Serum IL-17 is higher in patients with MSG-GCs |
| Peripheral blood | • Altered Treg cell percentage (increased, decreased, or comparable percentages with respect to HDs)<br>• Inverse correlation between the percentage of Treg cells and CRP, ESR, RF, and IgG<br>• No differences in Treg cell percentage according to ESSDAI and SSDAI<br>• Expansion of functionally suppressive CD25low/-GITR+ T cells<br>• Suppressive CD25low/-GITR+ T cell percentages are expanded in inactive pSS | • Increase of circulating CD4+Th17 cells<br>• Increase of circulating IL-17 + DN T cells |

CRP, C-reactive protein; DN, double negative; ESSDAI, EULAR Sjögren's syndrome disease activity index; ESR, erythrocyte sedimentation rate; EULAR, European League Against Rheumatism; FoxP3, forkhead box protein P3; GITR, glucocorticoid-induced tumor necrosis factor receptor–related protein; GC, germinal center; HD, healthy donor; IgG, immunoglobulin G; IL, interleukin; MSG, minor salivary gland; NA, not available; RF, rheumatoid factor; SSDAI, Sjögren's syndrome disease activity index; Th17, IL-17 producing T helper cells; Treg, T regulatory cells.

responses,[28] but IL-17 is also a leading player in pathological conditions, including cancer and autoimmune disorders.[29] Although several cell types such as neutrophils, mast cells, and natural killer cells are able to produce IL-17,[30] the main cellular source of this cytokine in both physiological and pathological conditions is represented by T lymphocytes. The specific T-cell subset able to secrete IL-17 was identified in 2005 and subsequently named Th17.[31] The polarization of naive T cells toward a Th17 phenotype is a complex multistep process orchestrated by several soluble mediators. The first event, namely the upregulation of the retinoic acid orphan receptor (ROR)γt transcriptional factor, is driven by IL-6, TGF-β, and IL-21. Then the polarization is fostered by IL-6 and IL-1β and, finally, IL-23 stabilizes the Th17 phenotype.[32] Besides IL-17, Th17 cells are able to secrete also IL-21 and IL-22, the former acting as paracrine stimulus to further boost Th17 cells.

The first evidence that IL-17 and therefore IL-17–producing cells may be involved in SS pathogenesis dates back to 2008, when Nguyen et al. described a consistent expression of this cytokine in MSGs of mice with experimental sialadenitis and SS patients.[33] Data from animal models also revealed that while IL-17 knock-out mice do not develop sialadenitis after immunization with salivary peptides,[34] RORγt transgenic mice spontaneously develop sialadenitis-like SS.[35] Interestingly, RORγt transgenic mice also display a lower proportion of circulating Treg cells. This evidence suggests that an imbalance between the Treg and Th17 arm of the immune system is a key event in the pathogenesis of SS.

It is interesting that, at least in mice, Th17 lymphocytes can also act as B-cell helpers.[36] Indeed, they induce a pronounced antibody response and are crucial in germinal center (GC) formation.[37]

It is noteworthy that also most of the cytokines that support the Th17 phenotype as well as other Th17-cell products, including IL-6, IL-21, IL-22, and IL-23 and their receptors, are consistently expressed in MSGs of patients with SS.[33,38–43] Subsequent studies revealed that glandular IL-17 and IL-21 expression appears to be linked to the extent of local inflammation, being directly correlated with the focus score and the Chisholm and Mason score.[44–46] IL-17 is also upregulated in SS biological fluids such as serum,[33,39,44–46] saliva,[47] and tears,[39,48–50] thereby supporting not only a local activity at glandular sites but also a systemic role of this cytokine (Table 13.1). It is worth mentioning that although the main source of glandular and circulating IL-17 in SS is represented by CD4+ and, to a lesser extent, CD8+ T lymphocytes,[51,52] recent data suggest that also a subset of CD3+ T lymphocytes, lacking CD4 and CD8 molecules on the cell surface (double negative), as well as mast cells, participate in such a balance.[41,53,54] Taken together, the available data regarding the IL-17 axis in SS indicate that this system has a clear pathogenic role. Moreover, the lack of any association between IL-17/Th17 cells and the clinical picture or disease activity further underscores their involvement in the induction and maintenance of the disease independently of the different clinical features.

## 4. FOLLICULAR T HELPER CELLS IN SJÖGREN'S SYNDROME

Follicular T helper (Tfh) cells are a specialized T-lymphocyte subset crucial for B-cell help in secondary lymphoid organs.[55,56] The commitment of a naive T cell toward a Tfh phenotype starts in the T-cell area of secondary lymphoid organs where dendritic cells (DCs) induce antigen priming and provide costimulatory signals such as the interaction between inducible T-cell costimulator (ICOS) and ICOS ligand. These initial events lead to the upregulation of the Tfh-specific transcription factor B-cell lymphoma 6 (BCL6). BCL6 drives the upregulation of CXCR5, the receptor of CXCL13, on the cell surface of pre-Tfh cells that are now allowed to migrate to the border between the B- and T-cell area.[57–61] In this site, the interaction between Tfh cells and B lymphocytes triggers a cascade of events culminating in antibody production and the formation of GCs. It should be noted, however, that the cross-talk between Tfh cells and B cells is mutual and provides Tfh cells with the costimulatory signals needed to enter the GCs. Within GCs, BCL6 is also upregulated by B lymphocytes resulting in increased proliferation, somatic hypermutation mediated by activation-induced cytidine deaminase, and differentiation of centroblasts into centrocytes. GC-Tfh cells, together with follicular DCs, also mediate immunoglobulin class-switch recombination in centrocytes, resulting in their differentiation into high-affinity memory B cells and long-lived plasma cells.[62] The peculiar functional features of Tfh cells allowed the speculation of an involvement of this T-cell subset in the pathogenesis of autoimmune diseases.[63] As far as SS is concerned, Tfh-related molecules have been identified within the mononuclear cell infiltrate of MSGs and found to be associated to a more severe glandular inflammation, including the presence of ectopic GCs.[64] Moreover, an expansion of circulating Tfh cells has been reported in the PB of SS patients and, interestingly, this increase was mainly evident in patients with extraglandular manifestations.[65] Given the aforementioned role of Tfh cells in the induction of GCs, these observations fit with the evidence that SS patients displaying ectopic GCs in MSGs experience a more severe disease phenotype.[66] Finally, the polarization of naive T cells into Tfh cells seems to occur at glandular level and to be orchestrated by salivary gland epithelial cells.[67] It is evident, therefore, that Tfh cells represent another pebble in the mosaic of SS pathogenesis, although additional studies are required to shed additional light on this issue and, possibly, provide the rationale for their therapeutic targeting.

## 5. T HELPER 22 AND T HELPER 9 CELLS

Besides Treg, Th17, and Tfh cells, in the last decade, additional T-cell subsets characterized by a peculiar set of surface marker and the production of specific cytokines have been identified. Among these, Th22 and Th9 cells are those best characterized.[68,69] IL-22 is involved in the pathogenesis of psoriasis, rheumatoid arthritis,[70] and probably also SS.[40] In the latter, innate lymphoid cells rather than T lymphocytes appear to be the more consistent source of IL-22 at the glandular level. It should be kept in mind, however, that Th17 and Thf cells can also produce IL-22, thereby rendering this issue more complex. To date, however, detailed studies regarding Th22 cells in SS are not yet available. Similarly, IL-9 and therefore IL-9–producing T lymphocytes (Th9), have been extensively investigated in autoimmune diseases, including rheumatoid arthritis,[71] but no data are available for SS.

# 6. CONCLUDING REMARKS

In the last two decades, a growing number of studies have shed some light on the role of novel T-cell subpopulations in the pathogenesis of SS. Although several aspects need to be clarified and some results may appear contradictory, the majority of studies agree on their possible targeting for therapeutic purposes. The use of novel technologies may help to further elucidate the T-cell–mediated mechanisms occurring in vivo and leading to the induction and perpetuation of the disease.

# REFERENCES

1. Fox RI, Adamson 3rd TC, Fong S, Young C, Howell FV. Characterization of the phenotype and function of lymphocytes infiltrating the salivary gland in patients with primary Sjögren syndrome. *Diagn Immunol* 1983;**1**:233–9.
2. Adamson 3rd TC, Fox RI, Frisman DM, Howell FV. Immunohistologic analysis of lymphoid infiltrates in primary Sjögren's syndrome using monoclonal antibodies. *J Immunol* 1983;**130**:203–8.
3. Boumba D, Skopouli FN, Moutsopoulos HM. Cytokine mRNA expression in the labial salivary gland tissues from patients with primary Sjögren's syndrome. *Br J Rheumatol* 1995;**34**:326–33.
4. Grant CR, Liberal R, Mieli-Vergani G, Vergani D, Longhi MS. Regulatory T-cells in autoimmune diseases: challenges, controversies and yet-unanswered questions. *Autoimmun Rev* 2015;**14**(2):105–16.
5. Sakaguchi S, Sakaguchi N, Asano M, Itoh M, Toda M. Immunologic self-tolerance maintained by activated T cells expressing IL-2 receptor alpha-chains (CD25): breakdown of a single mechanism of self-tolerance causes various autoimmune disease. *J Immunol* 1995;**155**:1151–64.
6. Dieckmann D, Plottner H, Berchtold S, Berger T, Schuler G. Ex vivo isolation of CD4(+) CD25(+) T cells with regulatory properties from human blood. *J Exp Med* 2001;**193**:1303–10.
7. Geiger TL, Tauro S. Nature and nurture in FoxP3(+) regulatory T cell development, stability, and function. *Hum Immunol* 2012;**73**:232–9.
8. Valzasina B, Piconese S, Guiducci C, Colombo MP. Tumor-induced expansion of regulatory T cells by conversion of CD4+CD25− lymphocytes is thymus and proliferation independent. *Cancer Res* 2006;**66**:4488–95.
9. Passerini L, Santoni de Sio FR, Roncarolo MG, Bacchetta R. Forkhead box P3: the peacekeeper of the immune system. *Int Rev Immunol* 2014;**33**(2):129–45.
10. Ramsdell F, Ziegler SF. FoxP3 and scurfy: how it all began. *Nat Rev Immunol* 2014;**14**(5):343–9.
11. Gottenberg JE, Lavie F, Abbed K, Gasnault J, Le Nevot E, Delfraissy JF, et al. CD4 CD25 high regulatory T cells are not impaired in patients with primary Sjögren's syndrome. *J Autoimmun* 2005;**24**(3):235–42.

12. Li X, Li X, Qian L, Wang G, Zhang H, Wang X, et al. T regulatory cells are markedly diminished in diseased salivary glands of patients with primary Sjögren's syndrome. *J Rheumatol* 2007;**34**(12):2438–45.

13. Liu MF, Lin LH, Weng CT, Weng MY. Decreased CD4+CD25+bright T cells in peripheral blood of patients with primary Sjögren's syndrome. *Lupus* 2008;**17**(1):34–9.

14. Miyara M, Amoura Z, Parizot C, Badoual C, Dorgham K, Trad S, et al. Global natural regulatory T cell depletion in active systemic lupus erythematosus. *J Immunol* 2005;**175**(12):8392–400.

15. Christodoulou MI, Kapsogeorgou EK, Moutsopoulos NM, Moutsopoulos HM. FoxP3+ T-regulatory cells in Sjögren's syndrome: correlation with the grade of the autoimmune lesion and certain adverse prognostic factors. *Am J Pathol* 2008;**173**(5):1389–96.

16. Szodoray P, Papp G, Horvath IF, Barath S, Sipka S, Nakken B, et al. Cells with regulatory function of the innate and adaptive immune system in primary Sjögren's syndrome. *Clin Exp Immunol* 2009;**157**(3):343–9.

17. Sarigul M, Yazisiz V, Bassorgun CI, Ulker M, Avci AB, Erbasan F, et al. The numbers of FoxP3+ Treg cells are positively correlated with higher grade of infiltration at the salivary glands in primary Sjögren's syndrome. *Lupus* 2010;**19**(2):138–45.

18. Banica L, Besliu A, Pistol G, Stavaru C, Ionescu R, Forsea AM, et al. Quantification and molecular characterization of regulatory T cells in connective tissue diseases. *Autoimmunity* 2009;**42**(1):41–9.

19. Furuzawa-Carballeda J, Hernández-Molina G, Lima G, Rivera-Vicencio Y, Férez-Blando K, Llorente L. Peripheral regulatory cells immunophenotyping in primary Sjögren's syndrome: a cross-sectional study. *Arthritis Res Ther* 2013;**15**(3):R68.

20. Alunno A, Petrillo MG, Nocentini G, Bistoni O, Bartoloni E, Caterbi S, et al. Characterization of a new regulatory CD4+ T cell subset in primary Sjögren's syndrome. *Rheumatology (Oxford)* 2013;**52**(8):1387–96.

21. Nocentini G, Alunno A, Petrillo MG, Bistoni O, Bartoloni E, Caterbi S, et al. Expansion of regulatory GITR+CD25 low/-CD4+ T cells in systemic lupus erythematosus patients. *Arthritis Res Ther* 2014;**16**(5):444.

22. Zhang B, Zhang X, Tang FL, Zhu LP, Liu Y, Lipsky PE. Clinical significance of increased CD4 + CD25-FoxP3+ T cells in patients with new-onset systemic lupus erythematosus. *Ann Rheum Dis* 2008;**67**:1037–40.

23. van Amelsfort JM, Jacobs KM, Bijlsma JW, Lafeber FP, Taams LS. CD4(+)CD25(+) regulatory T cells in rheumatoid arthritis: differences in the presence, phenotype, and function between peripheral blood and synovial fluid. *Arthritis Rheum* 2004;**50**(9):2775–85.

24. Möttönen M, Heikkinen J, Mustonen L, Isomäki P, Luukkainen R, Lassila O. CD4+CD25+ T cells with the phenotypic and functional characteristics of regulatory T cells are enriched in the synovial fluid of patients with rheumatoid arthritis. *Clin Exp Immunol* 2005;**140**(2):360–7.

25. Gu C, Wu L, Li X. IL-17 family: cytokines, receptors and signaling. *Cytokine* 2013;**64**(2):477–85.

26. Rouvier E, Luciani MF, Mattei MG, Denizot F, Golstein P. CTLA-8, cloned from an activated T cell, bearing AU-rich messenger RNA instability sequences, and homologous to a herpesvirus saimiri gene. *J Immunol* 1993;**150**:5445–56.

27. Yao Z, Painter SL, Fanslow WC, Ulrich D, Macduff BM, Spriggs MK, et al. Human IL 17: a novel cytokine derived from T cells. *J Immunol* 1995;**155**:5483–6.

28. Milner JD, Brenchley JM, Laurence A, Freeman AF, Hill BJ, Elias KM, et al. Impaired T(H)17 cell differentiation in subjects with autosomal dominant hyper-IgE syndrome. *Nature* 2008;**452**:773–6.

29. van den Berg WB, McInnes IB. Th17 cells and IL-17 a focus on immunopathogenesis and immunotherapeutics. *Semin Arthritis Rheum* 2013;**43**(2):158–70.

30. Hueber AJ, Asquith DL, Miller AM, Reilly J, Kerr S, Leipe J, et al. Mast cells express IL-17A in rheumatoid arthritis synovium. *J Immunol* 2010;**184**(7):3336–40.

31. Harrington LE, Hatton RD, Mangan PR, Turner H, Murphy TL, Murphy KM, et al. IL 17 producing CD4+ effector T cells develop via a lineage distinct from the T helper type 1 and 2 lineages. *Nat Immunol* 2005;**6**:1123–32.

32. Noack M, Miossec P. Th17 and regulatory T cell balance in autoimmune and inflammatory diseases. *Autoimmun Rev* 2014;**13**(6):668–77.

33. Nguyen CQ, Hu MH, Li Y, Stewart C, Peck AB. Salivary gland tissue expression of interleukin-23 and interleukin-17 in Sjögren's syndrome: findings in humans and mice. *Arthritis Rheum* 2008;**58**(3):734–43.

34. Lin X, Rui K, Deng J, Tian J, Wang X, Wang S. Th17 cells play a critical role in the development of experimental Sjögren's syndrome. *Ann Rheum Dis* 2015;**74**(6):1302–10.

35. Iizuka M, Tsuboi H, Matsuo N, Asashima H, Hirota T, Kondo Y. A crucial role of RORγt in the development of spontaneous Sialadenitis-like Sjögren's syndrome. *J Immunol* 2015;**194**:56–67.

36. Mitsdoerffer M, Lee Y, Jäger A, Kim HJ, Korn T, Kolls JK, et al. Proinflammatory T helper type 17 cells are effective B-cell helpers. *Proc Natl Acad Sci USA* 2010;**107**(32):14292–7.

37. Hsu HC, Yang P, Wang J, Wu Q, Myers R, Chen J, et al. Interleukin 17–producing T helper cells and interleukin 17 orchestrate autoreactive germinal center development in autoimmune BXD2 mice. *Nat Immunol* 2008;**9**(2):166–75.

38. Katsifis GE, Rekka S, Moutsopoulos NM, Pillemer S, Wahl SM. Systemic and local interleukin-17 and linked cytokines associated with Sjögren's syndrome immunopathogenesis. *Am J Pathol* 2009;**175**(3):1167–77.

39. Kang KY, Kim HO, Kwok SK, Ju JH, Park KS, Sun DI, et al. Impact of interleukin-21 in the pathogenesis of primary Sjögren's syndrome: increased serum levels of interleukin-21 and its expression in the labial salivary glands. *Arthritis Res Ther* 2011;**13**(5):R179.

40. Ciccia F, Guggino G, Rizzo A, Ferrante A, Raimondo S, Giardina A, et al. Potential involvement of IL-22 and IL-22-producing cells in the inflamed salivary glands of patients with Sjögren's syndrome. *Ann Rheum Dis* 2012;**71**(2):295–301.

41. Ciccia F, Guggino G, Rizzo A, Alessandro R, Carubbi F, Giardina A, et al. Rituximab modulates IL-17 expression in the salivary glands of patients with primary Sjögren's syndrome. *Rheumatology (Oxford)* 2014;**53**(7):1313–20.

42. Mieliauskaite D, Dumalakiene I, Rugiene R, Mackiewicz Z. Expression of IL-17, IL-23 and their receptors in minor salivary glands of patients with primary Sjögren's syndrome. *Clin Dev Immunol* 2012;**2012**:187258.

43. Maehara T, Moriyama M, Hayashida JN, Tanaka A, Shinozaki S, Kubo Y, et al. Selective localization of T helper subsets in labial salivary glands from primary Sjögren's syndrome patients. *Clin Exp Immunol* 2012;**169**(2):89–99.

44. Fei Y, Zhang W, Lin D, Wu C, Li M, Zhao Y, et al. Clinical parameter and Th17 related to lymphocytes infiltrating degree of labial salivary gland in primary Sjögren's syndrome. *Clin Rheumatol* 2014;**33**(4):523–9.

45. Reksten TR, Jonsson MV, Szyszko EA, Brun JG, Jonsson R, Brokstad KA. Cytokine and autoantibody profiling related to histopathological features in primary Sjögren's syndrome. *Rheumatology (Oxford)* 2009;**48**(9):1102–6.

46. Alunno A, Bistoni O, Caterbi S, Bartoloni E, Cafaro G, Gerli R. Serum interleukin-17 in primary Sjögren's syndrome: association with disease duration and parotid gland swelling. *Clin Exp Rheumatol* 2015;**33**(1):129.

47. Ohyama K, Moriyama M, Hayashida JN, Tanaka A, Maehara T, Ieda S, et al. Saliva as a potential tool for diagnosis of dry mouth including Sjögren's syndrome. *Oral Dis* 2015;**21**(2):224–31.

48. Lee SY, Han SJ, Nam SM, Yoon SC, Ahn JM, Kim TI, et al. Analysis of tear cytokines and clinical correlations in Sjögren syndrome dry eye patients and non-Sjögren syndrome dry eye patients. *Am J Ophthalmol* 2013;**156**(2):247–53.e1.

49. Tan X, Sun S, Liu Y, Zhu T, Wang K, Ren T, et al. Analysis of Th17-associated cytokines in tears of patients with dry eye syndrome. *Eye (Lond)* 2014;**28**(5):608–13.

50. Chung JK, Kim MK, Wee WR. Prognostic factors for the clinical severity of keratoconjunctivitis sicca in patients with Sjögren's syndrome. *Br J Ophthalmol* 2012;**96**(2):240–5.

51. Sakai A, Sugawara Y, Kuroishi T, Sasano T, Sugawara S. Identification of IL-18 and Th17 cells in salivary glands of patients with Sjögren's syndrome, and amplification of IL-17–mediated secretion of inflammatory cytokines from salivary gland cells by IL-18. *J Immunol* 2008;**181**(4):2898–906.

52. Kwok SK, Cho ML, Her YM, Oh HJ, Park MK, Lee SY, et al. TLR2 ligation induces the production of IL-23/IL-17 via IL-6, STAT3 and NF-κB pathway in patients with primary Sjögren's syndrome. *Arthritis Res Ther* 2012;**14**(2):R64.

53. Alunno A, Bistoni O, Bartoloni E, Caterbi S, Bigerna B, Tabarrini A, et al. IL-17-producing CD4−CD8− T cells are expanded in the peripheral blood, infiltrate salivary glands and are resistant to corticosteroids in patients with primary Sjögren's syndrome. *Ann Rheum Dis* 2013;**72**(2):286–92.

54. Alunno A, Carubbi F, Bistoni O, Caterbi S, Bartoloni E, Bigerna B, et al. CD4(−)CD8(−) T-cells in primary Sjögren's syndrome: association with the extent of glandular involvement. *J Autoimmun* 2014;**51**:38–43.

55. Ma CS, Suryani S, Avery DT, Chan A, Nanan R, Santner-Nanan B, et al. Early commitment of naïve human CD4(+) T cells to the T follicular helper (T(FH)) cell lineage is induced by IL-12. *Immunol Cell Biol* 2009;**87**(8):590–600.

56. Schmitt N, Morita R, Bourdery L, Bentebibel SE, Zurawski SM, Banchereau J, et al. Human dendritic cells induce the differentiation of interleukin-21-producing T follicular helper-like cells through interleukin-12. *Immunity* 2009;**31**(1):158–69.

57. Kim CH, Rott LS, Clark-Lewis I, Campbell DJ, Wu L, Butcher EC. Subspecialization of CXCR5+ T cells: B helper activity is focused in a germinal center-localized subset of CXCR5+ T cells. *J Exp Med* 2001;**193**(12):1373–81.

58. Hardtke S, Ohl L, Förster R. Balanced expression of CXCR5 and CCR7 on follicular T helper cells determines their transient positioning to lymph node follicles and is essential for efficient B-cell help. *Blood* 2005;**106**(6):1924–31.

59. Haynes NM, Allen CD, Lesley R, Ansel KM, Killeen N, Cyster JG. Role of CXCR5 and CCR7 in follicular Th cell positioning and appearance of a programmed cell death gene-1 high germinal center-associated subpopulation. *J Immunol* 2007;**179**(8):5099–108.

60. Kroenke MA, Eto D, Locci M, Cho M, Davidson T, Haddad EK, et al. Bcl6 and Maf cooperate to instruct human follicular helper CD4 T cell differentiation. *J Immunol* 2012;**188**(8):3734–44.

61. Nurieva RI, Chung Y, Martinez GJ, Yang XO, Tanaka S, Matskevitch TD, et al. BCL6 mediates the development of T follicular helper cells. *Science* 2009;**325**(5943):1001–5.

62. Tangye SG, Ma CS, Brink R, Deenick EK. The good, the bad and the ugly: TFH cells in human health and disease. *Nat Rev Immunol* 2013;**13**(6):412–26.

63. Craft JE. Follicular helper T cells in immunity and systemic autoimmunity. *Nat Rev Rheumatol* 2012;**8**:337–47.

64. Szabo K, Papp G, Dezso B, Zeher M. The histopathology of labial salivary glands in primary Sjögren's syndrome: focusing on follicular helper T cells in the inflammatory infiltrates. *Mediators Inflamm* 2014;**2014**:631787.

65. Szabo K, Papp G, Barath S, Gyimesi E, Szanto A, Zeher M. Follicular helper T cells may play an important role in the severity of primary Sjögren's syndrome. *Clin Immunol* 2013;**147**:95–104.

66. Carubbi F, Alunno A, Cipriani P, Di Benedetto P, Ruscitti P, Berardicurti O, et al. Is minor salivary gland biopsy more than a diagnostic tool in primary Sjögren's syndrome? Association between clinical, histopathological, and molecular features: a retrospective study. *Semin Arthritis Rheum* 2014;**44**(3):314–24.

67. Gong YZ, Nititham J, Taylor K, Miceli-Richard C, Sordet C, Wachsmann D, et al. Differentiation of follicular helper T cells by salivary gland epithelial cells in primary Sjögren's syndrome. *J Autoimmun* 2014;**51**:57–66.

68. Trifari S, Kaplan CD, Tran EH, Crellin NK, Spits H. Identification of a human helper T cell population that has abundant production of interleukin 22 and is distinct from T(H)-17, T(H)1 and T(H)2 cells. *Nat Immunol* 2009;**10**:864–71.

69. Schmitt E, Klein M, Bopp T. Th9 cells, new players in adaptive immunity. *Trends Immunol* 2014;**35**(2):61–8.

70. Yang X, Zheng SG. Interleukin-22: a likely target for treatment of autoimmune diseases. *Autoimmun Rev* 2014;**13**:615–20.

71. Ciccia F, Guggino G, Rizzo A, Manzo A, Vitolo B, La Manna MP, et al. Potential involvement of IL-9 and Th9 cells in the pathogenesis of rheumatoid arthritis. *Rheumatology (Oxford)* 2015. http://dx.doi.org/10.1093/rheumatology/kev252.

Chapter 14

# B Lymphocytes in Primary Sjögren's Syndrome

## J.-O. Pers, P. Youinou

*EA2216, INSERM ESPRI, ERI29, Université de Brest, Brest, France; LabEx IGO, Brest, France*

Primary Sjögren's syndrome (pSS) is a chronic autoimmune systemic disease, characterized by a lymphoplasmacytic infiltration, causing a progressive destruction of epithelial cells (ECs) of lacrimal and salivary glands (SGs) and ending up with ocular and mouth dryness. Beyond these sicca symptoms, half of these patients develop extraglandular complications such as arthritis, lung interstitial disease, nervous system involvement, and/or tubular nephropathy.

A long-held wisdom has been that pSS proceeds from T lymphocytes, with B lymphocytes confined, under their strict control, to the production of antibodies (Abs). Recently, the physiology of B cells has been revolutionized by the attribution of a number of new functions. We have indeed seen ever-growing evidence that B cells do not have the exclusive rights to turn into plasma cells (PCs) as the way to manufacture and secrete anti-self Abs. Actually, their effects in the pathophysiology of pSS are so multiple that this pathology may now be regarded as a quintessential B-cell–induced autoimmune disease. Such considerations have provided the rationale for developing strategies aimed at depleting B cells to treat patients with pSS.

## 1. B-CELL HYPERACTIVITY IS A HALLMARK OF PRIMARY SJÖGREN'S SYNDROME

Under the pretext of their predominance over the B lymphocytes within the aggregates infiltrating patients' exocrine glands, T lymphocytes have long been endowed with a leading role in the pathophysiology of their disease.[1] In opposition to this paradigm, evidence has since been accumulating to highlight the dominant contribution of B lymphocytes. Not only do they produce autoAbs, but they also make several cytokines and act as antigen (Ag)-presenting cells. Furthermore, they may differentiate into two types of effector cells, Be1 producing T helper (Th) 1 cytokines and Be2 producing Th2 cytokines.[1] Noteworthy is that Be1 and Be2 have the capacity to initiate Th1 and Th2 polarization, respectively. Which cells trigger the others looks like a catch-22 problem. In addition, mice have been transfected

Sjögren's Syndrome. http://dx.doi.org/10.1016/B978-0-12-803604-4.00014-9

with the gene for the B-cell activating factor (BAFF) of the tumor necrosis factor (TNF) family, a cytokine that rescues from B cells in general apoptosis and autoreactive B cells in particular. These transgenic (Tg) mice develop autoimmune traits reminiscent of pSS.[2] The importance of BAFF is supported by the fact that patients with pSS parallel their serum levels of BAFF with the production of autoAbs.[3] Moreover, the distribution of mature B (Bm) cell subsets from Bm1 through Bm5 in the peripheral blood (PB) of patients with pSS is characterized by higher percentage of Bm2 and Bm2', compared with that of normal controls, as well as with control patients with other autoimmune diseases such as rheumatoid arthritis (RA) and systemic lupus erythematosus (SLE).[4] Finally, B-cell infiltrates may form ectopic germinal centers (GCs) in the SGs.[5] Thus B cells are deeply involved in the genesis of pSS and thereby hold promise as therapeutic targets.

## 2. B-CELL CLASSIFICATION ACCORDING TO THEIR ONTOGENIC STATE

B cells originate in the bone marrow (BM). As soon as they have productively rearranged their immunoglobulin (Ig) variable genes, pro–B cells proceed to the pre–B-cell stage. On their arrival to the spleen, immature B cells give rise to type–1, type–2, and possibly type 3 transitional B (BT) cells.[6] As BT cells, they are pushed into migrating from the BM to secondary lymphoid organs (SLOs). There they carry on maturing and are sustaining selection by Ags. As BT1, they present as CD20+CD5+CD10+/–CD21+/–CD23+/–IgM+IgD+/– and CD38+, but once they have evolved to BT2, they become CD20+CD5+/– CD21++CD23+/–IgM++IgD++ and CD38+/–. Importantly, these latter BT2 cells accumulate in the SGs of patients with pSS.[7] Let's come back to the SLO where BT2 cells differentiate either into circulating lymphocytes that, on their way, get organized as GCs, or into noncirculating lymphocytes that are prone to populate the marginal zone (MZ). Progression of these BT2 cells toward the MZ or GCs may be determined by the quality of their B-cell receptor (BCR)–evoked signals and the subsequent expression of the Notch proteins.[8] Alternatively, MZ B cells with mutated Ig genes, but without activation-induced cytidine deaminase, may have passed a GC response.[9] To end it up, the expression of sphingosine 1–phosphate receptor 1 on B lymphocytes does overcome the recruiting activity of the B-cell–attracting (BCA) chemokine 1 to the GCs, and thereby retain B cells inside the MZ.[10] In this regard, it is interesting that BCA-1 (CXCL13) is expressed in the lymphoid follicles,[11] and its receptor upregulated by B cells of pSS patients (Fig. 14.1).[12]

## 3. B LYMPHOCYTES IN SALIVARY GLANDS

In parallel with their decreased number of memory B cells in the PB, memory CD20+ CD27+ B cells settle down in the SGs, whereas nearby infiltrating B cells present as hyperreactive. This is indicated by elevated proportion and level of Ig with autoAb activity.[13] However, we have recently identified novel

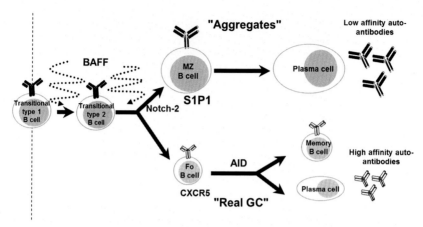

**FIGURE 14.1**    On their arrival from the bone marrow, immature B cells give rise to type 1 and type 2 transitional B cells. Only a minor fraction of immature B cells survive the shift from immature to the mature naive stage, so that the transitional B-cell compartment is widely believed to represent a negative selection checkpoint for autoreactive B cells. Importantly, B-cell activating factor (BAFF) facilitates the maintenance of B cells through this checkpoint. The consequence of a local excess of BAFF is that self-reactive B cells are unduly rescued from deletion and thereby offered the possibility to enter forbidden follicular (Fo) and marginal zone (MZ) niches. B lymphocytes differentiate into MZ or into Fo B cells, depending on the affinity of the B-cell receptors (BCRs) to their antigens (Ags). In salivary glands (SGs), a minority of B-cell clusters represent genuine germinal center (GC) cells, whereas the majority manifest features of being transitional B (BT) 2 and MZ cells. Interestingly, both types of B-cell "aggregates" include autoreactive B cells. *AID*, Activation-induced cytidine deaminase; *S1P1*, sphingosine 1-phosphate receptor 1.

transitional B cells, thus far misinterpreted because of their expression of CD27, which used to be viewed as associated with a memory B-cell phenotype. This subset of CD27+ transitional B cells has the capacity to produce high levels of interleukin (IL) 10 and the specificity to neutralize proinflammatory cytokines.[14] As a consequence, some of those CD27+ B cells found in the SGs of patients with pSS and described as memory B cells could in fact correspond to our transitional CD27+ B cells. In the inflammatory tissue, the distribution of PCs into producers of different Ig isotypes is altered. In patients, the IgG− and IgM− producing PCs predominate over those producing IgA, whereas in the controls, the main isotype selected by PCs is IgA.[15,16] B lymphocytes infiltrating SGs may be driven oligoclonal or monoclonal[17–19] and locally produce rheumatoid factor and anti-Ro/SSA and anti-La/SSB auto-Abs.[20,21] B cell clustering into aggregates and GC-like structures are detectable in up to one-third of the SG samples (Fig. 14.2) and coincide with elevated titers of rheumatoid factor, increased serum levels of IgG, and elevated focus score in the SGs.[22] The local high expression of BAFF by infiltrating mononuclear cells and ECs has been implicated in the expansion of autoreactive B lymphocytes, the altered B-cell differentiation and distribution, GC-like structure formation, and lymphoma transformation. In a retrospective study, it has been proposed that the presence of GC-like structures

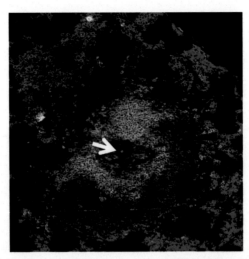

**FIGURE 14.2** Two-color immunofluorescence (FITC-conjugated anti-immunoglobulin D (IgD) and TRITC-conjugated anti-CD38 antibodies) staining of salivary gland biopsy of patient with primary Sjögren's syndrome (pSS). Ectopic germinal center (GC) (*arrow*) is shown as CD38-positive B cells surrounded by IgD-positive naive B cells. T-cell infiltrate (in red) corresponds to CD38-positive T cells.

in diagnostic SG biopsy might be used as a highly predictive marker for the development of non-Hodgkin lymphoma.[23]

Nonetheless, genuine GCs are less common in pSS than previously claimed. Notably, in patients' SGs aggregates, B cells lack the GC B-cell–associated CD10 and CD38 markers.[5] Furthermore, we didn't find the transcripts for activation-induced cytidine deaminase in most of the micro-dissected GC-like cell aggregates from SGs of pSS patients. Thus the presence of B-cell aggregates in the SGs does not necessarily mean that these are functional GCs.[5] On the other hand, immature pre-GC B cells have been identified in these SG aggregates.[7] BAFF produced in the nearby tissue encourages the formation of such aggregates. Immunohistological analyses of the primary effects after B-cell depletion by rituximab (RTX) in SGs have brought about relevant insights into the occurrence of B-cell abnormalities in pSS. After treatment with RTX, lymphocytic infiltrates of SGs were reduced, with decrease of the lymphoepithelial lesion and partial disappearance of GC-like structures.[24] Our group showed that, although the PB repopulation after RTX-induced B-cell elimination first mimics a second round of B-cell ontogeny, the characteristic abnormalities of circulating B-cell reoccur later. There is a predominance of naive B cells and a low number of memory B cells.[25] Memory and BT cells were the first B lymphocytes to repopulate the SGs. This sequence resembles the pathophysiology of memory B-cell accumulation and strongly suggests that the local micro-environment contributes to B-cell abnormalities in the disease.

## 4. B LYMPHOCYTES IN PERIPHERAL BLOOD

Increase of CD5+ B lymphocytes have been described in the PB and the SGs of the patients with pSS,[26] as well as those with RA or SLE.

In contrast, the distribution of B-cell subsets is markedly abnormal in the PB of patients with pSS, compared with those with RA or SLE. For example, as previously mentioned, memory B cells accumulate in target epithelial organs and form tertiary lymphoid structures, whereas their proportion is decreased in the PB[7,13] and those of transitional and naive B cells increased.[27] The developmental stages of GC B cells are based on the relative expression of IgD and CD38 on Bm lymphocytes[28] from naive cells (Bm1) just exiting the BM to memory B cells activated and differentiated by their specific Ag (Bm5). The development starts with CD38−IgD+ naive Bm1 that progresses into CD38+IgD+ Ag-activated Bm2, of which some become CD38++IgD+ Bm2′ GC founder cells. These differentiate into CD38++IgD−Bm3 centroblasts and Bm4 centrocytes. Finally, two types of B cells arise from GC reactions: CD38+IgD− early memory B lymphocytes that mature locally into CD38−IgD−Bm5 late memory B cells on the one hand, and CD38++IgD− plasmablasts on the other. They were first described by Odendahl et al.[29] and return to the BM where they differentiate into long-lived PCs. A few cells of each subset escape into the circulation from GCs. For unknown reasons, distribution of Bm cells is abnormal in the PB of patients with pSS.[13,30] Our group showed that a high (Bm2 + Bm2′)/ (eBm5 + Bm5) ratio (≥5) was strongly associated with a diagnosis of pSS, when compared with RA and SLE.[4]

In addition to this abnormal distribution, the membrane expression of CD72, a transmembrane lectin expressed throughout the period of B-cell maturation that can both positively and negatively modulate BCR-mediated signaling, is upregulated in B lymphocytes from pSS patients relative to those with RA or SLE.[31]

Here, we're going further in depth by exploring the regulatory B cells (Bregs). First studied in murine models of autoimmune diseases, a novel role has been ascribed to a subset of B cells, called Bregs. Although their phenotypic characterization is not completed in humans, strong evidence supports that they control the proliferation and differentiation of T cells[32] and dendritic cells.[33] We may assert that, in autoimmune diseases, Bregs play a central role in the dysregulation of the immune system, and thereby in the loss of tolerance.[34] Although we and others have demonstrated that these Breg cells were deficient in SLE, such was not the case in pSS.[32,35]

Based on flow cytometric staining of memory B cells with CD27 and IgD, a significant reduction of peripheral CD27+IgD+IgM+ memory B cells (having not undergone isotype switching) has been reported in patients with pSS, along with an enhanced surface-expression of HLA-DR, CD38, and CD95, as well as a reduced surface-expression of CD21, CXCR5, and inducible T-cell costimulator ligand.[36] This may reflect impaired differentiation and censoring mechanisms within SLOs and/or ectopic GCs. Classical memory B cells (CD27+IgD–IgM–) generated in GCs are markedly reduced in the PB of these patients, although they accumulated in inflamed tissues. Chemokine receptor–ligand interactions, especially CXCL12–CXCR4 and CXCL13–CXCR5 interactions may, at least in part, explain B-cell abnormalities in pSS and decrease of circulating memory B cells.[30]

## 5. INTRINSIC B-CELL DEFECTS

The cause of B-cell hyperactivity in pSS is not known, but at least three different intrinsic abnormalities have been identified. First, preswitch Ig transcripts are retained in circulating memory B cells, regardless of the advent or not of post-switch Ig transcripts. Secondly, the kinetics of BCR translocation to the lipid-rich membrane signaling microdomains, referred to as the lipid rafts (LRs), is altered in pSS.[27] There is evidence of prolonged translocation of the BCR into the LRs in B cells, resulting in inappropriately enhanced signaling. Thirdly, elevated serum and salivary levels of BAFF in pSS are responsible for B-cell survival and hyperactivity. The single-cell analysis technology has indeed enabled us to see that messenger RNA for BAFF exists in B cells from SGs. For this to occur, the downstream negative regulator of BAFF-mediated B-cell survival has to be inhibited.[37] Equally important in distinguishing the role of B cells in the pathogenesis of pSS is that BAFF potentiates the B-cell selection with the BCR complex,[38] and synergizes with IL-21 at that site.[39] Growing evidence suggests also that the signaling mechanisms that maintain B-cell fitness during selection at transitional stages, and survival after maturation, rely on cross-talk between BCR and one of the receptors for BAFF.[40] Of important note in this regard, is the fact that the preexisting levels of BAFF correlate inversely with the number of months B cells take to repopulate the PB of RTX-treated patients with pSS.[25] Supporting this concept are two observations: on the one hand that some patients resist RTX because of the local overexpression of BAFF in their SGs,[41] on the other that human CD20-Tg autoimmune-prone mice with elevated levels of BAFF resist the anti-CD20 monoclonal Ab RTX.[42] Thus B-cell infiltration would be modulated by BAFF in SGs,[43] but not in lupus nephritis.[44]

## 6. AUTOREACTIVITY-DRIVEN B LYMPHOCYTE PROLIFERATION

Autoreactive BT1 and BT2 lymphocytes may accumulate in an area resembling the splenic MZ, and hence serving as a fast track to autoimmunity. In SGs, this event is likely to happen, because SG-cell aggregates appear to primarily include BT2 and MZ-like B cells.[7] These clusters of MZ-like B cells serve as reservoirs for autoreactive B cells. Because of the permanent availability of autoAgs, a clone can be transformed and thereby become dominant. BAFF-Tg mice that lack MZ B cells develop nephritis but not sialadenitis.[44] These data demonstrate that the development of autoimmune epitheliitis requires the presence of MZ B cells.

The development of lymphoma may arise secondary to the autoimmune response. Sustained stimulation promotes the expansion of scarce clones and results in the outgrowth of monoclonal aggregates of B lymphocytes.[45] Thus B-cell transformation from the naive stage to a mature proliferating single clone through to a nonmalignant pseudolymphoma stage represents a continuum.

## 7. B-CELL–DERIVED CYTOKINES

Recent discoveries have unveiled new insights into B-cell–derived cytokines, including interferon (IFN) γ, and IL-4 that modulate the immune response.[46] They are likely to modulate some B cells' functions. Given the kinetics of B-cell generation and the cytokine profile of B lymphocytes, Th1 phenotype may be imprinted by Be1 cells through their expression of IL-2 and IFNγ by B cells. This is sustained by an IFNγ/IFNγ receptor autocrine loop. Conversely, Th2 cells induced naive B-cell polarization into Be2 cells, which produce IL-4 and IL-6 in the absence of GATA-3. In fact, the Th1/Th2 cytokine balance changes with the progress of immunopathological lesions.[47] Distinct populations of serum cytokines have also been found to differentiate patients from controls, and a given patient from another, depending on the presence or absence of extraglandular complications.[48] B-cell–produced cytokines may be classified as proinflammatory (IL-1, IL-6, TNF-α, and lymphotoxin-α), immunosuppressive cytokines (TGF-β and IL-10), or as hematopoietic growth factors (granulocyte/ monocyte-colony stimulating factor and IL-17).

The B-cell growth factor IL-14 has been extensively studied in animal models. Mice Tg for this cytokine develop clinical and immunological characteristics of pSS. In humans, the cells from patients express higher levels of IL-14 compared with controls.[49] Interestingly, IL-14 Tg mice develop clinical and immunological characteristic of pSS in the same order as human pathology (from early hypergammaglobulinemia to B-cell lymphoma), suggesting that this cytokine may play an essential role in pSS pathogenesis.

In pSS, IL-6 not only participates in the generation of Th17 cells but also activates local B cells in an autocrine manner. Th17 cells induced in the presence of IL-6 orchestrate the GC's development by autoreactive lymphocytes,[50] such as those that our group has described in SGs from these patients.[5] IL-6 contributes to the expression of recombination-activating gene. Results from our laboratory have shown that IL-6 signaling results in secondary Ab gene rearrangements, and, by doing so, favors the autoAb synthesis.[51]

## 8. INTERCONNECTIONS BETWEEN B- AND T-CELL CYTOKINE NETWORKS

Activated Th cells and activated B cells cross-talk with each other to regulate their reciprocal responses, inasmuch as Be cells modulate T-cell polarization. The factors that affect T-cell differentiation toward Th1 cells induce naive B cells to produce IFN-γ via activation of STAT-3, the phosphorylation of which is initiated by IL-12.[52] Once B cells have been induced to produce IFN-γ, Th1 is no longer required to maintain polarized Be cells. Aside from promoting Th1 cell polarization, Be1 cells amplify IFN-γ production by T cells via a TNF-α–mediated mechanism. Further, IL-10 produced by B cells suppresses IL-12 production by dendritic cells, thus blocking Th1 cell responses.

## 9. EPIGENETIC DYSREGULATIONS IN SALIVARY GLANDS IS ASCRIBED TO B CELLS

We have reported that global DNA methylation in patients with pSS was reduced in SGs, when comparing their biopsy sections with those of the controls. This defect was conserved when ECs eluted from the SGs were primarily cultured.[53] At the molecular level, global DNA demethylation of ECs was accounted for by a decrease in the methylating enzyme DNMT1 associated with an increase in its demethylating partner Gadd45-α. Our observations support an active DNA demethylation process in SG ECs from pSS patients. Furthermore, SG EC DNA methylation levels were inversely correlated with the severity of the disease, and the amount of infiltrating B cells. We further studied the contribution of B cells in the demethylation process in pSS patients treated with RTX, in the frame of our TEARS study.[53,54] Indeed, global DNA methylation levels were higher 4 months after B-cell depletion in comparison with the minor SG biopsy obtained at the initiation of RTX therapy, thus suggesting that DNA demethylation in ECs may be caused in part by infiltrating B cells. Our hypothesis was confirmed in vitro, revealing in coculture that B-cell–mediated DNA demethylation in ECs works through an alteration of the Erk/DNMT1 pathway.[55]

## 10. CONCLUSION

No doubt, the reader is now convinced that there is a striking revival of interest in B lymphocytes as contributors to the cause of pSS. There remain significant unmet needs in the current approaches to patient management. Still, this is palliative, aimed at diminishing symptoms, but new insights into B-cell behavior allow new approaches.[56] For example, treatments that target B lymphocytes for depletion are gaining in popularity.[57] The main randomized, placebo-controlled, parallel-group trial conducted by our group showed that RTX did not alleviate symptoms or disease activity at week 24, although it did so regarding some symptoms at earlier points.[58] Our results indicate that the endpoints used could have altered the efficacy of B-cell depletion in pSS.[59] These findings afford a rationale behind the therapeutic use of monoclonal Abs specific for B lymphocytes. Interestingly, the efficacy of B-cell depletion is dissociated from changes in levels of autoAbs because of the ongoing activity of long-lived PCs. Interesting as well is the reduction in the level of rheumatoid factor, generated by short-lived PCs.

In the absence of B cells upstream, these short-lived PCs are not produced anymore. It is all the more convincing that previous Abs aimed at killing the T cells have proved disappointing.[60] Finally, possibly in association with anti-B cell Abs, the therapeutic use of long-term treatment with antagonists of BAFF could also be beneficial in pSS.[61]

## REFERENCES

1. Daridon C, Devauchelle V, Hutin P, Le Berre R, Martins-Carvalho C, Bendaoud B, et al. Aberrant expression of BAFF by B lymphocytes infiltrating the salivary glands of patients with primary Sjögren's syndrome. *Arthritis Rheum* 2007;**56**:1134–44.
2. Groom J, Kalled SL, Cutler AH, Olson C, Woodcock SA, Schneider P, et al. Association of BAFF/BLyS overexpression and altered B cell differentiation with Sjögren's syndrome. *J Clin Invest* 2002;**109**:59–68.
3. Pers JO, Daridon C, Devauchelle V, Jousse S, Saraux A, Jamin C, et al. BAFF overexpression is associated with autoantibody production in autoimmune diseases. *Ann N Y Acad Sci* 2005;**1050**:34–9.
4. Binard A, Le Pottier L, Devauchelle-Pensec V, Saraux A, Youinou P, Pers JO. Is the blood B-cell subset profile diagnostic for Sjögren syndrome? *Ann Rheum Dis* 2009;**68**:1447–52.
5. Le Pottier L, Devauchelle V, Fautrel A, Daridon C, Saraux A, Youinou P, et al. Ectopic germinal centers are rare in Sjögren's syndrome salivary glands and do not exclude autoreactive B cells. *J Immunol* 2009;**182**:3540–7.
6. Palanichamy A, Barnard J, Zheng B, Owen T, Quach T, Wei C, et al. Novel human transitional B cell populations revealed by B cell depletion therapy. *J Immunol* 2009;**182**:5982–93.
7. Daridon C, Pers JO, Devauchelle V, Martins-Carvalho C, Hutin P, Pennec YL, et al. Identification of transitional type II B cells in the salivary glands of patients with Sjögren's syndrome. *Arthritis Rheum* 2006;**54**:2280–8.
8. Saito T, Chiba S, Ichikawa M, Kunisato A, Asai T, Shimizu K, et al. Notch2 is preferentially expressed in mature B cells and indispensable for marginal zone B lineage development. *Immunity* 2003;**18**:675–85.
9. Willenbrock K, Jungnickel B, Hansmann ML, Kuppers R. Human splenic marginal zone B cells lack expression of activation-induced cytidine deaminase. *Eur J Immunol* 2005;**35**:3002–7.
10. Cinamon G, Matloubian M, Lesneski MJ, Xu Y, Low C, Lu T, et al. Sphingosine 1-phosphate receptor 1 promotes B cell localization in the splenic marginal zone. *Nat Immunol* 2004;**5**:713–20.
11. Amft N, Bowman SJ. Chemokines and cell trafficking in Sjögren's syndrome. *Scand J Immunol* 2001;**54**:62–9.
12. Hansen A, Reiter K, Ziprian T, Jacobi A, Hoffmann A, Gosemann M, et al. Dysregulation of chemokine receptor expression and function by B cells of patients with primary Sjögren's syndrome. *Arthritis Rheum* 2005;**52**:2109–19.
13. Hansen A, Odendahl M, Reiter K, Jacobi AM, Feist E, Scholze J, et al. Diminished peripheral blood memory B cells and accumulation of memory B cells in the salivary glands of patients with Sjögren's syndrome. *Arthritis Rheum* 2002;**46**:2160–71.
14. Simon Q, Pers JO, Cornec D, Le Pottier L, Mageed R, Hillion S. In-depth characterization of CD24[high]CD38[high] transitional human B cells reveals different regulatory profiles. *J Allergy Clin Immunol* 2015.
15. Speight PM, Cruchley A, Williams DM. Quantification of plasma cells in labial salivary glands: increased expression of IgM in Sjögren's syndrome. *J Oral Pathol Med* 1990;**19**:126–30.

226    Sjögren's Syndrome

16. Matthews JB, Deacon EM, Wilson C, Potts AJ, Hamburger J. Plasma cell populations in labial salivary glands from patients with and without Sjögren's syndrome. *Histopathology* 1993;**23**:399–407.
17. Pablos JL, Carreira PE, Morillas L, Montalvo G, Ballestin C, Gomez-Reino JJ. Clonally expanded lymphocytes in the minor salivary glands of Sjögren's syndrome patients without lymphoproliferative disease. *Arthritis Rheum* 1994;**37**:1441–4.
18. Jordan R, Diss TC, Lench NJ, Isaacson PG, Speight PM. Immunoglobulin gene rearrangements in lymphoplasmacytic infiltrates of labial salivary glands in Sjögren's syndrome: a possible predictor of lymphoma development. *Oral Surg Oral Med Oral Pathol Oral Radiol Endod* 1995;**79**:723–9.
19. Stott DI, Hiepe F, Hummel M, Steinhauser G, Berek C. Antigen-driven clonal proliferation of B cells within the target tissue of an autoimmune disease: the salivary glands of patients with Sjögren's syndrome. *J Clin Invest* 1998;**102**:938–46.
20. Halse A, Harley JB, Kroneld U, Jonsson R. Ro/SS-A-reactive B lymphocytes in salivary glands and peripheral blood of patients with Sjögren's syndrome. *Clin Exp Immunol* 1999;**115**:203–7.
21. Salomonsson S, Jonsson MV, Skarstein K, Brokstad KA, Hjelmstrom P, Wahren-Herlenius M, et al. Cellular basis of ectopic germinal center formation and autoantibody production in the target organ of patients with Sjögren's syndrome. *Arthritis Rheum* 2003;**48**:3187–201.
22. Jonsson MV, Skarstein K, Jonsson R, Brun JG. Serological implications of germinal center-like structures in primary Sjögren's syndrome. *J Rheumatol* 2007;**34**:2044–9.
23. Theander E, Vasaitis L, Baecklund E, Nordmark G, Warfvinge G, Liedholm R, et al. Lymphoid organisation in labial salivary gland biopsies is a possible predictor for the development of malignant lymphoma in primary Sjögren's syndrome. *Ann Rheum Dis* 2011;**70**:1363–8.
24. Seror R, Sordet C, Guillevin L, Hachulla E, Masson C, Ittah M, et al. Tolerance and efficacy of rituximab and changes in serum B cell biomarkers in patients with systemic complications of primary Sjögren's syndrome. *Ann Rheum Dis* 2007;**66**:351–7.
25. Pers JO, Devauchelle V, Daridon C, Bendaoud B, Le Berre R, Bordron A, et al. BAFF-modulated repopulation of B lymphocytes in the blood and salivary glands of rituximab-treated patients with Sjögren's syndrome. *Arthritis Rheum* 2007;**56**:1464–77.
26. Youinou P, Mackenzie L, le Masson G, Papadopoulos NM, Jouquan J, Pennec YL, et al. CD5-expressing B lymphocytes in the blood and salivary glands of patients with primary Sjögren's syndrome. *J Autoimmun* 1988;**1**:185–94.
27. d'Arbonneau F, Pers JO, Devauchelle V, Pennec Y, Saraux A, Youinou P. BAFF-induced changes in B cell antigen receptor-containing lipid rafts in Sjögren's syndrome. *Arthritis Rheum* 2006;**54**:115–26.
28. Pascual M, Vicente M, Monferrer L, Artero R. The muscleblind family of proteins: an emerging class of regulators of developmentally programmed alternative splicing. *Differentiation* 2006;**74**:65–80.
29. Odendahl M, Jacobi A, Hansen A, Feist E, Hiepe F, Burmester GR, et al. Disturbed peripheral B lymphocyte homeostasis in systemic lupus erythematosus. *J Immunol* 2000;**165**:5970–9.
30. Bohnhorst JO, Thoen JE, Natvig JB, Thompson KM. Significantly depressed percentage of CD27+ (memory) B cells among peripheral blood B cells in patients with primary Sjögren's syndrome. *Scand J Immunol* 2001;**54**:421–7.
31. Smith AJ, Gordon TP, Macardle PJ. Increased expression of the B-cell-regulatory molecule CD72 in primary Sjögren's syndrome. *Tissue Antigens* 2004;**63**:255–9.
32. Lemoine S, Morva A, Youinou P, Jamin C. Human T cells induce their own regulation through activation of B cells. *J Autoimmun* 2011;**36**:228–38.
33. Morva A, Lemoine S, Achour A, Pers JO, Youinou P, Jamin C. Maturation and function of human dendritic cells are regulated by B lymphocytes. *Blood* 2012;**119**:106–14.

34. Jamin C, Morva A, Lemoine S, Daridon C, de Mendoza AR, Youinou P. Regulatory B lymphocytes in humans: a potential role in autoimmunity. *Arthritis Rheum* 2008;**58**:1900–6.
35. Blair PA, Norena LY, Flores-Borja F, Rawlings DJ, Isenberg DA, Ehrenstein MR, et al. CD19(+)CD24(hi)CD38(hi) B cells exhibit regulatory capacity in healthy individuals but are functionally impaired in systemic Lupus Erythematosus patients. *Immunity* 2010;**32**:129–40.
36. Hansen A, Dang MA, Reiter K, Frölich D, Lipsky PE, Dörner T. Peripheral CD27+IgD+IgM+ B cells in patients with primary Sjögren's syndrome and healthy donors. *Ann Rheum Dis* 2009;**68**(Suppl. 3).
37. Qian Y, Qin J, Cui G, Naramura M, Snow EC, Ware CF, et al. Act1, a negative regulator in CD40- and BAFF-mediated B cell survival. *Immunity* 2004;**21**:575–87.
38. Hase H, Kanno Y, Kojima M, Hasegawa K, Sakurai D, Kojima H, et al. BAFF/BLyS can potentiate B-cell selection with the B-cell coreceptor complex. *Blood* 2004;**103**:2257–65.
39. Ettinger R, Sims GP, Robbins R, Withers D, Fischer RT, Grammer AC, et al. IL-21 and BAFF/BLyS synergize in stimulating plasma cell differentiation from a unique population of human splenic memory B cells. *J Immunol* 2007;**178**:2872–82.
40. Khan WN. B cell receptor and BAFF receptor signaling regulation of B cell homeostasis. *J Immunol* 2009;**183**:3561–7.
41. Quartuccio L, Fabris M, Moretti M, Barone F, Bombardieri M, Rupolo M, et al. Resistance to rituximab therapy and local BAFF overexpression in Sjögren's syndrome: related myoepithelial sialadenitis and low-grade parotid B-cell lymphoma. *Open Rheumatol J* 2008;**2**:38–43.
42. Ahuja A, Shupe J, Dunn R, Kashgarian M, Kehry MR, Shlomchik MJ. Depletion of B cells in murine lupus: efficacy and resistance. *J Immunol* 2007;**179**:3351–61.
43. Jonsson MV, Szodoray P, Jellestad S, Jonsson R, Skarstein K. Association between circulating levels of the novel TNF family members APRIL and BAFF and lymphoid organization in primary Sjögren's syndrome. *J Clin Immunol* 2005;**25**:189–201.
44. Fletcher CA, Sutherland AP, Groom JR, Batten ML, Ng LG, Gommerman J, et al. Development of nephritis but not sialadenitis in autoimmune-prone BAFF transgenic mice lacking marginal zone B cells. *Eur J Immunol* 2006;**36**:2504–14.
45. Fridman WH. Factors controlling immunoglobulin production and B cell proliferation. *Bull Cancer* 1991;**78**:195–201.
46. Youinou P, Taher TE, Pers JO, Mageed RA, Renaudineau Y. B lymphocyte cytokines and rheumatic autoimmune disease. *Arthritis Rheum* 2009;**60**:1873–80.
47. Mitsias DI, Tzioufas AG, Veiopoulou C, Zintzaras E, Tassios IK, Kogopoulou O, et al. The Th1/Th2 cytokine balance changes with the progress of the immunopathological lesion of Sjögren's syndrome. *Clin Exp Immunol* 2002;**128**:562–8.
48. Szodoray P, Alex P, Brun JG, Centola M, Jonsson R. Circulating cytokines in primary Sjögren's syndrome determined by a multiplex cytokine array system. *Scand J Immunol* 2004;**59**:592–9.
49. Shen L, Suresh L, Li H, Zhang C, Kumar V, Pankewycz O, et al. IL-14 alpha, the nexus for primary Sjögren's disease in mice and humans. *Clin Immunol* 2009;**130**:304–12.
50. Hsu HC, Yang P, Wang J, Wu Q, Myers R, Chen J, et al. Interleukin 17-producing T helper cells and interleukin 17 orchestrate autoreactive germinal center development in autoimmune BXD2 mice. *Nat Immunol* 2008;**9**:166–75.
51. Hillion S, Dueymes M, Youinou P, Jamin C. IL-6 contributes to the expression of RAGs in human mature B cells. *J Immunol* 2007;**179**:6790–8.
52. Durali D, de Goer de Herve MG, Giron-Michel J, Azzarone B, Delfraissy JF, Taoufik Y. In human B cells, IL-12 triggers a cascade of molecular events similar to Th1 commitment. *Blood* 2003;**102**:4084–9.

53. Thabet Y, Le Dantec C, Ghedira I, Devauchelle V, Cornec D, Pers JO, et al. Epigenetic dysregulation in salivary glands from patients with primary Sjögren's syndrome may be ascribed to infiltrating B cells. *J Autoimmun* 2013;**41**:175–81.

54. Devauchelle-Pensec V, Pennec Y, Morvan J, Pers JO, Daridon C, Jousse-Joulin S, et al. Improvement of Sjögren's syndrome after two infusions of rituximab (anti-CD20). *Arthritis Rheum* 2007;**57**:310–7.

55. Konsta OD, Thabet Y, Le Dantec C, Brooks WH, Tzioufas AG, Pers JO, et al. The contribution of epigenetics in Sjögren's Syndrome. *Front Genet* 2014;**5**:71.

56. Edwards JC, Cambridge G. B-cell targeting in rheumatoid arthritis and other autoimmune diseases. *Nat Rev Immunol* 2006;**6**:394–403.

57. Blank M, Shoenfeld Y. B cell targeted therapy in autoimmunity. *J Autoimmun* 2007;**28**:62–8.

58. Devauchelle-Pensec V, Mariette X, Jousse-Joulin S, Berthelot JM, Perdriger A, Puechal X, et al. Treatment of primary Sjögren syndrome with rituximab: a randomized trial. *Ann Intern Med* 2014;**160**:233–42.

59. Cornec D, Devauchelle-Pensec V, Mariette X, Jousse-Joulin S, Berthelot JM, Perdriger A, et al. Development of the Sjögren's Syndrome Responder Index, a data-driven composite endpoint for assessing treatment efficacy. *Rheumatology* 2015;**54**:1699–708.

60. Ramos-Casals M, Brito-Zeron P. Emerging biological therapies in primary Sjögren's syndrome. *Rheumatology* 2007;**46**:1389–96.

61. De Vita S, Quartuccio L, Seror R, Salvin S, Ravaud P, Fabris M, et al. Efficacy and safety of belimumab given for 12 months in primary Sjögren's syndrome: the BELISS open-label phase II study. *Rheumatology* 2015.

Chapter 15

# Cytokines, Chemokines, and the Innate Immune System in Sjögren's Syndrome

## S. Appel
*University of Bergen, Bergen, Norway*

## R. Jonsson
*University of Bergen, Bergen, Norway; Haukeland University Hospital, Bergen, Norway*

## 1. INTRODUCTION

Cytokines are the mediators of the immune system. They are small proteins of around 25 kD that are produced in response to a stimulus (ie, invading microbes) by numerous cell types. They mediate and regulate immune responses, inflammatory reactions, wound healing, hematopoiesis, and chemotaxis, and can be divided into being proinflammatory or antiinflammatory. Their mechanism of action is via specific receptors and can either be autocrine (ie, on themselves), paracrine (ie, on cells in the vicinity), or endocrine (ie, spread via circulation to distant sites). Originally, they were named according to their functionality after either the cell type producing them (monokine and lymphokine) or the cell they acted upon [interleukin (IL): acting on leukocytes]. Cytokines can be divided into chemokines, interferons (IFNs), ILs, some colony-stimulating factors, and tumor necrosis factor (TNF). Chemokines are a certain subclass of cytokines. Approximately 50 different chemokines have been described so far, and they function as chemo-attractants, inducing cells recognizing them to migrate along the chemokine gradient. They determine, for example, the specific localization of lymphocytes and dendritic cells (DCs) in peripheral lymphoid organs. Chemokines can be divided into two different subclasses: CC chemokines with two neighboring cysteine residues close to the amino terminus, and CXC chemokines with two cysteine residues separated by another amino acid. CC chemokines are recognized by CC receptors (CCRs), whereas CXC chemokines are recognized by CXC receptor (CXCR) molecules.

In contrast to hormones, which are present at very low concentrations and are produced by specific cells, cytokines are present at higher (some even

Sjögren's Syndrome. http://dx.doi.org/10.1016/B978-0-12-803604-4.00015-0

picomolar) concentrations that can under certain circumstances increase dramatically. Moreover, a given cytokine can be secreted by several different cells, and several cytokines may act in similar ways, resulting in a certain redundancy of the system. In addition, one cytokine may affect different cell types in different ways (pleiotropy).

In most cases, there is not a single cytokine present, but multiple different ones acting either additively, synergistically or antagonistically to each other, leading to a complexity in the system that is difficult to analyze in in vitro systems.

The innate immune system is considered to be fast but rather nonspecific. It comprises physical barriers, such as epithelia, soluble molecules such as complement, and cellular components, such as leukocytes. Besides neutrophils, macrophages, DCs and natural killer (NK) cells, also the recently identified innate lymphoid cells (ILCs) possess important regulatory and effector functions in immunity and homeostasis.[1] Pathogens and tissue damage are detected by innate immune cells via pattern recognition receptors (PRRs). The first ones discovered and best characterized are Toll-like receptors (TLRs), which are present both on the cell surface and in endosomes.[2] Moreover, additional PRRs are present on the cell surface, such as C-type lectin receptors, and the cytosol, such as nonobese diabetic (NOD)-like receptors, and RIG-I–like receptors.[2]

## 2. CYTOKINES OF THE INNATE IMMUNE SYSTEM IN PRIMARY SJÖGREN'S SYNDROME

The production of cytokines and chemokines and their interplay are central parts of the regulation of immune responses. An imbalance of the cytokine network is commonly observed in patients with primary Sjögren's syndrome (pSS) and contributes to local as well as systemic aberrations of this disease.[3,4] One prominent pathway that has emerged in recent years as a result of expression profiling of salivary glands[5,6] and peripheral blood cells[7–9] from pSS patients as well as genome-wide association studies[10] is the type I IFN pathway.

### 2.1 Type I Interferon

As is true for several autoimmune diseases such as systemic lupus erythematosus (SLE), rheumatoid arthritis, and scleroderma,[11,12] approximately 50% of patients with Sjögren's syndrome (SS) have an activated type I IFN system.[13] This IFN signature is present in both blood[7–9] and salivary glands.[5,6] Human type I IFNs include 13 different types of IFN-α, IFN-β, IFN-ε, IFN-κ, and IFN-ω.[14] The many subtypes hamper an easy detection using enzyme-linked immunosorbent assay, as antibodies will only recognize specific subsets.

Type I IFNs are secreted as a result of infection. They serve three major purposes: (1) limiting the spreading of pathogens by inducing cell-intrinsic antimicrobial states in infected and neighboring cells, (2) enhancing antigen presentation and NK cell functions while restraining proinflammatory pathways by modulating innate immune responses, and (3) activating the adaptive immune system, resulting in antigen-specific T- and B-cell responses and immunological memory.[15]

Plasmacytoid DCs (pDCs) are the main type I IFN-producing cells upon viral infection.[16,17] Production of type I IFN is induced by pathogen components recognized by PRRs such as TLRs. Type I IFNs are recognized by a heterodimeric receptor comprised of two chains, IFNAR1 and IFNAR2. IFNAR signals through kinases Tyk2 and Jak1, members of the Janus family. This leads to the formation of STAT1-STAT2 heterodimers, which migrate to the nucleus where they will associate with IFN regulatory factor (IRF) 9 to form IFN-stimulated gene factor 3. This results in binding to upstream IFN-stimulated response elements, activating transcription of IFN-inducible genes.[18,19] Moreover, IFNAR also signals by activation and translocation of STAT1 homodimers, which bind to the promoters of IFN-γ–induced genes.[18,19] This effect of type I IFN results in the same gene expression pattern as IFN-γ.[20]

Interestingly, IFN-γ has been shown to be involved in the onset of SS-like disease in mouse models of the disease, as SS-prone mice lacking either IFN-γ or the IFN-γ receptor (NOD.IFN-γ$^{-/-}$ and NOD.IFN-γR$^{-/-}$) do not develop sialadenitis.[21] They have an increased IFN-γ and Stat1 activity already at birth, suggesting that IFN-γ has a critical role in disease initiation.

Several polymorphisms in the type I IFN pathway have been shown to be associated with pSS and other autoimmune diseases.[22,23] Surprisingly, lower IFN-α production of pDC was associated with the SLE risk variant of the *IRF5* CGGGG indel.[24]

## 2.2 Tumor Necrosis Factor

TNF is a key activator of the nuclear factor (NF)-κB pathway. It belongs to the TNF superfamily with 19 ligands and 29 receptors identified in humans.[25] TNF forms homotrimers and can signal via two different receptors, either membrane-bound or soluble via TNF receptor (TNFR) 1, and membrane-bound only via TNFR2.[26–28] TNFR1 is widely expressed on a variety of cells, whereas expression of TNFR2 is restricted to cells of the immune system. Originally, TNF was recognized to have tumor suppressive properties, because it can induce apoptosis in certain cell types (hence the name),[27] and it is one of the cytokines responsible for acute phase reaction and septic shock.[29] Upon binding of the TNF homotrimer, the receptor forms a trimer leading to potential activation of several signaling pathways.[28,30] Recruitment of TNF-receptor associated factor 2 will either lead to activation of NF-κB or the mitogen-activated protein kinase (MAPK), c-Jun N-terminal kinase.[28] Moreover, TNF can also, via TNFR1, lead to death signaling via caspases.[30] With regard to inflammation, NF-κB activation is considered to be the most important pathway. In pSS patients, elevated levels of TNF-α are detected both systemically and locally in the salivary glands.[4,31] However, several clinical trials using anti-TNF targeted therapies in pSS resulted in a lack of beneficial effects.[32] Polymorphisms in the

TNF-α induced protein 3 interacting protein (TFIP) 1 gene have recently been reported to be associated with autoantibody positive pSS patients.[33] TFIP1 is, in interaction with A20, a negative regulator of TNF-α activated NF-κB signaling. A more individualized anti-TNF therapy might therefore be beneficial for a certain subgroup of patients.

## 2.3 B-Cell Activating Factor

B-cell activating factor (BAFF) increases survival and differentiation of B cells.[34] BAFF can signal either via B-cell maturation antigen (BCMA), transmembrane activator and calcium-modulator and cyclophilin ligand interactor (TACI), or BAFF-receptor (BAFF-R). While TACI is expressed mainly on memory B cells and activated T cells, BAFF-R and BCMA are predominantly expressed on B cells. TACI and BAFF-R have been implicated in isotype switching.[35] Elevated serum and salivary gland levels of BAFF have been detected in patients with pSS,[34,36,37] and plasma levels correlate with hypergammaglobulinemia.[38] Moreover, besides having SLE-like features, BAFF transgenic mice develop sialadenitis with reduction of saliva production reminiscent of SS.[39]

Interestingly, BAFF expression correlates with an activated type I IFN system.[8,40]

Because of the critical role of BAFF in B-cell survival and activation and the correlation of increased BAFF levels and development of lymphoma,[41] the effect of BAFF blockade in pSS patients using a monoclonal antibody has been analyzed in a clinical trial with promising results.[42] Most of the patients achieved the primary endpoint and the treatment was safe with few side effects.[42] Moreover, anti-BAFF treatment restored B-cell frequencies and function in these patients,[43] making this a promising treatment option for pSS patients that has to be evaluated in larger clinical trials.

Lymphotoxin α (LTA) is another member of the TNF superfamily associated with SS.[44,45] Association of several polymorphisms in the *LTA/LTB/TNF* region has been observed with anti-SSA and anti-SSB positive patients.[46] CXCL13, a chemokine important for B-cell homing and lymph node development, is regulated by LT, and is elevated in serum and saliva of pSS patients.[47] In NOD mice, CXCL13 blockade before disease onset, either directly or via anti-LT treatment, results in reduction of B-cell infiltrations in the salivary glands and partial restoration of salivary flow.[47–49]

## 2.4 Interleukin-6

Another cytokine, elevated both systemically and locally in pSS patients, is IL-6.[4,50] This complex inflammatory cytokine can signal via a membrane bound (IL-6R; "classical") and a soluble (sIL-6R; "trans-signaling") receptor, resulting in different outcomes. Although both pathways require binding of the IL-6/IL-6R complex to membrane-bound glycoprotein gp130, the following intracellular signaling cascades are far from being clear.[51] Several pathways have been shown to be involved in IL-6 signaling, the most investigated being the JAK/ STAT pathway, the MAPK cascade, and the PI3K cascade.[52,53] Whereas the classical activation (ie, membrane bound IL-6R) leads to activation of STAT3m, resulting in antiinflammatory, regenerative, and protective function, the transactivation (ie, sIL-6R) has been described to have an activating effect on the immune system with proinflammatory functions.[52,54] Not surprisingly, IL-6 signaling is tightly regulated. Especially the metalloprotease ADAM17 is thought to have an important role in balancing proinflammatory and antiinflammatory signaling of IL-6.[55] Because ADAM17 was originally found to cleave membrane-bound TNF-α precursor to release soluble TNF-α,[56,57] it was first termed *TNF-converting enzyme*. However, multiple other targets have been identified by now,[58] many of which are involved in inflammation and autoimmunity. In SS, it has been shown that ADAM17-dependent epidermal growth factor receptor signaling increases proinflammatory cytokine production by salivary gland epithelial cells that could be reduced by inhibiting ADAM17.[59]

Whereas IL-6R expression is limited to mainly hepatocytes, neutrophils, monocytes, and CD4+ T cells,[60,61] gp130 is expressed ubiquitously.[62] Normally, IL-6 concentrations in blood are very low, whereas sIL-6R and soluble gp130 are present in high concentrations. This is thought to act as a buffer for IL-6, with IL-6R being the limiting factor.[52]

Adding to the complexity of IL-6 signaling, both gp130 and IL-6R are activated by cytokines of the IL-12 family.[63]

## 2.5 Interleukin-1

Fatigue is a major reason for the disability and reduced quality of life reported by many pSS patients.[3] A possible connection to sickness behavior (ie, drowsiness, loss of appetite, decreased activity, and social exploration in response to infection and inflammation) described in animals was postulated to be the IL-1 system.[64] IL-1 was the first member of the interleukin family to be described, and has been shown to be a central mediator of inflammation.[65] The IL-1 family is growing steadily, and with the discovery of ILCs, the IL-1 system has gained even more in complexity.[65,66] IL-1 is a proinflammatory cytokine that exists in two forms, IL-1α and IL-1β, encoded by two distinct genes.[67] A membrane bound form of IL-1a is present on activated monocytes, whereas an IL-1a precursor is present in epithelial layers of the gastrointestinal tract, lung, liver, kidney, endothelial cells, and astrocytes. Upon necrosis, this precursor is released and acts as an "alarmin" to initiate a cascade of cytokines and chemokines.[65] IL-1b is mainly secreted by monocytes, macrophages, DCs, and microglia upon activation of TLRs, complement, or other cytokines such as TNF or IL-1.[65,68] In contrast to the already active IL-1a precursor, the IL-1b precursor is inactive and needs cleavage by caspase-1 to be activated. As a prerequisite, caspase-1 needs to be generated first by cleavage of procaspase-1 by the inflammasome.[69] Both IL-1a and IL-1b bind to IL-1R1 and IL-1R2. Another member of the IL-1 family, IL-1RA, is an endogenous antagonist of the IL-1R1. The blocking function of this molecule has been exploited for neutralization of IL-1, eg, for the treatment of rheumatological and inflammatory diseases.[70] Anakinra was also used in a randomized clinical trial with pSS patients, with the main intention to treat fatigue in these patients.[71] Even though no statistically significant difference in fatigue score was observed upon IL-1R1 blockade, this might be attributed to inclusion of too few patients.[71] Other members of the IL-1 family have also been implicated in the pathogenesis of SS.[72,73]

In addition to the previously mentioned cytokines, numerous others have been suggested to be involved in the pathogenesis of pSS, eg, as IL-17.[74,75] So far, little is known about the involvement of ILCs in the pathogenesis of SS. However, because of their role in immune homeostasis, a dysfunction of these cells could well result in autoimmunity.[76] Recently, it was shown that ILCs also have an effect on B cells, resulting in enhanced antibody production.[77] Moreover, a polymorphism in the activating receptor NCR3/NKp30 associated with pSS has suggested involvement of NK cells.[78]

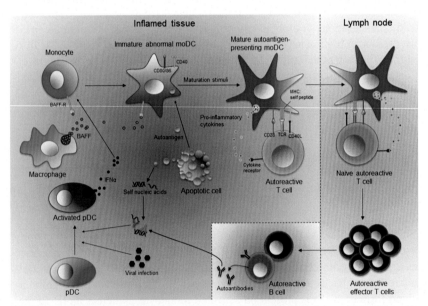

**FIGURE 15.1** Potential interplay of various factors of the immune system in the pathogenesis of primary Sjögren's syndrome (pSS). An initial trigger (viral infection and immune complexes) activates plasmacytoid dendritic cell *(pDCs)*, leading to secretion of type I interferon (IFN). This inflammatory setting stimulates monocytes to become monocyte-derived DCs. In presence of B-cell activating factor (BAFF) and autoantigens, these cells mature and present autoantigens in a proinflammatory cytokine-rich environment, stimulating autoreactive T and B cells. Autoantibodies will in turn assemble into immune complexes, stimulating pDCs to produce even more type I IFN, completing the vicious cycle. *BAFF-R*, BAFF receptor, *MHC*, major histocompatibility complex; *moDC*, monocyte-derived DC; *TCR*, T-cell receptor. *Adapted from Røise D. The impact of BAFF on the development of monocyte-derived dendritic cells in patients with rheumatic autoimmune diseases [Master thesis]. Bergen, Norway: University of Bergen; 2015. Conceptual design by Petra Vogelsang.*

# 3. CONCLUSION

In conclusion, the cytokine system is very complex with a multitude of interactions and interference. Because of the activated type I IFN system in many pSS patients, it is conceivable that a viral infection initiates a cascade of events in genetically predisposed individuals, resulting in activation of pDCs and presentation of auto-antigens on activated DCs, leading to activation of autoreactive T and B cells in lymph nodes. Production of autoantibodies and generation of immune complexes will further enhance pDC activation and type I IFN production (Fig. 15.1). These events might take place long before the disease manifestation, because autoantibodies related to pSS are detectable up to decades before symptoms develop.[79,80]

# REFERENCES

1. Hazenberg MD, Spits H. Human innate lymphoid cells. *Blood* 2014;**124**:700–9.
2. Kawai T, Akira S. Toll-like receptors and their crosstalk with other innate receptors in infection and immunity. *Immunity* 2011;**34**:637–50.
3. Jonsson R, Vogelsang P, Volchenkov R, Espinosa A, Wahren-Herlenius M, Appel S. The complexity of Sjögren's syndrome: novel aspects on pathogenesis. *Immunol Lett* 2011;**141**:1–9.
4. Roescher N, Tak PP, Illei GG. Cytokines in Sjögren's syndrome. *Oral Dis* 2009;**15**:519–26.
5. Bave U, Nordmark G, Lovgren T, Ronnelid J, Cajander S, Eloranta ML, et al. Activation of the type I interferon system in primary Sjögren's syndrome: a possible etiopathogenic mechanism. *Arthritis Rheum* 2005;**52**:1185–95.
6. Hjelmervik TO, Petersen K, Jonassen I, Jonsson R, Bolstad AI. Gene expression profiling of minor salivary glands clearly distinguishes primary Sjögren's syndrome patients from healthy control subjects. *Arthritis Rheum* 2005;**52**:1534–44.
7. Wildenberg ME, Helden-Meeuwsen CG, van de Merwe JP, Drexhage HA, Versnel MA. Systemic increase in type I interferon activity in Sjögren's syndrome: a putative role for plasmacytoid dendritic cells. *Eur J Immunol* 2008;**38**:2024–33.
8. Brkic Z, Maria NI, van Helden-Meeuwsen CG, van de Merwe JP, van Daele PL, Dalm VA, et al. Prevalence of interferon type I signature in CD14 monocytes of patients with Sjögren's syndrome and association with disease activity and BAFF gene expression. *Ann Rheum Dis* 2013;**72**:728–35.
9. Emamian ES, Leon JM, Lessard CJ, Grandits M, Baechler EC, Gaffney PM, et al. Peripheral blood gene expression profiling in Sjögren's syndrome. *Genes Immun* 2009;**10**:285–96.
10. Lessard CJ, Li H, Adrianto I, Ice JA, Rasmussen A, Grundahl KM, et al. Variants at multiple loci implicated in both innate and adaptive immune responses are associated with Sjögren's syndrome. *Nat Genet* 2013;**45**:1284–92.
11. Higgs BW, Liu Z, White B, Zhu W, White WI, Morehouse C, et al. Patients with systemic lupus erythematosus, myositis, rheumatoid arthritis and scleroderma share activation of a common type I interferon pathway. *Ann Rheum Dis* 2011;**70**:2029–36.
12. Hagberg N, Ronnblom L. Systemic lupus erythematosus: a disease with a dysregulated type I interferon system. *Scand J Immunol* 2015;**82**:199–207.
13. Brkic Z, Versnel MA. Type I IFN signature in primary Sjögren's syndrome patients. *Expert Rev Clin Immunol* 2014;**10**:457–67.
14. Platanias LC. Mechanisms of type-I– and type-II–interferon–mediated signalling. *Nat Rev Immunol* 2005;**5**:375–86.

15. Ivashkiv LB, Donlin LT. Regulation of type I interferon responses. *Nat Rev Immunol* 2014;**14**:36–49.

16. Fitzgerald-Bocarsly P, Dai J, Singh S. Plasmacytoid dendritic cells and type I IFN: 50 years of convergent history. *Cytokine Growth Factor Rev* 2008;**19**:3–19.

17. Colonna M, Trinchieri G, Liu YJ. Plasmacytoid dendritic cells in immunity. *Nat Immunol* 2004;**5**:1219–26.

18. Trinchieri G. Type I interferon: friend or foe? *J Exp Med* 2010;**207**:2053–63.

19. Decker T, Muller M, Stockinger S. The yin and yang of type I interferon activity in bacterial infection. *Nat Rev Immunol* 2005;**5**:675–87.

20. van Boxel-Dezaire AH, Rani MR, Stark GR. Complex modulation of cell type-specific signaling in response to type I interferons. *Immunity* 2006;**25**:361–72.

21. Cha S, Brayer J, Gao J, Brown V, Killedar S, Yasunari U, et al. A dual role for interferon-gamma in the pathogenesis of Sjögren's syndrome-like autoimmune exocrinopathy in the non-obese diabetic mouse. *Scand J Immunol* 2004;**60**:552–65.

22. Miceli-Richard C, Comets E, Loiseau P, Puechal X, Hachulla E, Mariette X. Association of an IRF5 gene functional polymorphism with Sjögren's syndrome. *Arthritis Rheum* 2007;**56**:3989–94.

23. Nordmark G, Kristjansdottir G, Theander E, Eriksson P, Brun JG, Wang C, et al. Additive effects of the major risk alleles of *IRF5* and *STAT4* in primary Sjögren's syndrome. *Genes Immun* 2009;**10**:68–76.

24. Berggren O, Alexsson A, Morris DL, Tandre K, Weber G, Vyse TJ, et al. IFN-α production by plasmacytoid dendritic cell associations with polymorphisms in gene loci related to autoimmune and inflammatory diseases. *Hum Mol Genet* 2015;**24**:3571–81.

25. Aggarwal BB. Signalling pathways of the TNF superfamily: a double-edged sword. *Nat Rev Immunol* 2003;**3**:745–56.

26. Locksley RM, Killeen N, Lenardo MJ. The TNF and TNF receptor superfamilies: integrating mammalian biology. *Cell* 2001;**104**:487–501.

27. West NR, McCuaig S, Franchini F, Powrie F. Emerging cytokine networks in colorectal cancer. *Nat Rev Immunol* 2015;**15**:615–29.

28. Wajant H, Pfizenmaier K, Scheurich P. Tumor necrosis factor signaling. *Cell Death Differ* 2003;**10**:45–65.

29. Mannel DN, Echtenacher B. TNF in the inflammatory response. *Chem Immunol* 2000;**74**:141–61.

30. Chen G, Goeddel DV. TNF-R1 signaling: a beautiful pathway. *Science* 2002;**296**:1634–5.

31. Szodoray P, Alex P, Brun JG, Centola M, Jonsson R. Circulating cytokines in primary Sjögren's syndrome determined by a multiplex cytokine array system. *Scand J Immunol* 2004;**59**:592–9.

32. Sada PR, Isenberg D, Ciurtin C. Biologic treatment in Sjögren's syndrome. *Rheumatology* 2015;**54**:219–30.

33. Nordmark G, Wang C, Vasaitis L, Eriksson P, Theander E, Kvarnstrom M, et al. Association of genes in the NF-κB pathway with antibody-positive primary Sjögren's syndrome. *Scand J Immunol* 2013;**78**:447–54.

34. Szodoray P, Jonsson R. The BAFF/APRIL system in systemic autoimmune diseases with a special emphasis on Sjögren's syndrome. *Scand J Immunol* 2005;**62**:421–8.

35. Castigli E, Wilson SA, Scott S, Dedeoglu F, Xu S, Lam KP, et al. TACI and BAFF-R mediate isotype switching in B cells. *J Exp Med* 2005;**201**:35–9.

36. Mariette X, Roux S, Zhang J, Bengoufa D, Lavie F, Zhou T, et al. The level of BLyS (BAFF) correlates with the titre of autoantibodies in human Sjögren's syndrome. *Ann Rheum Dis* 2003;**62**:168–71.

37. Lavie F, Miceli-Richard C, Quillard J, Roux S, Leclerc P, Mariette X. Expression of BAFF (BLyS) in T cells infiltrating labial salivary glands from patients with Sjögren's syndrome. *J Pathol* 2004;**202**:496–502.

38. Szodoray P, Jellestad S, Alex P, Zhou T, Wilson PC, Centola M, et al. Programmed cell death of peripheral blood B cells determined by laser scanning cytometry in Sjögren's syndrome with a special emphasis on BAFF. *J Clin Immunol* 2004;**24**:600–11.

39. Groom J, Kalled SL, Cutler AH, Olson C, Woodcock SA, Schneider P, et al. Association of BAFF/BLyS overexpression and altered B cell differentiation with Sjögren's syndrome. *J Clin Invest* 2002;**109**:59–68.

40. Ittah M, Miceli-Richard C, Eric Gottenberg J, Lavie F, Lazure T, Ba N, et al. B cell-activating factor of the tumor necrosis factor family (BAFF) is expressed under stimulation by interferon in salivary gland epithelial cells in primary Sjögren's syndrome. *Arthritis Res Ther* 2006;**8**:R51.

41. Quartuccio L, Salvin S, Fabris M, Maset M, Pontarini E, Isola M, et al. BLyS upregulation in Sjögren's syndrome associated with lymphoproliferative disorders, higher ESSDAI score and B-cell clonal expansion in the salivary glands. *Rheumatology* 2013;**52**:276–81.

42. Mariette X, Seror R, Quartuccio L, Baron G, Salvin S, Fabris M, et al. Efficacy and safety of belimumab in primary Sjögren's syndrome: results of the BELISS open-label phase II study. *Ann Rheum Dis* 2015;**74**:526–31.

43. Pontarini E, Fabris M, Quartuccio L, Cappeletti M, Calcaterra F, Roberto A, et al. Treatment with belimumab restores B cell subsets and their expression of B cell activating factor receptor in patients with primary Sjögren's syndrome. *Rheumatology* 2015;**54**:1429–34.

44. Kramer JM. Early events in Sjögren's Syndrome pathogenesis: the importance of innate immunity in disease initiation. *Cytokine* 2014;**67**:92–101.

45. Shen L, Suresh L, Wu J, Xuan J, Li H, Zhang C, et al. A role for lymphotoxin in primary Sjögren's disease. *J Immunol* 2010;**185**:6355–63.

46. Bolstad AI, Le Hellard S, Kristjansdottir G, Vasaitis L, Kvarnstrom M, Sjowall C, et al. Association between genetic variants in the tumour necrosis factor/lymphotoxin alpha/lymphotoxin beta locus and primary Sjögren's syndrome in Scandinavian samples. *Ann Rheum Dis* 2012;**71**:981–8.

47. Kramer JM, Klimatcheva E, Rothstein TL. CXCL13 is elevated in Sjögren's syndrome in mice and humans and is implicated in disease pathogenesis. *J Leukoc Biol* 2013;**94**:1079–89.

48. Fava RA, Kennedy SM, Wood SG, Bolstad AI, Bienkowska J, Papandile A, et al. Lymphotoxin-beta receptor blockade reduces CXCL13 in lacrimal glands and improves corneal integrity in the NOD model of Sjögren's syndrome. *Arthritis Res Ther* 2011;**13**:R182.

49. Gatumu MK, Skarstein K, Papandile A, Browning JL, Fava RA, Bolstad AI. Blockade of lymphotoxin-beta receptor signaling reduces aspects of Sjögren's syndrome in salivary glands of non-obese diabetic mice. *Arthritis Res Ther* 2009;**11**:R24.

50. Halse A, Tengner P, Wahren-Herlenius M, Haga H, Jonsson R. Increased frequency of cells secreting interleukin-6 and interleukin-10 in peripheral blood of patients with primary Sjögren's syndrome. *Scand J Immunol* 1999;**49**:533–8.

51. Dittrich A, Hessenkemper W, Schaper F. Systems biology of IL-6, IL-12 family cytokines. *Cytokine Growth Factor Rev* 2015;**26**:595–602.

52. Schaper F, Rose-John S. Interleukin-6: biology, signaling and strategies of blockade. *Cytokine Growth Factor Rev* 2015;**26**:475–87.

53. Eulenfeld R, Dittrich A, Khouri C, Muller PJ, Mutze B, Wolf A, et al. Interleukin-6 signalling: more than Jaks and STATs. *Eur J Cell Biol* 2012;**91**:486–95.

54. Scheller J, Chalaris A, Schmidt-Arras D, Rose-John S. The pro- and anti-inflammatory properties of the cytokine interleukin-6. *Biochim Biophys Acta* 2011;**1813**:878–88.

55. Scheller J, Chalaris A, Garbers C, Rose-John S. *ADAM17*: a molecular switch to control inflammation and tissue regeneration. *Trends Immunol* 2011;**32**:380–7.

56. Black RA, Rauch CT, Kozlosky CJ, Peschon JJ, Slack JL, Wolfson MF, et al. A metalloproteinase disintegrin that releases tumour-necrosis factor-alpha from cells. *Nature* 1997;**385**:729–33.

57. Moss ML, Jin SL, Milla ME, Bickett DM, Burkhart W, Carter HL, et al. Cloning of a disintegrin metalloproteinase that processes precursor tumour-necrosis factor-alpha. *Nature* 1997;**385**:733–6.

58. Lisi S, D'Amore M, Sisto M. *ADAM17* at the interface between inflammation and autoimmunity. *Immunol Lett* 2014;**162**:159–69.

59. Sisto M, Lisi S, D'Amore M, Lofrumento DD. The metalloproteinase *ADAM17* and the epidermal growth factor receptor (EGFR) signaling drive the inflammatory epithelial response in Sjögren's syndrome. *Clin Exp Med* 2015;**15**:215–25.

60. Gauldie J, Richards C, Harnish D, Lansdorp P, Baumann H. Interferon beta 2/B-cell stimulatory factor type 2 shares identity with monocyte-derived hepatocyte-stimulating factor and regulates the major acute phase protein response in liver cells. *Proc Natl Acad Sci USA* 1987;**84**:7251–5.

61. Oberg HH, Wesch D, Grussel S, Rose-John S, Kabelitz D. Differential expression of CD126 and CD130 mediates different STAT-3 phosphorylation in CD4+CD25- and CD25high regulatory T cells. *Int Immunol* 2006;**18**:555–63.

62. Hibi M, Murakami M, Saito M, Hirano T, Taga T, Kishimoto T. Molecular cloning and expression of an IL-6 signal transducer, gp130. *Cell* 1990;**63**:1149–57.

63. Rose-John S, Scheller J, Schaper F. "Family reunion": a structured view on the composition of the receptor complexes of interleukin-6-type and interleukin-12-type cytokines. *Cytokine Growth Factor Rev* 2015;**26**:471–4.

64. Harboe E, Tjensvoll AB, Vefring HK, Goransson LG, Kvaloy JT, Omdal R. Fatigue in primary Sjögren's syndrome: a link to sickness behaviour in animals? *Brain Behav Immun* 2009;**23**:1104–8.

65. Garlanda C, Dinarello CA, Mantovani A. The interleukin-1 family: back to the future. *Immunity* 2013;**39**:1003–18.

66. Spits H, Artis D, Colonna M, Diefenbach A, Di Santo JP, Eberl G, et al. Innate lymphoid cells: a proposal for uniform nomenclature. *Nat Rev Immunol* 2013;**13**:145–9.

67. Nicklin MJ, Weith A, Duff GW. A physical map of the region encompassing the human interleukin-1 alpha, interleukin-1 beta, and interleukin-1 receptor antagonist genes. *Genomics* 1994;**19**:382–4.

68. Dinarello CA. Interleukin-1 in the pathogenesis and treatment of inflammatory diseases. *Blood* 2011;**117**:3720–32.

69. Martinon F, Burns K, Tschopp J. The inflammasome: a molecular platform triggering activation of inflammatory caspases and processing of proIL-$\beta$. *Mol Cell* 2002;**10**:417–26.

70. Cavalli G, Dinarello CA. Treating rheumatological diseases and co-morbidities with interleukin-1 blocking therapies. *Rheumatology* 2015;**54**:2134–44.

71. Norheim KB, Harboe E, Goransson LG, Omdal R. Interleukin-1 inhibition and fatigue in primary Sjögren's syndrome: a double blind, randomised clinical trial. *PLoS One* 2012;**7**:e30123.

72. Ciccia F, Accardo-Palumbo A, Alessandro R, Alessandri C, Priori R, Guggino G, et al. Interleukin-36$\alpha$ axis is modulated in patients with primary Sjögren's syndrome. *Clin Exp Immunol* 2015;**181**:230–8.

73. Ciccia F, Guggino G, Rizzo A, Bombardieri M, Raimondo S, Carubbi F, et al. Interleukin (IL)-22 receptor 1 is over-expressed in primary Sjögren's syndrome and Sjögren-associated non-Hodgkin lymphomas and is regulated by IL-18. *Clin Exp Immunol* 2015;**181**:219–29.

74. Katsifis GE, Rekka S, Moutsopoulos NM, Pillemer S, Wahl SM. Systemic and local interleukin-17 and linked cytokines associated with Sjögren's syndrome immunopathogenesis. *Am J Pathol* 2009;**175**:1167–77.

75. Nguyen CQ, Hu MH, Li Y, Stewart C, Peck AB. Salivary gland tissue expression of interleukin-23 and interleukin-17 in Sjögren's syndrome: findings in humans and mice. *Arthritis Rheum* 2008;**58**:734–43.

76. McKenzie AN, Spits H, Eberl G. Innate lymphoid cells in inflammation and immunity. *Immunity* 2014;**41**:366–74.

77. Magri G, Miyajima M, Bascones S, Mortha A, Puga I, Cassis L, et al. Innate lymphoid cells integrate stromal and immunological signals to enhance antibody production by splenic marginal zone B cells. *Nat Immunol* 2014;**15**:354–64.

78. Rusakiewicz S, Nocturne G, Lazure T, Semeraro M, Flament C, Caillat-Zucman S, et al. NCR3/NKp30 contributes to pathogenesis in primary Sjögren's syndrome. *Sci Transl Med* 2013;**5**:195ra96.

79. Jonsson R, Theander E, Sjostrom B, Brokstad K, Henriksson G. Autoantibodies present before symptom onset in primary Sjögren syndrome. *JAMA* 2013;**310**:1854–5.

80. Theander E, Jonsson R, Sjostrom B, Brokstad K, Olsson P, Henriksson G. Prediction of Sjögren's syndrome years before diagnosis and identification of patients with early onset and severe disease course by autoantibody profiling. *Arthritis Rheumatol* 2015;**67**:2427–36.

81. Røise D. *The impact of BAFF on the development of monocyte-derived dendritic cells in patients with rheumatic autoimmune diseases* [Master thesis]. Bergen, Norway: University of Bergen; 2015.

Chapter 16

# Autoantibodies and Autoantigens in Sjögren's Syndrome

R.I. Fox, C.M. Fox
*Scripps Memorial Hospital and Research Foundation, La Jolla, CA, United States*

## 1. BACKGROUND OF AUTOANTIBODIES SSA/B

Initial pioneering studies in systemic lupus erythematosus (SLE) noticed that patient sera could react with the nucleus of acetone-fixed nucleated cells using an immunofluorescent assay (IFA) (Fig. 16.1).[1,2] A series of different patterns of reactivity (ie, diffuse, fine-speckled, large-speckled, etc.) were noted and associated with distinct clinical features. The autoantibodies that produced each pattern were named by investigators at Rockefeller Institute for the initials of the patient who donated that serum sample (ie, patient Ro or La). However, in a different laboratory, the antibodies that reacted with the same antigens were called *SSA* or *SSB* for Sjögren's-associated antigen A or B. The use of specific terminology "Ro/La or SS-A/SS-B" is quite inconsistent in published papers and thus confusing to readers. For example, the name for the same antigen (ie, Ro or SS-A) may be used interchangeable in the same sentence or paragraph for no apparent reason except historical associations with particular reported symptoms.

The relationship with Sjögren's syndrome (SS) was initially noted by Tan et al.,[1] leading to the terms *SSA* and *SSB*. The same antibodies were associated with a subset of SLE by Reichlin et al.[3] and were termed *Ro* and *La*.

- For simplicity, I will use the terminology *Ro/SSA* and *La/SSB*.
- For the constituent molecules of *Ro/SSA*, I will use the terminology *Ro62* and *Ro50*.

The Ro/SSA antigen was initially identified by a line on Ouchterlony plates, and subsequently shown by immunoprecipitation or Western blot analysis to result from reactivity with a 60 kD (Ro60) and/or 52 kD (Ro52) molecules.[4–11] Exchange of sera samples indicates La/SSB antibodies identified by Ro antibodies, or the identical molecules.

Sjögren's Syndrome. http://dx.doi.org/10.1016/B978-0-12-803604-4.00016-2

## Staining pattern produced by anti-Ro52 antibodies

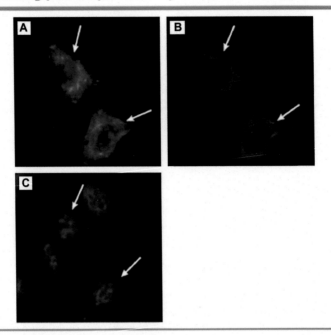

FIGURE 16.1   Example of an antinuclear antibody (ANA) assay as detected by immunofluorescent method where speckled nuclear particles are the location of Ro/SSA antigen. The substrate was the Hep2000 cell, which has been transfected with the Ro/SSA antigen to ensure its sensitivity to this labile antigen, is the best method for gold standard of detection. Human serum containing antibodies directed against Ro52 stained the cytoplasm of HEp-2 cells. To demonstrate the cytoplasmic staining pattern produced by these antibodies, a plasmid encoding Ro52 fused to green fluorescent protein (GFP) was expressed in HEp-2 cells and was stained with mouse anti-GFP (green, panel A). Two of the five cells in the field were successfully transfected with the plasmid (indicated by *white arrows*). Human anti-Ro52 antibodies stained the cytoplasm of all the HEp-2 cells in the field, but staining was especially intense in cells overexpressing Ro52-GFP (red, panel B). DAPI staining (blue) in panel C indicates the location of nuclei. *DAPI*, 4′,6′-diamidino-2-phenylindole.

It has been shown that most anti-Ro60 positive sera also react with a structurally unrelated Ro52 (26, 34, 35). There has been report of association of Ro60 and Ro52 via direct protein–protein interaction[12]; however, the interaction may be weak or transient, and was not observed by other investigators.[13]

This Ro60 binds to a family of small RNA molecules called *hYRNA* that have important functions in "quality control" and processing of RNAs. The cellular function for YRNAs remains unknown, but Ro60 protein is postulated to play roles in small RNA quality control and the enhancement of cell survival after exposure to ultraviolet irradiation. These are shown schematically in a crystallographic form binding to hYRNA in Fig. 16.2.

Perhaps the most interesting and pathogenetically important feature of the Ro62 molecule is its ability to withstand apoptotic degradation, maintain its binding to hYRNA, and migrate into the surface apoptotic bleb of dying cells,

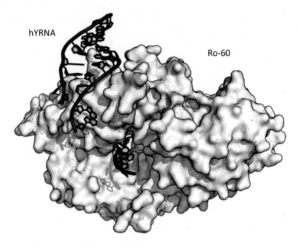

Schematic representation of hYRNA1 binding to Ro60

**FIGURE 16.2** Structure of Ro60 and Ro52 binding to hYRNA. This frame shows schematic binding of Ro60 and Ro52 proteins to hYRNA. The Ro60 kD is shown in white, while the Ro52 is shown in gray. Ro60 lacks caspase-sensitive sites and thus resists apoptotic cleavage. Ro52 may also have important roles in the regulation of inflammation. Ro52 adds an ubiquitin molecule to activated inhibitor of nuclear factor κB (NF-κB) kinase subunit β (IKKB). Ro52 also inhibits inflammation by targeting interferon regulatory factors (IRF) 3and 7 for ubiquitin-mediated degradation.

where it will be phagocytosed by macrophages and subsequently play a role in the perpetuation of the autoimmune process (described in the following).[14]

Another interesting feature of autoantibodies, including anti-Ro/SSA and anti-La/SSB, is their ability to bind near the "active" site of the target protein and to recognize conserved amino acid or structural motifs in patients with different ethnic backgrounds and their different human leukocyte antigen–antigen D–related (HLA-DR) genotypes.[2,15–17]

The antibody to La/SSB binds to a distinct 45 kD molecule that is loosely associated with the Ro/hYRNA complex. La/SSB is involved in diverse aspects of RNA metabolism, including binding and protecting 3′ UUU (OH) elements of newly RNA polymerase III-transcribed RNA, processing 5′ and 3′ ends of pretransfer (pre-tRNA) precursors, acting as an RNA chaperone and binding viral RNAs associated with hepatitis C virus.

## 2. METHODS OF DETECTION OF ANTINUCLEAR ANTIBODIES AND Ro/SSA AND La/SSB

The "gold standard" of detection of antinuclear antibodies (ANAs) is the IFA, originally using a cell line (Hep2). After many years of propagation in vitro, these Hep2 cell lines were determined to have been cross-contaminated by a myriad of other cell lines such as HeLa. Thus a standardized Hep cell line called *Hep2 2000* was suggested and its use as a standardized substrate is strongly advised.[18] This cell line has been transfected with Ro (60 and 52 kD) genes.

The problem in clinical practice is that not all laboratories use the same method, and different methods give different results.[19] One of the earliest examples of this laboratory "error" was the syndrome of "subacute" lupus characterized by a rash of erythema annulare. The patient would have a "negative" result for ANA, but a positive result for SSA antibody.[20] Because the Ro/SSA is a nuclear component, it is logically impossible for both tests to be correct. The most common explanation was the lability of the Ro/SSA antigen to fixation process during preparation of slides for IFA. When correctly fixed slides were used, the entire syndrome of "subacute lupus" disappeared.

In an effort to cut costs of laboratory evaluation, the IFA method of ANA detection has been replaced in many laboratories by an enzyme-linked immunosorbent assay (ELISA) method. Depending on the quality of the extract used for ELISA, differing results may be obtained. Thus the rheumatologist may obtain a negative ANA result in an ELISA test *in the same sample that yields a positive IFA in a different laboratory*. Similarly, the finding of a negative ANA by ELISA may accompany a report of positive antibodies to Ro/SSA on the same sample. This is logically inconsistent and indicates that one of the two assays is incorrect.

It is important for the rheumatologist and other physicians to recognize that the ANA by ELISA method in most clinical laboratories is "geared" to detect SLE sera, and thus may miss the patient who has only the Ro/SSA antibody or the anticentromere antibody (ACA).

This interesting discrepancy in results of ANA testing was actually the subject for a *New England Journal of Medicine* "Clinical Pathology Correlation" case study.[21] The diagnosis of SLE/SS was excluded on the basis of a negative ELISA, and the correct diagnosis was only made when IFA detection was used to detect positive ANA and then the antibody to Ro/SSA antigen.

In a clinical world where diagnosis is often made or excluded on the basis of a laboratory test, the type of test used to support a diagnosis is rarely recorded. The standard positive sera provided to the laboratory for ANA generally are derived from an SLE patient who has very high titers of anti-DNA antibodies. A positive standard sample containing only antibody to Ro/SSA is rarely included. Unless specifically requested, the large clinical laboratory rarely runs an antibody test for Ro/SSA and La/SSB or ACA unless the screening ANA is positive.

The problem of standardization has further been exacerbated in the United States by the proliferation of individual rheumatologists who run the ANA and Ro/SSA tests in their office laboratories, presumably as a method of obtaining increased revenue.

The importance of this simple but important diagnostic "pitfall" in diagnosis of SS deserves repetition:

- If the ANA by ELISA is negative, then an anti-Ro/SSA test is not routinely run, because the "full panel" is only run as a reflex response to the positive ANA.
- This simple laboratory artifact may bias entire disease registries and population studies.
- Perhaps the most important "simple" change in identifying SS patients would be the standardization of ANA by IFA or ELISA tests.

## 3. DETECTION OF SPECIFIC ANTIBODIES TO Ro/SSA AND La/SSB

Ro60 and Ro52 may be prepared by recombinant methods or by affinity columns. They may be detected either separately or in combination. Similarly, antibodies to La (45 kD), ACA, and rheumatoid factor (RF) are done by different methods. Although large laboratories attempt standardization by exchange of substrate and positive blood samples, there remains continued and significant variation in the results based on the substrate preparation and detection methods.

## 4. SIMPLE MODEL FOR THE ROLE OF Ro/SSA AND La/SSB IN PATHOGENESIS AND AS A POSSIBLE TARGET FOR THERAPY

Gordon et al.[22] initially proposed division of the steps for the pathogenesis of Ro/SSA and La/SSB in SS:

1. the initiation of autoimmunity, probably by an intercurrent viral infection that included damage to epithelial cells;
2. infiltration of the glands by lymphocytes and the diversification of autoantibodies to apoptosis-associated antigens;
3. the antibody-mediated tissue injury that perpetuated the cycle of apoptosis and further lymphoid infiltration;
4. the escape of particular lymphoid B-cell clones to lymphoma.

In the initiation step, the key finding is that intracellular autoantigens, including Ro/SSA and La/SSB, are clustered in membrane blebs (apoptotic blebs) at the surface of apoptotic cells. It has been proposed that apoptotic cells serve as a source of immunogen of intracellular proteins for the production of autoantibodies. Redistribution of Ro/SSA and La/SSB polypeptide into the blebs may produce neoepitopes by mechanisms such as oxidation, proteolytic cleavage, or conformational changes, and these have been termed "apotopes."

However, the resistance to apoptotic degradation can be only part of the story. It is known that SS is strongly associated with particular HLA-DR alleles.[23] This association may be different among divergent ethnic populations. In Caucasians, extended HLA-DR3/DQ1 haplotype and in Han Chinese or Japanese SS patients, a different HLA-DR haplotype, even though similar Ro/SSA epitopes, are recognized.[24]

The production of autoantibodies to Ro/SSA and La/SSB in SS patients was strongly linked to these same HLA-DR/DQ alleles over 40 years ago.[25–27] More recently, genome-wide association studies (GWASs) have further extended this result to include other loci associated with SS (and thus autoantibody to Ro/SSA), including genes associated with interferon (IFN) type 1 gene signature and B-cell stimulating factors[28,29] (Table 16.1).

Taken together, their findings suggest a simplified model that includes the Ro/SSA antigen that can bind to: (1) anti-Ro/SSA antibody, (2) the hYRNA that can bind to Toll-like receptors (TLRs), and (3) particular HLA-DR antigens associated with SS. Details of findings are as follows:

- an environmental agent or genetic tendency for initial damage to the lacrimal or salivary gland; indirect evidence suggesting a potential role for Epstein-Barr virus, a related virus, an endogenous viral fragment, or perhaps production of a microRNA in this initial damage;
- apoptosis of the glandular tissues with resistance of the Ro/SSA antigen from degradation and migration of the Ro/SSA–hYRNA complex into the apoptotic bleb;
- binding of the anti-Ro/SSA antibody to the Ro/SSA–hYRNA complex;
- phagocytosis of the Ro/SSA antigen (bound to hYRNA) by macrophages or antigen-presenting cells (APCs) where its normal fate would be enzymatic degradation;
- entry of the immune complex (antibody to Ro/SSA–Ro/SSA–hYRNA) to be into the lysosome or antigen-binding compartments of the macrophage;

**TABLE 16.1 Additional SNPs That Have Been Associated With Antibody to Ro/SSA**

| | | | |
|---|---|---|---|
| IL-10 | Promoter-1082<br>Promoter-819<br>Promoter-592 | SNP G/A<br>SNP C/T<br>SNP C/A | pSS |
| IL-1Ra | Intron-2 | IL1RN*2 | pSS |
| IL-6 | Promoter-174 | SNP G/C | IL-6 level, not pSS |
| TNF-α | TNFa | TNFa10 | pSS with arthritis or with anti-Ro/SSA |
| Ro52 | Intron 3 (137 bp upstream from exon 4) | SNP C/T | Anti-Ro52 in SS |
| TAP2 | Codon 577 | TAP2*Bky2 | pSS and anti-Ro/SSA |
| GSTM1 | GSTM1 | Homozygous null genotype | pSS and anti-Ro/SSA |
| MBL | MBL codon 54 | Wild-type allele<br>Homozygous mutant allele | pSS<br>Lupus and<br>SS and RA |
| Fas gene | MBL promoter enhancer region-671<br>IVS2nt176<br>IVS5nt82 | SNP G/G<br>SNP C/T<br>SNP C/G | pSS |

GSTM1, Glutathione S-transferase M1; IL, interleukin; MBL, mannose-binding lectin; pSS, primary Sjögren's syndrome; R, receptor; RA, rheumatoid arthritis; SNP, single nucleotide polymorphism; SS, Sjögren's syndrome; TNF, tumor necrosis factor.

- entry into other compartments of the macrophage by the complex because of the Fc receptors on the lysosomal membrane that bind to the Fc on the anti-Ro/SSA antibody;
- Ro/SSA antigen degraded into a peptide that is able to bind to the specific HLA-DR antigen for presentation to T helper cells that drive B-cell autoantibody production;
- hYRNA (containing both single- and double-stranded RNA regions) in the same lysosomal compartments, able to activate TLR to generate type 1 and γ IFN signatures;
- activated TLRs and activated T helper cells drive B cells to release further cytokines, form immune complexes, and eventually drive lymphocyte "aggressive" behavior as a result of continued antigen-driven processes;
- the role of other factors including hormonal status and local glandular factors in perpetuating this cycle.

In the particular case of antibodies to Ro/SSA and La/SSB, the immune complex of antibody/protein/hYRNA was historically first identified but later shown to play a plausible pathogenetic role (Figs. 16.3–16.6).

The hYRNA has single- and double-stranded regions that may appear similar to APCs as viral pathogens. To provide immediate and strong immune response to these viral challenges, the innate system has developed a family of TLRs that generate potent type 1 IFN and later type 2 IFNγ responses.

To protect delicate areas (such as eye or mouth) from indiscriminate destruction from these innate immune responses, natural evolution has cleverly "hidden" these TLRs inside lysosomal compartments of APCs, where they are not exposed to the direct liberation of RNA debris of dying cells. Thus

hYRNA has single and double stranded domains that
could trick body into thinking it was an RNA virus

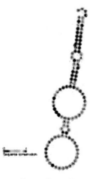

FIGURE 16.3   hYRNA family contains at least four members. These hYRNAs have single- and double-stranded RNA regions that have the ability to bind to Toll-like receptors (TLRs) 7 and 9. hYRNA1 has additional nucleotides form a "tail" binding to the lowest loop. This tail contains double stranded sequences shown schematically to the left of the lowest loop. This "tail" region of hYRNA1 is the structure where Ro60 binds.

| Unique ID | N =8 Control | Focus score Low N =8 | High N =8 | Salivary flow Normal N =6 | Decreased |
|---|---|---|---|---|---|
| hsa-miR-150 | 3.2 | 122.4 | 931.3 | – | – |
| hsa-miR-650 | 4.6 | 7.2 | 49.3 | – | – |
| hsa-miR-142-5p | 221.6 | 442.5 | 2,067.8 | – | – |
| hsa-miR-135b | 1.0 | 8.0 | 31.8 | – | – |
| hsa-miR-330 | 1.6 | 3.3 | 11.7 | – | – |
| hsa-miR-513 | 3.7 | 60.4 | 189.5 | – | – |
| hsa-miR-342 | 61.5 | 175.5 | 530.5 | – | – |
| hsa-miR-501 | 2.9 | 6.9 | 20.6 | – | – |
| hsa-miR-126* | 1.0 | 55.9 | 162.0 | – | – |
| ebv-miR-BART19 | 5.2 | 482.4 | 1,206.8 | – | – |
| hsa-miR-765 | – | – | – | 37.0 | 91.1 |
| hsa-miR-181a | – | – | – | 113.6 | 210.5 |
| hsa-miR-766 | – | – | – | 13.4 | 42.4 |
| hsa-miR-335 | – | – | – | 407.4 | 231.5 |
| hsa-miR-16 | – | – | – | 1,883.7 | 2,973.8 |
| hsa-miR-671 | – | – | – | 32.0 | 108.0 |
| hsa-miR-663 | – | – | – | 43.2 | 156.2 |
| hsa-miR-340 | – | – | – | 10.6 | 2.7 |
| hsa-miR-155 | – | – | – | 171.2 | 436.5 |

**FIGURE 16.4**   MicroRNA's have predicted structure similar to hYRNA and have been found in SS salivary glands.

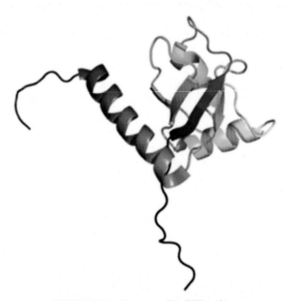

**FIGURE 16.5**   Structure of La/SSB antigen.

- La/SSB is an interferon-inducible protein that belongs to the "tripartite motif" family of proteins.
- The protein localizes to the cytoplasm and functions as an E3 ubiquitin ligase, an enzyme that adds ubiquitin molecules to target proteins.
- The N-terminus of the protein contains an "La" RNA-binding domain and an adjacent RNA recognition motif (RRM), which cooperate to bind RNA.
- The C-terminus of the protein contains a second RRM followed by a short basic motif ("SBF" domain) and a nuclear localization sequence.
- The N-terminal portion of La/SSB mediates the interaction with the 3' end of RNA polymerase III transcripts.
- La participates in the processing of small, noncoding RNAs such as ribosomal 5S RNA.

## SS-A Antibody perpetuates Pathogenesis

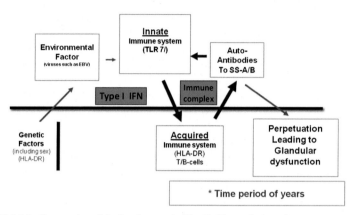

FIGURE 16.6  Proposed model of pathogenesis. The Ro60 protein is resistant to apoptosis and migrates into apoptotic blebs together with its associated hYRNA. In genetically susceptible individuals, an IgG antibody binds to the Ro/SSA–hYRNA complex. The Fc portion of the anti-Ro60 antibody binds to the Fc receptor on either dendritic cells, macrophages, or B cells to allow their internalization into the lysosome or other intracytoplasmic compartments. Within the cytoplasmic compartment of these dendritic-like cells, the hYRNA (containing both single- and double-stranded regions) are able to bind to Toll-like receptor *(TLR)* 7 or 9. The binding to the TLR receptor initiates a cascade of cytokines, including type 1 interferons and other factors that perpetuate activation of both T-helper and B-cell responses. *EBV*, Epstein-Barr virus; *HLA-DR*, human leukocyte antigen–antigen D related; *IFN*, interferon.

a rate-limiting step in the inflammatory response is the ability of autoantigens to gain entry into the cytoplasmic component, where they can stimulate and perpetuate autoimmune responses that eventuate in an autoimmune disease.

This "perfect" storm occurs in SS patients with:

- a positive antibody to Ro/SSA;
- Ro/SSA that binds to hYRNA in the apoptic bleb;
- antibody to Ro/SSA forming an immune complex with Ro/SSA–hYRNA;
- internalization of the immune complex into the phagocytic or dendritic cell through its Fc receptor;
- delivery of the immune complex to the intracytoplasmic TLRs;
- stimulation of TLR 7/9 by the single- and double-stranded RNA components to generate a type 1 and type 2 IFN signature;
- further activation of local T cells and B cells that result in cytokine production and continued antibody to Ro/SSA.

The genes predisposing to this model have been identified in recent GWAS studies (see Table 16.1).

The steps in this pathogenesis are shown in Fig. 16.1.

## 5. MAPPING OF ANTIGENIC EPITOPES ON Ro/SSA AND La/SSB

In genetically susceptible individuals, autoantibodies to "self"-antigens may result from the failure of thymiclike mechanisms to remove all T cells with the ability to respond to self-antigens. In this mechanism, the generation of nontolerized epitopes of Ro/SSA and La/SSB may initiate an autoimmune response, particularly in situations of increased apoptosis or where the clearance of apoptotic cells is impaired.[30,31]

However, the incomplete apoptotic destruction of Ro/SSA may allow the creation of "neo-epitopes." To date, there are several interesting reports on apotopes and posttranslational modification of Ro60 and La.[32–34] The epitopes on Ro60 remain relatively stable but the repertoire of autoantibodies in a single SS patient continues to evolve to higher affinity and possibly to include new cross-specificities.[35] In this regard, a recent abstract presented evidence that an antibody to Ro60 could bind to and block the functional action of the muscarinic 3 receptor (M3R).

Traditional mapping techniques of ELISA or immunoblotting have identified three immunodominant epitopes of La/SSB: LaA (aa1-107), LaC (aa111-242), and LaL2/3 (aa346-408). Passive transfer of immunoglobulin (Ig) G specific for LaA and LaC could bind cell membrane of apoptotic cells in a murine xenograft model, and identical findings were observed in cultured human fetal cardiocytes rendered apoptotic in vitro.[36,37]

Therefore LaA and LaC are exposed as apotopes, whereas the LaL2/3 epitope remains masked, presumably by maintaining an intracellular location in apoptotic cells. Furthermore, sera from mothers of infants with congenital heart block (CHB) react with LaA and LaC, indicating that these apotopes may be targets of maternal autoantibodies.[36,37]

In contrast to Ro60, Ro52 has been reported not to be detected on cell surface of early and late apoptotic cells using human Jurkat and HeLa cell lines.[32] This contrasts with earlier studies, in which surface binding of anti-Ro52 antibodies to apoptotic fetal cardiocytes and impairment of their clearance were reported.

Once the initiation step of autoantibodies production is established, it has been thought that intrastructural–intermolecular epitope spreading occurs for the diversification of the anti-Ro/SSA and anti-La/SSB autoimmune response.[38]

Spreading of the immune response appears to be a common theme in autoimmune diseases. The clustering of autoantibody specificity in patients with SS is thought to arise through a process of B-cell epitope spreading between components of Ro/SSA and La/SSB ribonucleoprotein complexes after the initiation of immunity to a single component of this structure.[39] Such spreading has been reported in mice immunized with Ro/SSA or La/SSB proteins or corresponding shorter synthetic peptides and rabbits after immunization with Ro60 peptide.[40] A similar type of epitope spreading in humans has been suggested to provide the bridge between initial viral infection and induction of SS in genetically predisposed individuals.[41]

# 6. La/SSB ANTIBODY

SSB/La is a distinct 47 kD protein (see Fig. 16.2B) and associates with a variety of small RNAs derived from RNA polymerase III, including Ro hYRNAs, pre-5S RNA, and pre-tRNA as well as many viral RNAs of the *TRIM* family.[42] The La/SSB protein has been described to have multiple functions, including as a transcription termination factor for RNA polymerase and a factor in mediating the correct ribosome translational start sites.

Anti-Ro/SSA antibodies, reflecting the physical association of these molecules in the Ro and La ribonucleoprotein particle complex, almost invariably accompany anti-La/SSB antibodies, but anti-Ro/SSA antibodies commonly occur in the absence of anti-La/SSB antibodies.

Of interest, immunization of animals with Ro60/hYRNA complexes can lead to the development of antibody to La/SSB.[39] This suggests a process of epitope spreading in this animal model, although patients who are Ro/SSA(+) and La/SSB(−) initially in their clinical course do not subsequently develop antibody to La/SSB later in their clinical course.

In 2006, the laboratories of Kamitani and Wahren-Herlenius independently reported that Ro52 is an E3 ubiquitin ligase.[43] Thus it is possible that Ro60 and/or La/SSB are substrates for Ro52-mediated ubiquitinylation and somehow they are stabilized during certain disease states, and the complexes contribute to the formation of autoantibodies to these components.

# 7. ANTIBODY TO Ro/SSA AND CHB

After the establishment of the autoimmune response, some pathological autoantibodies may subsequently have the capability of causing tissue destruction. Although a mechanism of the tissue destruction of anti-Ro/SSA and anti-La/SSB autoantibodies has not been elucidated, some new observations concerned with the tissue destruction of anti-Ro/SSA and anti-La/SSB autoantibodies have been reported in the CHB model.[43]

In a fetus diagnosed with isolated CHB, evaluation of the maternal serum almost invariably reveals the presence of autoantibodies against Ro/SSA and La/SSB in vitro, and in vivo studies suggest that one pathogenic cascade linking the antibodies to eventual scarring may be induced via apoptosis.

Clancy RM et al.[44] reported that nuclear injury and the translocation of Ro/SSA and La/SSB antigens to the fetal cardiomyocyte plasma membrane were common downstream events of Fas and tumor necrosis factor (TNF) receptor ligation, requiring caspase activation. These investigators also showed that cultured fetal cardiomyocyte-expressed phosphatidylserine receptors (PSRs) are known to mediate phagocytosis of apoptotic cells. The phagocytic uptake was blocked by anti-PSR antibodies, and was significantly inhibited after preincubation of apoptotic cardiomyocytes with IgG from an anti-Ro/SSA and anti-La/SSB autoantibody–positive mother of a CHB child.

## 8. ANTI-Ro/SSA ANTIBODIES PRECEDE DEVELOPMENT OF CLINICAL MANIFESTATIONS

In recent elegant studies, Theander et al. have shown that antibodies to ANA or Ro60 may precede the development of clinical SS symptoms by up to 20 years. They first identified SS patients in their Scandinavian cohort.[45,46]

One hundred and seventeen of these SS patients had serum samples that had been collected from healthy Swedish individuals as part of a long-term health study program. They compared them to serum samples from healthy individuals who had not developed SS at a median age of 6 years, but with some samples up to 20 years before clinical diagnosis. This finding mirrors similar observations in SLE, where autoantibodies preceded clinical features by over 8 years but the majority of ANA-positive individuals did not develop clinical SLE.[47]

This bank of "normal sera" allowed them to assess an increased risk of development of SS in asymptomatic individuals who had a positive ANA or Ro60 test.[47] They could calculate a Bayesian risk of development of SS about 25% if anti-Ro60 was present in the preclinical sample. This value is roughly comparable to the risk assessed in identical twins discordant for SLE, or development of SS in mothers who deliver babies with neonatal heart block anti-Ro60 antibodies.

## 9. OTHER AUTOANTIBODIES ASSOCIATED WITH SS

RF is typically an IgM antibody directed against the Fc binding portion of the IgG molecule.[48] This antibody is associated with rheumatoid arthritis (RA) but also occurs in the absence of anti–citrullinated protein antibodies (anti-CCPs) or radiographic evidence of RA. Of importance, particular idiotypic or germline-conserved sequences in the heavy and light chain of RF were initially identified in patients with Waldenström macroglobulinemia and mixed cryoglobulinemia. These conserved sequences and idiotypes are also preferentially expressed in SS patients[49,50] and contribute to the occurrence of type II mixed cryoglobulinemia and lymphoma.[48,51,52]

In addition to the anti-Ro/SSA and anti-La/SSB antibodies, a series of other antibodies have been associated with SS and may play a significant role in either pathogenesis or diagnosis. These include antibodies to the acetylcholine receptor, fodrin, Golgi proteins, and other proteins found in salivary glands.

Two additional autoantigens, α-fodrin[53] and M3R,[54,55] were identified more recently as targets for SS-specific autoantibodies.

Although the interests of many researchers have focused on these autoantibodies, they have not yet been established as SS-specific autoantibodies for clinical diagnostic use.

Furthermore, there have been many reports of other less prevalent autoantibodies such as nuclear mitotic apparatus protein,[56,57] members of Golgi autoantigen protein family, poly-adenosine triphosphate ribose polymerase,[58]

90-kDa nucleolar organizer region protein (NOR90/hUBF),[59] p80-coilin,[60] nuclear autoantigen 14 kD (NA14),[61] and many others that have been described in SS.

Some of the controversies regarding anti-M3R autoantibodies lie in their prevalence and specificity. The prevalence of these receptors ranged anywhere from 9% to 90%, depending upon the sensitivity of assay systems developed and targeted epitopes on M3R.[62–64] ELISA (or its variants) has been the most common screening method for this antibody, and linear peptides were not suitable for detection or inhibition studies, indicating that the M3R epitope is discontinuous or conformational.

In fact, the highest prevalence originated from a study utilizing glutathione S-transferase (GST)–fusion recombinant peptides, allowing dimerization of linear peptides, thus maintaining a native tertiary structure found in-vivo.[65]

Although the critical epitope(s) of M3R have not been clearly defined to date, the dominant epitope was presumed to be present in the second extracellular cellular loop (aa213-228), where a receptor and ligand binding site is located.[66]

However, later studies pointed out other potential epitopes, such as the third extracellular loop (aa514-527)[67] or second extracellular loop encompassing the transmembrane domain (aa213-237),[68] as M3R epitopes. More importantly, it is still questionable as to whether anti-M3R binding is specific to M3R, as indicated by a study where antipeptide M3R (aa208-228) antibodies strongly bind to M1R.[69]

Nonetheless, full mapping of M3R epitopes, improvement of sensitivity/specificity of assays, proper and well-defined selection of disease and healthy controls, and large patient-oriented studies will allow more consistent findings and thorough information on prevalence and specificity.

## 10. ANTI–α-FODRIN ANTIBODIES

α-Fodrin belongs to the α-spectrin family and has been known, alternatively, as *nonerythroid α-spectrin* (also called *calspectin* or *α-spectrin* ΠΣ1).[70]

In humans, four spectrin genes have been identified, including α- and β-spectrin genes. Genes for nonerthyroid fodrin encode proteins and are approximately 60% identical to their erythroid counterparts. α-Fodrin is expressed ubiquitously in nonerythroid tissues, and is similar to erythroid spectrin in some respects, including immunochemical reactivity, rodlike appearance on electron microscopy, tetramer formation, and ability to bind actin and ankyrin.[71] Unlike erythroid spectrin, α-fodrin is not uniformly distributed along the cell membrane.

Although the current understanding of the function of α-fodrin is incomplete, it has been suggested that α-fodrin maintains the spatial organization of specialized membrane proteins and mediate their attachment to the actin cytoskeleton.[71] Interestingly, α-fodrin is known to associate with membrane ion channels and pumps such as $Na^+/K^+$ adenosine triphosphatase in salivary glands via various ankyrin species.[72]

In mice, α-fodrin is a 240 kDa protein forming a heterodimer with β-fodrin, and it has been shown that α-fodrin is cleaved by caspase 3 into small fragments of 150 and 120. Subsequently, Yanagi et al. reported that, in nonobese diabetic mice, specific autoantibody production was found against 120 kDa α-fodrin and that it was closely related to autoimmune sialadenitis, which resembles human SS.[73]

In humans, it has also been reported that anti–α-fodrin antibody is predominantly detected in the sera from SS patients compared with SLE patients, suggesting that anti–α-fodrin autoantibody is valuable for the diagnosis of SS.[74] Although antibody against β-fodrin also has been described in the sera of SS patients, clinical associations have not been reported.[75]

The incidence of anti–α-fodrin antibodies in SS varies between 40% and 70%,[76] although anti–α-fodrin autoantibodies originally were described as SS-specific autoantibodies. Recent data have shown that anti–α-fodrin autoantibodies are present in 10% to 30% of patients with active inflammatory diseases such as RA or SLE, and 2% of healthy blood donors.[76]

In summary, current opinion supports a 2008 study using 321 primary SS patients where investigators reported that antibodies to α-fodrin were not diagnostically superior to conventional anti-Ro/SSA and anti-La/SSB testing.[77]

## 11. ANTIBODIES TO NA14

Chan et al. reported a novel class of coiled-coil–rich proteins that are recognized as cytoplasmic organelle-associated autoantigens in systemic autoimmune diseases.[78] These include a family of Golgi complex autoantigens known as "golgins" (such as giantin, golgin-245, Golgi-associated microtubule-binding protein [GMAP-210], golgin-95/GM130, golgin-160, and golgin-97); endosomal proteins EEA1 and CLIP-170; and centrosomal proteins pericentrin, ninein, Cep250, and Cep110.

## 12. NUCLEAR AUTOANTIGEN 14 kD

NA14 was originally identified as a novel coiled-coil autoantigen recognized by an autoimmune serum from a patient with SS.[61] In fact, the same SS patient serum was used to screen a complementary DNA library, and another coiled-coil–rich GMAP-210 was cloned and characterized.[79]

In a study of multiple patients with autoimmune diseases, the prevalence of anti-NA14 was 18/132 (13.6%) in primary SS, 0/50 (0%) in secondary SS, 2/100 (2%) in SLE, 1/43 (2.3%) in systemic sclerosis (SSc), 0/54 (0%) in RA, and 1/29 (3.4%) in polymyositis/dermatomyositis.[60] Anti-NA14 antibody positive sera were observed most often in primary SS. Interestingly, none of the secondary SS patients had autoantibodies to NA14. This data showed that anti-NA14 antibodies appeared independent of anti-Ro/SSA anti-La/SSB antibodies, and 36.4% (4/11) of anti-NA14 positive sera was negative for anti-Ro/SSA and anti-La/SSB antibodies.

## 13. SUMMARY

Several of the key take-home points for clinicians are researchers are summarized in Table 16.2.

*Antibodies to Ro/SSA and La/SSB are now a criterion for primary SS.* The ability of this antigen to withstand apoptotic degradation and bind hYRNA has led to a plausible hypothesis for its role in pathogenesis through stimulation of TLRs.

*The distinction between primary SS, SLE, and RA has been difficult using serological methods alone.* Indeed, one recent study indicated that over 50% of patients classified as SLE were actually suffering from SS when minor salivary gland biopsies and ophthalmological examinations were performed.

This is important, because many SS patients with extraglandular manifestations are not currently included in our clinical studies. Thus our failure to develop novel therapies is partly the result of misclassification of SS patients who have extraglandular manifestations as a misunderstanding of anti-Ro/SSA antibody serology.

*RF is commonly found in SS patients, and patients are erroneously treated for RA with TNF inhibitors,* which may exacerbate the SS or lymphomagenesis predilection. The presence of RF may be associated with mixed cryoglobulinemia and increased risk of lymphoma.

*About 20% of SS patients are negative for antibodies to Ro/SS-A and La/SSB antigens or RF.* Many of these patients have ACAs but do not fulfill the criteria for SSc. Nevertheless, these ACA patients appear to form a subgroup with a higher incidence of Raynaud phenomena and increased fibrosis on their lip biopsy, two features that are found in the limited SSc population (ie, calcinosis cutis, Raynaud phenomenon, esophageal dysfunction, sclerodactyly, and telangiectasia [CREST]) subgroup.

*Recent candidates for early diagnosis of SS include parotid specific protein 1.* It has been proposed that this antibody may precede the evolution of clinical SS by many years. However, the sensitivity and specificity of these tests has not yet been verified, and no conclusions about its predictive values should be concluded, despite its vigorous sales marketing campaign.

Even in the case of Ro/SSA and La/SSB positivity that has been considered criteria for diagnosis of SS, the proportion of antibody-positive patients who later develop SS may only be in the 18% to 25% range after 10 years of follow-up observation.

**TABLE 16.2  Key Points About Autoantibodies in Sjögren's Syndrome**

1. **Ro/SSA contains two chains called Ro60 and Ro52** that are noncovalently bound to a transfer RNA-like structure called *hYRNA*.
2. **hYRNA contains both single- and double-stranded RNA regions that could be "mistaken" for viral sequences by Toll-like receptors** (TLRs) 7 and 9 if they were able to gain access to the lysosomal compartment of phagocytic or dendritic cells, initiating a cascade of cytokines leading to a type 1 interferon signature.
3. **Ro/SSA is resistant to normal apoptotic degradation**, and along with its bound hYRNA, migrates to the surface "apoptotic bleb."
4. **Antibodies to Ro/SSA and La/SSB is part of the current criteria for diagnosis of SS.** However, the presence of these antibodies is neither necessary, nor sufficient, to make the diagnosis of SS.
5. **In large population studies of normal individuals, antibody to Ro/SSA occurs in approximately 0.5%.** In retrospective studies of SS patients, the antibody to Ro/SSA precedes clinical features by 8 to 20 years.
6. **The presence of anti-Ro/SSA antibody increases the preclinical individual's chance of developing SS to 18% to 25% over a 20-year follow-up period.** This calls for caution about "overdiagnosis" of SS, and creating unnecessary anxiety for the patient is important.
7. **Over 50% of SS patients are mislabeled**, most commonly as systemic lupus erythematosus (SLE) or rheumatoid arthritis (RA), even in rheumatology clinics.
8. **RF may be associated with type II mixed cryoglobulinemia** and increased risk of lymphoma.
9. **(ACAs) may be found in 8% to 10% of SS patients where patients have incidence of Raynaud phenomenon and increased glandular fibrosis**, yet the patients do not fulfill diagnostic criteria for scleroderma (SSc).
10. **The overlap with SLE is common and points out that SLE is composed of a series of subsets**, including one characterized by anti-Ro/SSA antibodies.
11. **The failure to recognize SS patients (ie, mislabeled as RA or SLE) has impeded clinical studies.** The SS patients most likely to respond to immodulating agents are those with extraglandular manifestations, and they not enrolled owing to their misdiagnosis.
12. **Other autoantibodies such as antibody to muscarinic M3 receptor are intriguing, and would help to explain the organ specific features of SS.** However, it is unclear whether they are present in human SS (although clearly present in animal models) and whether they are primary or secondary events.
13. **Antibodies for "early" diagnosis, such as parotid specific protein (PSP), have been aggressively marketed recently through optometrists for dry-eye patients.** The sensitivity and specificity of these tests needs further evaluation before any recommendations can be made.

*Therefore caution in advising patients who are found to have this antibody on "general screening" must be advised* because a putative diagnosis of SS may interfere with their choices in family planning and career, and cause unnecessary anxiety.

## ABBREVIATIONS

**ACA** Anticentromere antibody, generally associated with SSc but also found in a subset of SS patients.

**ANA** Antinuclear antibody, initially detected by immune fluorescent method and more recently by ELISA method; these methods may not give similar result.

**APC** Antigen-presenting cell, contains lysosomal organelles, which contain Toll-like receptors

**CCP** Citrullinated protein antibody

**CHB** Congenital heart block, occurring predominantly in infants and may be caused by antibody to Ro/SSA.

**ELISA** Enzyme-linked immunosorbent assay

**GMAP-210** Golgi-associated microtubule-binding protein

**GWAS** Genome-wide association study

**HLA-DR** Human leukocyte antigen–antigen D related

**IFA** Immune fluorescent assay

**IFN** Interferon

**Ig** Immunoglobulin

**M3R** Muscarinic 3 receptor, plays a role in neural innervation of lacrimal and salivary glands

**NA14** Nuclear autoantigen 14 kD

**PSP** Parotid specific protein, an antigen expressed in rodent glands, but not in human glands, that may react with human sera and proposed as a preclinical marker for SS

**PSR** Phosphatidylserine receptors

**RA** Rheumatoid arthritis

**RF** Rheumatoid factor, an antibody that reacts with the Fc portion of IgG antibody associated with anti-CCP in RA patients

**Ro52** A component of the Ro/SSA antigen, a distinct molecule with 52 kD molecular weight that may be loosely associated with Ro60 antigen

**Ro60** One component of Ro/SSA with 60 kD molecular weight

**SLE** Systemic lupus erythematosus

**SS** Sjögren's syndrome, may be primary SS or secondary SS, which refers to the overlap of sicca symptoms to patients with another well-defined disorder such as SLE, SSc, or RA

**SSA** Original nuclear antigen defined by Ouchterlony immunodiffusion method and that gives a speckled pattern on ANAs by IFA

**SSc** Systemic sclerosis, scleroderma that may be limited or diffuse

**TLR** Toll-like receptor

**TNF** Tumor necrosis factor

**tRNA** Transfer RNA

## REFERENCES

1. Martinez-Lavin M, Vaughan J, Tan E. Autoantibodies and the spectrum of Sjögren's syndrome. *Ann Intern Med* 1979;**91**:185–90.

2. Tan EM. Autoantibodies to nuclear antigens (ANA): their immunobiology medicine. *Adv Immunol* 1982;**33**:167–240.

3. Wasicek C, Reichlin M. Clinical and serological differences between systemic lupus erythematosus patients with antibodies to Ro versus patients with antibodies to Ro and La. *J Clin Invest* 1982;**69**:835.

4. Ben-Chetrit E, Chan EKL, Sullivan KF, Tan EM. A 52 kD protein is a novel component of the SS-A-Ro antigenic particle. *J Exp Med* 1988;**167**:1560–71.

5. Chan EK, Sullivan KF, Tan EM. Ribonucleoprotein SS-B/La belongs to a protein family with consensus sequence for RNA-binding. *Nucleic Acids Res* 1989;**17**:2233–44.

6. Chan EKL, Sullivan KF, Fox RI, Tan EM. Sjögren's syndrome nuclear antigen B (La): cDNA cloning, structural domains, and autoepitopes. *J Autoimmun* 1989;**2**:321–7.

7. Tan EM. Antinuclear antibodies: diagnostic markers for autoimmune diseases and probes for cell biology. *Adv Immunol* 1989;**44**:93–151.

8. Chan EK, Tan EM, Ward DC, Matera AG. Human 60-kDa SS-A/Ro ribonucleoprotein auto-antigen gene (SSA2) localized to 1q31 by fluorescence in situ hybridization. *Genomics* 1994;**23**:298–300.

9. Tan E. Autoimmunity and apoptosis. *J Exp Med* 1994;**179**:1083–6.

10. Tan E, Muro Y, Pollard K. Autoantibody-defined epitopes on nuclear antigens are conserved, conformation-dependent and active site regions. *Clin Exp Rheumatol* 1994;**12**: S27–31.

11. Tan EM. Autoantibodies: what do they recognize? *Verh Dtsch Ges Pathol* 1996;**80**:1–11.

12. Slobbe R, Pluk W, Van Venrooij W, Pruijn G. Ro ribonucleoprotein assembly in vitro: identification of RNA-protein and protein-protein interactions. *J Mol Biol* 1992;**227**:361–6.

13. Boire G, Gendron M, Monast N, Bastin B, Menard H. Purification of antigenically intact Ro ribonucleoproteins: biochemical and immunological evidence that the 52-kD protein is not a Ro protein. *Clin Exp Immunol* 1995;**100**:489.

14. Bolstad AI, Jonsson R. The role of apoptosis in Sjögren's syndrome. *Ann Med Interne (Paris)* 1998;**149**:25–9.

15. Tan EM, Vaughan JH. *Antinuclear antibodies: significance of biochemical specificities in immunopathology of the skin.* 1973.

16. Chan EK, Francoeur AM, Tan EM. Epitopes, structural domains, and asymmetry of amino acid residues in SS-B/La nuclear protein. *J Immunol* 1986;**136**:3744.

17. Tan EM, Muro Y, Pollard KM. Autoantibody-defined epitopes on nuclear antigens are conserved, conformation-dependent and active site regions. *Clin Exp Rheumatol* 1994;**12**(Suppl. 11):S27–31.

18. Peene I, Van Ael W, Vandenbossche M, Vervaet T, Veys E, De Keyser F. Sensitivity of the HEp-2000 substrate for the detection of anti-SSA/Ro60 antibodies. *Clin Rheumatol* 2000; **19**:291–5.

19. Tan EM, Smolen JS, McDougal JS, Butcher BT, Conn D, Dawkins R, et al. A critical evaluation of enzyme immunoassays for detection of antinuclear autoantibodies of defined specificities. I. Precision, sensitivity, and specificity. *Arthritis Rheum* 1999;**42**:455–64.

20. Vazquez-Doval J, Ruiz de Erenchun F, Sanchez-Ibarrola A, Contreras F, Soto de Delas J, Quintanilla E. Subacute cutaneous lupus erythematosus: clinical, histopathological and immunophenotypical study of five cases. *J Investig Allergol Clin Immunol* 1992;**2**:27–32.

21. Cabot RC, Stone JH, Bloch DB, Sepehr A. Case 5-2009: a 47-year-old woman with a rash and numbness and pain in the legs. *New Eng J Med* 2009;**360**:711–20.

22. Gordon TP, Bolstad AI, Rischmueller M, Jonsson R, Waterman SA. Autoantibodies in primary Sjögren's syndrome: new insights into mechanisms of autoantibody diversification and disease pathogenesis. *Autoimmunity* 2001;**34**:123–32.

23. Fox RI. Sjögren's syndrome. *Lancet* 2005;**366**:321–31.

24. Kang HI, Fei H, Fox RI. Comparison of genetic factors in Chinese, Japanese and Caucasoid patients with Sjögren's syndrome. *Arthritis & Rheum* 1991;**34**. S41 (Supplement).

25. Harley JB, Alexander EL, Bias WB, Fox OF, Provost TT, Reichlin M, et al. Anti-Ro (SS-A) and Anti-La (SS-B) in patients with Sjögren's syndrome. *Arthritis Rheum* 1986;**29**:196–206.

26. Arnett F. Histocompatibility typing in the rheumatic diseases: diagnostic and prognostic implications. *Med Clin North Am* 1994;**20**:371–87.

27. Arnett F, Reichlin M. Lupus hepatitis: an under-recognized disease feature associated with autoantibodies to ribosomal P. *Am J Med* 1995;**99**:465–72.
28. Lessard CJ, Li H, Adrianto I, Ice JA, Rasmussen A, Grundahl KM, et al. Variants at multiple loci implicated in both innate and adaptive immune responses are associated with Sjögren's syndrome. *Nat Genet* 2013;**45**:1284–92.
29. Li H, Ice JA, Lessard CJ, Sivils KL. Interferons in Sjögren's syndrome: genes, mechanisms, and effects. *Front Immunol* 2013;**4**:290.
30. Rosen A, Casciola-Rosen L, Ahearn J. Novel packages of viral and self-antigens are generated during apoptosis. *J Exp Med* 1995;**181**:1557–61.
31. Pan ZJ, Davis K, Maier S, Bachmann MP, Kim-Howard XR, Keech C, et al. Neo-epitopes are required for immunogenicity of the La/SS-B nuclear antigen in the context of late apoptotic cells. *Clin Exp Immunol* 2006;**143**:237–48.
32. Reed JH, Neufing PJ, Jackson MW, Clancy RM, Macardle PJ, Buyon JP, et al. Different temporal expression of immunodominant Ro60/60 kDa-SSA and La/SSB apotopes. *Clin Exp Immunol* 2007;**148**:153–60.
33. Terzoglou AG, Routsias JG, Moutsopoulos HM, Tzioufas AG. Post-translational modifications of the major linear epitope 169-190aa of Ro60 kDa autoantigen alter the autoantibody binding. *Clin Exp Immunol* 2006;**146**:60–5.
34. Terzoglou AG, Routsias JG, Avrameas S, Moutsopoulos HM, Tzioufas AG. Preferential recognition of the phosphorylated major linear B-cell epitope of La/SSB 349-368 aa by anti-La/SSB autoantibodies from patients with systemic autoimmune diseases. *Clin Exp Immunol* 2006;**144**:432–9.
35. Reed JH, Gordon TP. Autoimmunity: Ro60-associated RNA takes its toll on disease pathogenesis. *Nat Rev Rheum* 2015.
36. Tsay GJ, Chan EK, Peebles CL, Pollard KM, Tan EM. An immunoassay differentiating sera with antibodies to Sm alone, antibodies to Sm/RNP complex, and antibodies to RNP alone. *Arthritis Rheum* 1987;**30**:389–96.
37. Neufing PJ, Clancy RM, Jackson MW, Tran HB, Buyon JP, Gordon TP. Exposure and binding of selected immunodominant La/SSB epitopes on human apoptotic cells. *Arthritis Rheum* 2005;**52**:3934–42.
38. Gordon TP, Kinoshita G, Cavill D, Keech C, Farris A, Kaufman K, et al. Restricted specificity of intermolecular spreading to endogenous La (SS-B) and 60 kDa Ro (SS-A) in experimental autoimmunity. *Scand J Immunol* 2002;**56**:168–73.
39. Scofield RH, Kaufman KM, Baber U, James JA, Harley JB, Kurien BT. Immunization of mice with human 60-kD Ro peptides results in epitope spreading if the peptides are highly homologous between human and mouse. *Arthritis Rheum* 1999;**42**:1017–24.
40. Scofield RH, Henry WE, Kurien BT, James JA, Harley JB. Immunization with short peptides from the sequence of the systemic lupus erythematosus-associated 60-kDa Ro autoantigen results in anti-Ro ribonucleoprotein autoimmunity. *J Immunol* 1996;**156**:4059–66.
41. Igoe A, Scofield RH. Autoimmunity and infection in Sjögren's syndrome. *Curr Opin Rheumatol* 2013;**25**:480.
42. Kurien B, Dsouza A, Igoe A, Lee YJ, Maier-Moore JS, Gordon T, et al. Immunization with 60 kD Ro peptide produces different stages of preclinical autoimmunity in a Sjögren's syndrome model among multiple strains of inbred mice. *Clin Exp Immunol* 2013;**173**:67–75.
43. Oke V, Wahren-Herlenius M. The immunobiology of Ro52 (TRIM21) in autoimmunity: a critical review. *J Autoimmun* 2012;**39**:77–82.
44. Reed JH, Sim S, Wolin SL, Clancy RM, Buyon JP. Ro60 requires Y3 RNA for cell surface exposure and inflammation associated with cardiac manifestations of neonatal lupus. *J Immunol* 2013;**191**:110–6.

45. Konsta OD, Le Dantec C, Charras A, Brooks WH, Arleevskaya MI, Bordron A, et al. An in silico approach reveals associations between genetic and epigenetic factors within regulatory elements in B cells from primary Sjögren's syndrome patients. *Front Immunol* 2015;**6**.

46. Theander E, Jonsson R, Sjöström B, Brokstad K, Olsson P, Henriksson G. Prediction of Sjögren's syndrome years before diagnosis and identification of patients with early onset and severe disease course by autoantibody profiling. *Arthritis Rheumatol* 2015;**67**:2427–36.

47. Arbuckle MR, McClain MT, Rubertone MV, Scofield RH, Dennis GJ, James JA, et al. Development of autoantibodies before the clinical onset of systemic lupus erythematosus. *N Engl J Med* 2003;**349**:1526–33.

48. Fong S, Chen PP, Fox RI, Goldfien RD, Silverman GJ, Radoux V, et al. Rheumatoid factors in human autoimmune disease: their origin, development and function. *Pathol Immunopathol Res* 1986;**5**:305–16.

49. Fox RI, Fong S, Chen PP, Kipps TJ. Autoantibody production in Sjögren's syndrome: a hypothesis regarding defects in somatic diversification of germ line encoded genes. *In Vivo* 1988;**2**:47–56.

50. Kipps TJ, Tomhave E, Chen PP, Fox RI. Molecular characterization of a major autoantibody-associated cross-reactive idiotype in Sjögren's syndrome. *J Immunol* 1989;**142**:4261–8.

51. Fong S, Chen PP, Gilbertson TA, Weber JR, Fox RI, Carson DA. Expression of three cross-reactive idiotypes on rheumatoid factor autoantibodies from patients with autoimmune diseases and seropositive adults. *J Immunol* 1986;**137**:122–8.

52. Fox RI, Chen PP, Carson DA, Fong S. Expression of a cross reactive idiotype on rheumatoid factor in patients with Sjögren's syndrome. *J Immunol* 1986;**136**:477–83.

53. Haneji N, Nakamura T, Takio K, Yanagi K, Higashiyama H, Saito I, et al. Identification of alpha-fodrin as a candidate autoantigen in primary Sjögren's syndrome. *Science* 1997;**276**:604–7.

54. Bacman S, Sterin-Borda L, Camusso JJ, Arana R, Hubscher O, Borda E. Circulating antibodies against rat parotid gland M3 muscarinic receptors in primary Sjögren's syndrome. *Clin Exp Immunol* 1996;**104**:454–9.

55. Beroukas D, Goodfellow R, Hiscock J, Jonsson R, Gordon TP, Waterman SA. Up-regulation of M3-muscarinic receptors in labial salivary gland acini in primary Sjögren's syndrome. *Lab Invest* 2002;**82**:203–10.

56. Chan EK, Damoiseaux J, Carballo OG, Conrad K, de Melo Cruvinel W, Francescantonio PL, et al. Report of the first international consensus on standardized nomenclature of antinuclear antibody HEp-2 cell patterns 2014–2015. *Front Immunol* 2015;**6**.

57. Price CM, Mccarty GA, Pettijohn DE. NuMA protein is a human autoantigen. *Arthritis Rheum* 1984;**27**:774–9.

58. Griffith KJ, Chan EK, Lung CC, Hamel JC, Guo X, Miyachi K, et al. Molecular cloning of a novel 97-kD Golgi complex autoantigen associated with Sjögren's syndrome. *Arthritis Rheum* 1997;**40**:1693–702.

59. Chan E, Imai H, Hamel JC, Tan E. Human autoantibody to RNA polymerase I transcription factor hUBF: molecular identity of nucleolus organizer region autoantigen NOR-90 and ribosomal RNA transcription upstream binding factor. *J Exp Med* 1991;**174**:1239–44.

60. Andrade L, Chan E, Raska I, Peebles CL, Roos G, Tan EM. Human autoantibody to a novel protein of the nuclear coiled body: immunological characterization and cDNA cloning of p.80-coilin. *J Exp Med* 1991;**173**:1407–19.

61. Ramos-Morales F, Infante C, Fedriani C, Bornens M, Rios RM. NA14 is a novel nuclear autoantigen with a coiled-coil domain. *J Biol Chem* 1998;**273**:1634–9.

62. Kovács L, Fehér E, Bodnár I, Marczinovits I, Nagy GM, Somos J, et al. Demonstration of autoantibody binding to muscarinic acetylcholine receptors in the salivary gland in primary Sjögren's syndrome. *Clin Immunol* 2008;**128**:269–76.

63. Cha S, Singson E, Cornelius J, Yagna JP, Knot HJ, Peck AB. Muscarinic acetylcholine type-3 receptor desensitization due to chronic exposure to Sjögren's syndrome-associated autoantibodies. *J Rheumatol* 2006;**33**:296–306.

64. Cavill D, Waterman SA, Gordon TP. Failure to detect antibodies to extracellular loop peptides of the muscarinic M3 receptor in primary Sjögren's syndrome. *J Rheumatol* 2002;**29**:1342–4.

65. Kovacs L, Marczinovits I, György A, Tóth GK, Dorgai L, Pál J, et al. Clinical associations of autoantibodies to human muscarinic acetylcholine receptor 3213–228 in primary Sjögren's syndrome. *Rheumatology* 2005;**44**:1021–5.

66. Cavill D, Waterman SA, Gordon TP. Antibodies raised against the second extracellular loop of the human muscarinic M3 receptor mimic functional autoantibodies in Sjögren's syndrome. *Scand J Immunol* 2004;**59**:261–6.

67. Koo N-Y, Li J, Hwang SM, Choi SY, Lee SJ, Oh SB, et al. Functional epitope of muscarinic type 3 receptor which interacts with autoantibodies from Sjögren's syndrome patients. *Rheumatology* 2008;**47**:828–33.

68. Naito Y, Matsumoto I, Wakamatsu E, Goto D, Sugiyama T, Matsumura R, et al. Muscarinic acetylcholine receptor autoantibodies in patients with Sjögren's syndrome. *Ann Rheum Dis* 2005;**64**:510–1.

69. Schegg V, Vogel M, Didichenko S, Stadler MB, Beleznay Z, Gadola S, et al. Evidence that anti-muscarinic antibodies in Sjögren's syndrome recognise both M3R and M1R. *Biologicals* 2008;**36**:213–22.

70. Winkelmann JC, Forget BG. Erythroid and nonerythroid spectrins. *Blood* 1993;**81**:3173–85.

71. Bennett V. Spectrin-based membrane skeleton: a multipotential adaptor between plasma membrane and cytoplasm. *Physiol Rev* 1990;**70**:1029–65.

72. Koob R, Zimmermann M, Schoner W, Drenckhahn D. Colocalization and coprecipitation of ankyrin and Na+, K+-ATPase in kidney epithelial cells. *Eur J Cell Biol* 1988;**45**:230–7.

73. Maruyama T, Saito I, Hayashi Y, Kompfner E, Fox RI, Burton DR, et al. Molecular analysis of the human autoantibody response to α-fodrin in Sjögren's syndrome reveals novel apoptosis-induced specificity. *Am J Pathol* 2004;**165**:53–61.

74. Watanabe T, Tsuchida T, Kanda N, Mori K, Hayashi Y, Tamaki K. Anti–α-Fodrin antibodies in Sjögren syndrome and lupus erythematosus. *Arch Dermatol* 1999;**135**:535–9.

75. Kuwana M, Okano T, Ogawa Y, Kaburaki J, Kawakami Y. Autoantibodies to the amino-terminal fragment of β-fodrin expressed in glandular epithelial cells in patients with Sjögren's syndrome. *J Immunol* 2001;**167**:5449–56.

76. Witte T, Matthias T, Bierwirth J, Schmidt RE. Antibodies against alpha-fodrin are associated with sicca syndrome in the general population. *Ann N Y Acad Sci* 2007;**1108**:414–7.

77. Locht H, Pelck R, Manthorpe R. Diagnostic and prognostic significance of measuring antibodies to alpha-fodrin compared to anti-Ro-52, anti-Ro-60, and anti-La in primary Sjögren's syndrome. *J Rheumatol* 2008;**35**:845–9.

78. Chan EK, Fritzler MJ. Golgins: coiled-coil-rich proteins associated with the Golgi complex. *Electron J Biotechnol* 1998;**1**:01–20.

79. Infante C, Ramos-Morales F, Fedriani C, Bornens M, Rios RM. GMAP-210, a cis-Golgi network-associated protein, is a minus end microtubule-binding protein. *J Cell Biol* 1999;**145**: 83–98.

Chapter 17

# Outcome Measures in Sjögren's Syndrome and Perspectives in Clinical Trial Design

R. Felten, J. Sibilia, J.-E. Gottenberg
*Strasbourg University Hospital, Strasbourg, France*

## 1. CURRENT OUTCOME MEASURES IN PRIMARY SJÖGREN'S SYNDROME

### 1.1 Symptoms

Evaluation of the three main symptoms of primary Sjögren's syndrome (pSS): dryness, pain, and fatigue, is pivotal, because these concerns are shared by all patients with pSS, in contrast to systemic complications, which affect approximately 30% of patients. Individual visual analog scales (VASs), ie, pain and fatigue VASs, represent the only way to assess patients' symptoms. Early randomized clinical trials in pSS evaluating infliximab[1] or etanercept[2] defined the primary outcome criteria as a decrease in patients' VAS score (pain, fatigue, and dryness). Recently, the European League Against Rheumatism (EULAR) Sjögren's Syndrome Patient-Related Index (ESSPRI) was internationally validated.[3] This patient-related outcome is very simple to score (it is the mean of VAS pain, fatigue, and dryness) and sensitive to change. The ESSPRI allows patients to be divided into different disease activity subsets. In addition, it has recently been shown that patients' minimal clinically important improvement (MCII) corresponds to a decrease of at least 15% of the ESSPRI baseline value or a decrease of at least one point (on a 10-point score).[4] Consequences of these symptoms on quality of life (QOL) can be assessed using QOL scales such as the Short Form-36 and on depression by the Health Assessment Questionnaire score. Fatigue and dryness can also be studied more in-depth by using fatigue scores such as the Functional Assessment of Chronic Illness Therapy[5] and the Profile of Fatigue and Discomfort-Sicca Symptoms Inventory questionnaires.[6,7]

Sjögren's Syndrome. http://dx.doi.org/10.1016/B978-0-12-803604-4.00017-4

## 1.2 Systemic Complications

Evaluation of systemic complications used to be very complicated in pSS. There was no consensus on the definition of systemic complications and there were no available scores. Patients were divided into patients with only glandular symptoms and patients with extraglandular involvement. However, the latter term was not clearly defined either. An international task force addressed this important issue and consensually defined each feature of systemic disease activity. Its objective was to set up a scale which was easy to score, sensitive to change, and capable of discriminating activity from damage. Parotid gland swelling and some biological parameters [cytopenia, elevated immunoglobulin (Ig) G, decreased complement levels, cryoglobulinemia] were also considered to mirror systemic involvement. This effort resulted in the EULAR Sjögren's Syndrome Disease Activity Index (ESSDAI),[8] composed of 12 domains, including one biological domain. Each domain is rated according to the severity of the involvement (no involvement; low, moderate, or high disease activity). The score was developed through the evaluation of the activity of 702 clinical vignettes based on 96 real patients. These vignettes were used to analyze a large number of cases with all possible systemic complications of the disease. The weights of each domain were obtained with multiple regression models using the physician global assessment of disease activity as a gold standard. The ESSDAI is effectively easy to score and sensitive to changes of disease activity. It has already been used in clinical trials (both in open trials and retrospectively in controlled trials) and is the main outcome criteria chosen in ongoing and forthcoming randomized clinical trials. A glossary explaining the way to correctly rate the ESSDAI is now available.[9] The ESSDAI allows patients to be divided into different disease activity subgroups.[4] Low systemic activity is defined by an ESSDAI of less than 5, moderate activity by an ESSDAI of greater or equal to 5 and lower or equal to 13, and high activity by an ESSDAI of greater or equal to 14. In addition, it was recently shown that MCII corresponds to a decrease of at least three points of the baseline value of ESSDAI.[4] A clinical ESSDAI, without the biological domain, was recently proposed to offer the possibility of scoring systemic disease activity immediately after clinical examination and to evaluate the clinical effect of some biological drugs independently of their effect on IgG, cryoglobulinemia, or complement.[10]

Given the previous paragraph, the ESSDAI definitively represents a great achievement for clinical trials. It has already been adopted and used in different ongoing or forthcoming clinical trials. In these trials, an ESSDAI equal to or greater than 5 or 6 is required as inclusion criteria. The primary outcome is either a decrease of at least three points or a change in ESSDAI. Nonetheless, using the ESSDAI as a primary outcome criteria has some limitations:

- Some of its highly weighted domains refer to pulmonary or peripheral nerve involvement where discriminating activity from damage is complicated.
- Two domains (hematological and biological domains) are purely biological.

**TABLE 17.1** Proposal for a Sjögren's Syndrome Response Index (Used in the Ongoing Randomized Placebo Controlled Trial of Tocilizumab)

ESSDAI decrease greater than or equal to 3 points from baseline

No new ESSDAI domain of moderate or high activity

No worsening greater than 1 point on a 10-point physician global assessment of systemic disease activity

*ESSDAI*, EULAR Sjögren's Syndrome Disease Activity Index.

- The glandular domain requires the evaluation of the size of the parotid glands, which is complicated from a clinical point of view.
- The ESSDAI score might decrease if the activity of a domain of high weight improves while the activity of another domain of lower weight increases.
- The ESSDAI evaluation does not take into account the clinician's global assessment.

To circumvent some of these limitations, we proposed to use a Sjögren's Syndrome Response Index in the tocilizumab multicenter placebo controlled trial, defined in Table 17.1.

## 1.3 Objective Assessment of Dryness (Tear and Saliva Secretion)

### 1.3.1 Oral Dryness

For oral dryness, unstimulated and stimulated salivary flow can be used and provide additional information on salivary function. These tests are very easy to perform.

#### 1.3.1.1 Unstimulated Salivary Flow

Unstimulated salivary flow is assessed by asking the patient to expectorate all saliva possible over 15 min without gustatory provocation. A volume of <1.5 mL of saliva in 15 min is considered abnormal.[11]

#### 1.3.1.2 Stimulated Salivary Flow

Different ways to stimulate salivary flow had been described and used in different studies. The first one consists of measuring stimulated salivary flow after stimulation with 0.1 mL of an ophthalmic 5% pilocarpine solution (5 mg pilocarpine)[12] administered sublingually. Stimulated saliva can also be collected after a 10-min stimulation of salivary glands. The salivary glands are stimulated with citric acid solution (2%), and a cotton swab is applied to the lateral borders of the tongue every 30 s.[13] Finally, another way to perform this is to ask the patient to chew on wax or gum for 1 min and to collect the volume of saliva expectorated during this time. Significant dryness is defined as an expectoration of <0.6 mL of saliva in 1 min.

Compared with unstimulated salivary flow, stimulated salivary flow appeared to be more associated with inflammation (according to the focus score).[12,14] In patients with sicca without Sjögren's syndrome (SS), the unstimulated salivary flow rate appeared to be more often abnormal as compared with the stimulated salivary flow rate.[14] In two studies (one evaluating rituximab[13] and the other an ongoing trial with baminercept), stimulated salivary flow was chosen as the primary outcome criteria.

### 1.3.2 Ocular Dryness

Ocular dryness can be assessed using the Schirmer test. This test is easy to perform but poorly reproducible. Conversely, the other tests have less variability but are more time-consuming and require an ophthalmologist.

#### 1.3.2.1 Schirmer Test

Standardized Schirmer strips are bent at the notch and placed carefully over the lower lid margin as far toward the temporal angle of the lids as possible. The patient is instructed to keep her/his eyelids closed during the test. Strips remain in place for 5 min, or until they are completely saturated with tears. After 5 min, wetting of the strips is measured using the millimeter scale on each strip. It is generally agreed that a Schirmer I test of 5 mm or less in 5 min is abnormal, but the results are variable.[15,16]

#### 1.3.2.2 Ocular Staining Score

Recently, a combination of lissamine green and fluorescein staining [Ocular Surface Score (OSS)] was proposed by the Sjögren's International Collaborative Clinical Alliance (SICCA) research groups[17] and included in the new preliminary American College of Rheumatology classification criteria for SS.[18] The association of both tests is of high interest, because they actually explore corneal and conjunctival dryness in a complementary way.

##### 1.3.2.2.1 Corneal Fluorescein Staining Pattern (Step 1 of the OSS SICCA Grading) Each cornea is examined at the slit lamp using the cobalt blue filter. Punctate epithelial erosions (PEEs) that stain with fluorescein are counted and scored. If there is no PEE, the score is 0. If one to five PEEs are seen, the corneal score is 1; 6 to 30 PEEs are scored as 2; and >30 PEEs are scored as 3. An additional point is added if: (1) PEEs occurred in the central 4-mm diameter portion of the cornea, (2) one or more filaments are observed anywhere on the cornea, or (3) one or more patches of confluent staining, including linear stains, are found anywhere on the cornea. The maximum possible score for each cornea is 6.

##### 1.3.2.2.2 Conjunctival Lissamine Green Staining Pattern (Step 2 of the OSS SICCA Grading) After the external examination, one drop of 1% lissamine green dye is applied to the inferior conjunctival fornix of both eyes. The conjunctivae are examined with the slit lamp at ×10 magnification, using a neutral-density filter over the light source to avoid blanching of the conjunctiva. In the OSS, grade 0 is defined as zero to nine dots of lissamine green staining of the interpalpebral bulbar

conjunctiva (nasal and temporal bulbar conjunctivae graded separately); grade 1 is defined by the presence of 10 to 32 dots; grade 2 by 33 to 100 dots; and grade 3 by >100 dots. Because of the difficulty of counting individual dots in a moving eye at the slit lamp, any area of confluent staining ≥4 mm² is considered to be >100 dots. Nasal and temporal areas of the conjunctiva are graded separately with a maximum score of 3 for each area or a total maximum score of 6 for each eye (nasal plus temporal). The total OSS for each eye is the summation of the fluorescein score for the cornea and the lissamine green scores for the nasal and temporal bulbar conjunctiva. Therefore the maximum possible score for each eye is 12.

An abnormal OSS is defined as being a score of 3 or above.

### 1.4 Other Potential Outcome Measures

The role of salivary gland ultrasonography[19,20] or magnetic resonance imaging [21,22] in the assessment of disease activity remains to be defined. Whole-body[23] and salivary positron emission tomography–computed tomography need to be further evaluated.

## 2. PERSPECTIVES IN CLINICAL TRIAL DESIGN

### 2.1 Complexity of Designing a Clinical Trial in pSS

First, clinical involvement of the disease encompasses a wide spectrum of manifestations. Some patients with systemic complications might not suffer from dryness. The majority of patients with pSS do not have systemic complications. It is therefore clear that the ESSDAI and ESSPRI capture different aspects of the disease and are not correlated.[24] In addition, symptoms of dryness are poorly associated with objective assessments of dryness (Fig. 17.1).

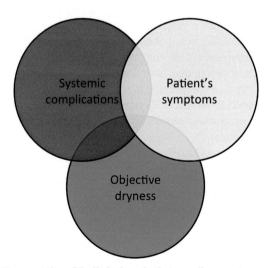

**FIGURE 17.1** Representation of the limited overlap between disease outcome measures in pSS.

The predominant dryness site (oral, ocular, cutaneous, vaginal) differs from patient to patient. Furthermore, the severity of dryness might change over time. Thus some groups include in clinical trials only patients with recent disease onset and persistent salivary flow (>0.15 mL/min). Focusing on one specific disease outcome results in restricting the inclusion criteria of clinical trials and loss of clinical relevance of the results of clinical trials in common practice. For instance, the choice of the ESSDAI as primary outcome criteria excludes patients without systemic involvement and complicates the recruitment of patients. Alternatively, focusing on symptoms by the choice of the ESSPRI as primary outcome criteria limits the interpretation of the effect of a drug on systemic complications as a result of methodological considerations. It should be borne in mind that patients who are mainly symptomatic for dryness, pain, and fatigue might have a lower incidence of systemic complications. Last, to choose salivary flow as primary outcome criteria, as in some trials which evaluate biological agents, excludes the more severe patients (with no saliva at all) and patients with long-standing disease (as aforementioned) and limits the potential conclusions on their effect on systemic complications.

The choice of outcome criteria obviously depends on the drugs evaluated. Of course, for a sialagogue, analysis of salivary flow would make perfect sense. For a targeted therapy, expected to improve different aspects of the disease (dry symptoms but also saliva and tear secretion, fatigue, pain, and systemic complications), there is no clear rationale for the preference of one outcome criteria over another.

## 2.2 Perspectives for a New Composite Outcome Criteria

The first possibility would be to define response as a significant improvement of the ESSDAI score (greater than or equal to three points) and/or of the ESSPRI score (greater than or equal to one point), significant improvement of the stimulated whole salivary flow, and/or significant improvement in the tear secretion (assessed by the Schirmer test or OSS). Such a proposal could raise very difficult methodological concerns regarding the different population samples to include in order to interpret the results on each component of the composite outcome criteria. In addition, adopting such a clinical trial design may not allow the conclusion that the drug investigated has a global effect on the different aspects of the disease (it would only mean that the drug evaluated has an effect on systemic complications or on symptoms).

The second, more realistic possibility would be to create a new composite score taking into account all of these aspects. To achieve this goal, different approaches could be hypothesized:

- Integrate all these components (ESSPRI, ESSDAI, salivary flow, tear secretion) using a mathematical formula, as follows: ESSPRI + ESSDAI + OSS − Salivary flow, or ESSPRI + ESSDAI-Schirmer test-salivary flow. This approach again raises methodological concerns, because the range of these different scores differs widely (the ESSDAI ranges from 0 to 133, the ESSPRI from 0 to 10, the OSS from 0 to 12, and the salivary flow from 0 to a few mL/min). In

**TABLE 17.2** Proposal Method for Designing a Composite Outcome Criteria Integrating A Patient's Symptoms, Systemic Complications, and Objective Assessment of Dryness

Gold Standard:

• Either the patient's global assessment

OR

• Mean of patient's and physician's global assessment

Variables integrated in the multivariable analyses:
• ESSPRI
• ESSDAI
• OSS or Schirmer test
• Stimulated salivary flow

addition, such a global score implies that each of its components has an equal consequence on patients' global assessment and QOL, and on the clinician's global assessment and the clinician's adaptation of therapy.

• Use the patient's global assessment or the mean of the patient's global assessment and the physician's global assessment as the gold standards and calculate the respective weights of the ESSPRI, ESSDAI, salivary flow, and OSS/Schirmer test in a multiple regression analysis (Table 17.2).

The advantage of this approach is that it takes into account the patient's and the clinician's global assessment in order to weigh the respective importance of symptoms, systemic complications, and salivary and lacrimal function. Because we have most of this data already collected in cohorts and clinical trials, such statistical analyses can be rapidly performed to test these different models. The recent examples of the ESSPRI and the ESSDAI that have been widely adopted in clinical trials show the importance of addressing the complicated issue of a composite score through a joint effort by patients with pSS and the international community of clinicians devoted to the disease.

## REFERENCES

1. Mariette X, Ravaud P, Steinfeld S, Baron G, Goetz J, Hachulla E, et al. Inefficacy of infliximab in primary Sjögren's syndrome: results of the randomized, controlled Trial of Remicade in Primary Sjögren's Syndrome (TRIPSS). *Arthritis Rheum* 2004;**50**:1270–6.
2. Sankar V, Brennan MT, Kok MR, Leakan RA, Smith JA, Manny J, et al. Etanercept in Sjögren's syndrome: a twelve-week randomized, double-blind, placebo-controlled pilot clinical trial. *Arthritis Rheum* 2004;**50**:2240–5.
3. Seror R, Ravaud P, Mariette X, Bootsma H, Theander E, Hansen A, et al. EULAR Sjögren's Syndrome Patient Reported Index (ESSPRI): development of a consensus patient index for primary Sjogren's syndrome. *Ann Rheum Dis* 2011;**70**:968–72.

4. Seror R, Bootsma H, Saraux A, Bowman SJ, Theander E, Brun JG, et al. Defining disease activity states and clinically meaningful improvement in primary Sjögren's syndrome with EULAR primary Sjögren's syndrome disease activity (ESSDAI) and patient-reported indexes (ESSPRI). *Ann Rheum Dis* 2014;**75**(2):382–9.

5. Hewlett S, Dures E, Almeida C. Measures of fatigue: Bristol Rheumatoid Arthritis Fatigue Multi-Dimensional Questionnaire (BRAF MDQ), Bristol Rheumatoid Arthritis Fatigue Numerical Rating Scales (BRAF NRS) for Severity, Effect, and Coping, Chalder Fatigue Questionnaire (CFQ), Checklist Individual Strength (CIS20R and CIS8R), Fatigue Severity Scale (FSS), Functional Assessment Chronic Illness Therapy (Fatigue) (FACIT-F), Multi-Dimensional Assessment of Fatigue (MAF), Multi-Dimensional Fatigue Inventory (MFI), Pediatric Quality of Life (PedsQL) Multi-Dimensional Fatigue Scale, Profile of Fatigue (ProF), Short Form 36 Vitality Subscale (SF-36 VT), and Visual Analog Scales (VAS). *Arthritis Care Res* 2011;**63**(Suppl. 11):S263–86.

6. Pillemer SR, Smith J, Fox PC, Bowman SJ. Outcome measures for Sjögren's syndrome, April 10–11, 2003, Bethesda, Maryland, USA. *J Rheumatol* 2005;**32**:143–9.

7. Bowman SJ, Booth DA, Platts RG, Group US. Measurement of fatigue and discomfort in primary Sjögren's syndrome using a new questionnaire tool. *Rheumatology* 2004;**43**:758–64.

8. Seror R, Ravaud P, Bowman SJ, Baron G, Tzioufas A, Theander E, et al. EULAR Sjögren's Syndrome Disease Activity Index: development of a consensus systemic disease activity index for primary Sjogren's syndrome. *Ann Rheum Dis* 2010;**69**:1103–9.

9. Seror R, Bowman SJ, Brito-Zeron P, Theander E, Bootsma H, Tzioufas A, et al. EULAR Sjögren's Syndrome Disease Activity Index (ESSDAI): a user guide. *RMD Open* 2015;**1**:e000022.

10. Seror R, Meiners P, Baron G, Bootsma H, Bowman SJ, Vitali C, et al. Development of clinESSDAI score (Clinical EULAR Sjögren's Syndrome Disease Activity Index) without the biological domain: a tool for biological studies. *Ann Rheum Dis* 2016. http://dx.doi.org/10.1136/annrheumdis-2015-208504.

11. Skopouli FN, Siouna-Fatourou HI, Ziciadis C, Moutsopoulos HM. Evaluation of unstimulated whole saliva flow rate and stimulated parotid flow as confirmatory tests for xerostomia. *Clin Exp Rheumatol* 1989;**7**:127–9.

12. Rosas J, Ramos-Casals M, Ena J, García-Carrasco M, Verdu J, Cervera R, et al. Usefulness of basal and pilocarpine-stimulated salivary flow in primary Sjögren's syndrome: correlation with clinical, immunological and histological features. *Rheumatology* 2002;**41**:670–5.

13. Meijer JM, Meiners PM, Vissink A, Spijkervet FKL, Abdulahad W, Kamminga N, et al. Effectiveness of rituximab treatment in primary Sjögren's syndrome: a randomized, double-blind, placebo-controlled trial. *Arthritis Rheum* 2010;**62**:960–8.

14. Bookman AAM, Shen H, Cook RJ, Bailey D, McComb RJ, Rutka JA, et al. Whole stimulated salivary flow: correlation with the pathology of inflammation and damage in minor salivary gland biopsy specimens from patients with primary Sjögren's syndrome but not patients with sicca. *Arthritis Rheum* 2011;**63**:2014–20.

15. Van Bijsterveld OP. Diagnostic tests in the sicca syndrome. *Arch Ophthalmol (Chic Ill: 1960)* 1969;**82**:10–4.

16. Lemp MA. Report of the National Eye Institute/Industry workshop on clinical trials in dry eyes. *CLAO J* 1995;**21**:221–32.

17. Whitcher JP, Shiboski CH, Shiboski SC, Heidenreich AM, Kitagawa K, Zhang S, et al. A simplified quantitative method for assessing keratoconjunctivitis sicca from the Sjögren's syndrome international registry. *Am J Ophthalmol* 2010;**149**:405–15.

18. Shiboski SC, Shiboski CH, Criswell LA, Baer AN, Challacombe S, Lanfranchi H, et al. American College of Rheumatology classification criteria for Sjögren's syndrome: a data-driven, expert consensus approach in the Sjögren's International Collaborative Clinical Alliance cohort. *Arthritis Care Res* 2012;**64**:475–87.

19. Baldini C, Luciano N, Tarantini G, Pascale R, Sernissi F, Mosca M, et al. Salivary gland ultrasonography: a highly specific tool for the early diagnosis of primary Sjögren's syndrome. *Arthritis Res Ther* 2015;**17**:146.

20. Takagi Y, Sumi M, Nakamura H, Sato S, Kawakami A, Nakamura T. Salivary gland ultrasonography as a primary imaging tool for predicting efficacy of xerostomia treatment in patients with Sjögren's syndrome. *Rheumatology* 2015;**55**(2):237–45.

21. Regier M, Ries T, Arndt C, Cramer MC, Graessner J, Reitmeier F, et al. Sjögren's syndrome of the parotid gland: value of diffusion-weighted echo-planar MRI for diagnosis at an early stage based on MR sialography grading in comparison with healthy volunteers. *RöFo Fortschritte Auf Dem Geb Röntgenstrahlen Nukl* 2009;**181**:242–8.

22. Ding C, Xing X, Guo Q, Liu D, Guo Y, Cui H. Diffusion-weighted MRI findings in Sjögren's syndrome: a preliminary study. *Acta Radiol* September 2, 2015 [Epub ahead of print].

23. Cohen C, Mekinian A, Uzunhan Y, Fauchais A-L, Dhote R, Pop G, et al. 18F-fluorodeoxyglucose positron emission tomography/computer tomography as an objective tool for assessing disease activity in Sjögren's syndrome. *Autoimmun Rev* 2013;**12**:1109–14.

24. Seror R, Gottenberg JE, Devauchelle-Pensec V, Dubost JJ, Le Guern V, Hayem G, et al. European League Against Rheumatism Sjögren's Syndrome Disease Activity Index and European League Against Rheumatism Sjögren's Syndrome Patient-Reported Index: a complete picture of primary Sjögren's syndrome patients. *Arthritis Care Res* 2013;**65**:1358–64.

Chapter 18

# Novel Therapeutic Strategies in Sjögren's Syndrome: B-Cell Targeting

**F. Carubbi**
*University of L'Aquila, L'Aquila, Italy; ASL 1Avezzano-Sulmona-L'Aquila, L'Aquila, Italy*

**P. Cipriani, R. Giacomelli**
*University of L'Aquila, L'Aquila, Italy*

## 1. THERAPEUTIC POTENTIAL FOR B-CELL MODULATION IN SJÖGREN'S SYNDROME

Critical dysregulated immune pathways, including the key role of B cells as well as the ectopic lymphoneogenesis, are involved in primary Sjögren's syndrome (pSS) pathogenesis. B cells may provide a critical link between the development of tertiary lymphoid tissue within target tissues and the propagation of the autoimmune process. Although the peculiar role of B cells in autoimmunity is the production of autoantibodies, some data suggests that B cells may also exert additional pivotal functions such as antigen presentation and release of specific cytokines with immune regulatory, proinflammatory, polarizing, and tissue-organizing functions. In particular, a growing body of evidence has pointed out that B cells play a central role in the development, maintenance, and progression of the disease, with multiple roles at different points of pSS pathophysiology.[1] B-lymphocyte hyperactivity, minor salivary gland (MSG) infiltration, and the development of B-cell follicles containing germinal center (GC)–like structures, represent the hallmarks of the disease.[2] Excessive B-cell activation is responsible for a number of the extraglandular manifestations and serological features of pSS, including hypergammaglobulinemia, cryoglobulinemia, elevated levels of free light chains and $\beta$2-microglobulin, presence of anti-Ro/SSA and anti-La/SSB autoantibodies or rheumatoid factor (RF), hypocomplementemia, hypergamma-globulinemic purpura, arthritis, vasculitis, neuropathy, and glomerulonephritis.[3] Finally, prolonged B-cell survival and aberrant B-cell activity may lead to the development of non-Hodgkin lymphoma in 5% of pSS patients.[4]

Sjögren's Syndrome. http://dx.doi.org/10.1016/B978-0-12-803604-4.00018-6

273

Most pSS patients have a clinical pattern mainly dominated by severe dryness, fatigue, and pain, which although not life threatening, seriously impacts the quality of life. In contrast, systemic involvement plays a key role in the disease prognosis. In particular, Ioannidis et al. first proposed a prognostic classification, dividing pSS patients into two groups according to the presence or absence of risk factors, such as palpable purpura and low C4 levels.[5] Recently, Baldini et al. found that low C3/C4, hypergammaglobulinemia, RF, and cryoglobulinemia are markers of severity in pSS, and the prevalence of the high-risk pSS patient subset for severe systemic manifestations was about 15%.[6] Quartuccio et al. demonstrated for the first time that among pSS patients with salivary swelling, only those with low C4, cryoglobulins, anti-La/SSB antibodies, and leukopenia had an increased risk of lymphoma evolution.[7] This data suggests three important concepts: (1) the subset of patients at high risk of systemic complications is specifically characterized by an active serological profile, suggestive for B-cell chronic activation; (2) serological markers of disease severity should be considered in the management of pSS; and (3) patients with this clinical or immunological higher risk pattern should receive closer follow-up observation and an earlier and more aggressive immunosuppressive treatment.

Recent systematic reviews highlighted the lack of evidence-based recommendations for the majority of the drugs commonly employed in the spectrum of extraglandular involvement and, at last, pSS may be still considered an orphan disease.[8-12] Besides conventional immunosuppressive compounds, efficacy of targeted therapies in other systemic autoimmune diseases such as rheumatoid arthritis and systemic lupus erythematosus (SLE) suggested their possible use in pSS as well. Indeed, the treatment with immunosuppressive and biological agents in pSS is mainly based on their efficacy in the aforementioned conditions, expert opinion, and uncontrolled studies. Although many clinical manifestations may be shared among different systemic autoimmune diseases, it should be kept in mind, however, that the underlying pathogenic mechanisms could be different. This data points out the need for randomized clinical trials to investigate the safety and efficacy of these drugs in pSS in order to provide solid scientific evidence. Taken together, the difficulty in building therapeutic recommendations in pSS may be related to the heterogeneity of the clinical picture, the common failure of first line treatments, the lack of scientific evidence for drugs licensed for other diseases, and, finally, the lack of innovative therapeutic compounds. The need for more effective therapies with less toxic side effects as well as new insights into B-cell roles in disease pathogenesis has propelled interest in targeted biological therapies on the basis of an expanding understanding about disease pathogenesis. In this context, specific therapies with monoclonal antibodies (mAbs) recognizing targets on B-cell membrane (anti-CD20, anti-CD22), interfering with B/T cells, or inhibiting cytokines in B-cell development or activation such as B-cell activating factor (BAFF) and interleukin (IL) 6 or organization of ectopic lymphoid structures as shown for lymphotoxin (LT) β[13] were proposed (Fig. 18.1).

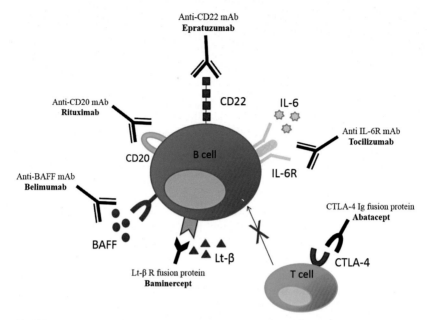

**FIGURE 18.1**    B-cell targeting therapies in primary Sjögren's syndrome. *BAFF*, B-cell activating factor; *CTLA-4*, cytotoxic T-lymphocyte antigen 4; *Ig*, immunoglobulin; *IL-6*, interleukin 6; *IL-6R*, interleukin 6 receptor; *LTβ*, lymphotoxin β; *LTβR*, lymphotoxin β receptor; *mAb*, monoclonal antibody.

## 2.  ANTI-CD20 ANTIBODIES IN pSS TREATMENT: THE ROLE OF RITUXIMAB

The CD20 (human B-lymphocyte–restricted differentiation antigen, Bp35) antigen is the most widely studied target for depleting B cells. This transmembrane molecule is found on the surface of most B cells, including pre-B and mature B lymphocytes, but not on stem cells, pro-B cells, normal plasma cells, or other normal tissues.[14] CD20 mediates activation, proliferation, and differentiation of B cells, and may participate in the generation of T-cell independent antibody response.[15] Many therapeutic mAbs targeting CD20 are currently available: rituximab (RTX), ocrelizumab, afutuzumab, ibritumomab tiuxetan, ofatumumab, TRU-015, tositumomab, and veltuzumab.[16] Generally, anti-CD20 mAbs are classified as type I (RTX-like) or type II (tositumomab-like), based on their ability to redistribute CD20 molecules in the plasma membrane and activate various effector functions. Type II mAbs are mostly employed in the treatment of B-cell malignancies owing to their longer depletion of B cells from the peripheral blood (PB) and secondary lymphoid organs. To date, the only anti-CD20 monoclonal antibody that has been tested in pSS is RTX.[17]

RTX, a chimeric (murine/human) mAb directly targeting CD20, prevents B-cell proliferation and induces depletion of circulating B cells from PB, salivary glands, and other target tissues by complement-mediated cytotoxicity, antibody-dependent cell-mediated cytotoxicity, or induction of apoptosis.[18]

Early studies on the efficacy of RTX reported the histological evidence of a B-cell depletion and a reduction in glandular inflammation combined with a disappearance of GCs.[19,20] It is worth noting that the histological findings paralleled the increase of parotid salivary flow and the normalization of the salivary sodium content, pointing out that the efficacy of B-cell depletion may also induce a potential glandular restoration in pSS.

The recovery of B-cell subsets after RTX treatment in pSS patients seemed to recapitulate B-cell ontogeny.[21] The first B cells appearing in PB are transitional type 1 (T1) B cells (CD19+CD5+IgD+CD38++) and plasmablasts (CD19+CD5−IgD−CD38++), followed by a further increased of naive B cells migrating from the bone marrow (BM). Memory B cells were detected early during repopulation, first in PB and only later in MSGs, although the number of memory B cells remained relatively lower in both PB and MSGs. Sequential MSG biopsies revealed that B cells were absent in these glands for 12 months, but they colonized the affected glands 24 months after RTX treatment. Memory and T1 B cells were the first B cells identified locally, and, interestingly, the GCs previously seen in the MSGs were no longer present after B-cell recovery. The sole difference among the treated patients was in the timing of B-cell reappearance and, in this respect, higher baseline serum levels of BAFF inversely correlated with the duration of B-cell depletion, which resulted in the reconstitution of the preexisting abnormalities in PB. Moreover, after RTX treatment, circulating CD19+ B-cells started to reappear at week 24 and were partially or fully reconstituted 36 to 48 weeks after treatment.[22] The large majority of the B cells that reappeared had a phenotype of transitional B cells and, interestingly, they did not derive from mature naive or memory peripheral B cells that were not depleted by RTX, but were newly generated B cells in the BM. In addition, the percentages and the absolute numbers of regulatory T (Treg) cells and effector T cells, as well as the ratio of effector T/Treg cells, did not significantly change after RTX treatment.

Beyond its direct activity on the B-cell compound, recent studies seem to further highlight the role of RTX in modifying the immunological microenvironment of inflamed salivary glands, suggesting new possible mechanisms: (1) reduction of the local expression of IL-22, interfering with the IL-22/IL-22RA1 axis, an important step in the emergence of T- and B-cell lymphoma[23]; (2) reduction of the expression of IL-17 and specifically induction of a pronounced apoptotic depletion of mast cells[24]; (3) reduction of serum levels of different molecules, including granulocyte macrophage colony-stimulating factor, IL-1Ra, IL-6, IL-10, interferon α, tumor necrosis factor (TNF) α, CCL4, and CXCL9, as indirect effects of B-cell depletion[25]; (4) induction of a significant decrease of inflammation proteins, cytokines, and growth factors released by epithelial cells, decreasing nuclear factor κB (NF-κB) activity and interrupting the NF-κB signaling pathway through the up-regulation of the Raf-1 kinase inhibitor protein[26]; and (5) interference with ectopic lymphoneogenesis not only by depleting B cells but also by tuning the delicate equilibrium between cells, molecules, and receptors, partially affecting the pro-B-cell inflammatory milieu.[27] Specifically, we recently showed a reduction of lymphocytic foci and in the Chisholm and Mason score in the majority of patients treated with RTX, providing additional insights in the biological effects of RTX.[27] MSGs of these patients presented, after 120 weeks of treatment, a nonspecific chronic sialadenitis pattern or a full restoration of glandular architecture associated to the disappearance of GC structures. Moreover, we observed a consistent reduction at messenger RNA (mRNA) levels of CXCR4 and CXCR5 associated to a parallel increase of the CXCL12 and CXCL13 mRNAs after anti-CD20 therapy. Although LTα and LTβ were markedly reduced by RTX, BAFF was not affected by the biological treatment. Finally, our study showed, at a histological and molecular level, the strong effect of RTX in dissolving the immunological organization of the affected tissues, which was not observed with disease-modifying antirheumatic drugs (DMARDs) therapy.

## 2.1 Clinical Effects of Rituximab in pSS

RTX was first tested in several open-label studies in pSS, which suggested an improvement of fatigue, sicca symptoms, glandular enlargement, and extraglandular manifestations. However, the duration of the clinical effects was rather variable among the studies and these effects partially overlapped PB B-cell depletion. Furthermore, retreatment with RTX resulted in a clinical and biological response comparable to the initial treatment. The two common infusion protocols are a low dose of 375 mg/m² weekly on days 0, 7, 12, and 21, or 1.000 mg on days 1 and 15. Although different dosing schedules for RTX have been used in different studies, it can be concluded that RTX induces effective depletion of circulating B cells in pSS patients and a B-cell subset reconstitution pattern with similar kinetics, independently of therapeutic strategies and different dosage.[21,28]

The first two small, double-blind, randomized studies showed a certain efficacy of RTX in pSS patients, namely an improvement of fatigue,[29] objective and subjective sicca symptoms,[30] and a significant reduction of the number of extraglandular manifestations.[30]

However, these results were not replicated in a recent larger placebo-controlled, double-blind trial, the French Tolerance and EfficAcy of Rituximab in Primary Sjögren Syndrome (TEARS) study.[31] Although the study failed to reach the primary end point (improvement of at least 30 mm in two of four visual analog scales [VASs] exploring global activity, fatigue, pain, and dryness between weeks 0 and 24), several secondary endpoints (dryness and fatigue scores, salivary flow rate, and laboratory response) were significantly improved in patients treated with RTX.

Another large randomized controlled trial, namely the Trial of Anti–B-cell Therapy in Patients with Primary Sjögren's Syndrome (TRACTISS) study, a phase III study, has been completed in the United Kingdom. The TRACTISS treatment regimen comprised two courses of either RTX or placebo, and the outcomes on fatigue, oral dryness, and other glandular manifestations are to be reported in autumn of 2015.[32] This study could further provide some information to evaluate the efficacy of RTX in pSS, particularly because the study design was intended to be closely aligned to that of the TEARS study, thus allowing subsequent data meta-analysis.

As far as systemic involvement was concerned, Gottenberg et al. demonstrated an improvement of systemic manifestations, including parotid swelling and pulmonary and articular involvement, 6 months after the first treatment cycle with RTX in a cohort of 78 pSS patients with systemic involvement or severe glandular involvement.[33] In addition, both the median European League Against Rheumatism (EULAR) Sjögren's Syndrome Disease Activity Index (ESSDAI) and the median daily dose of prednisone decreased 6 months after RTX administration. Similar results were also observed in uncontrolled studies, especially for articular, vascular, pulmonary, and neurological involvement.[17–34] Meiners et al. treated 28 pSS patients with RTX in order to evaluate the responsiveness of the EULAR Sjögren's Syndrome Patient Reported Index (ESSPRI) and ESSDAI.[35] They reported an improvement at week 16 in both ESSDAI and ESSPRI scores, concluding that both of these indexes, in particular the ESSDAI, display a good sensitivity to change concerning the disease activity after therapeutic intervention. Seror et al. reported a decrease in the daily dose of corticosteroids in pSS patients with systemic involvement after RTX treatment, highlighting the risk reduction of steroid-associated adverse events.[36] Finally, several studies reported significant reductions in analytical parameters such as erythrocyte sedimentation rate (ESR), C reactive protein, cryoglobulinemia, RF, $\beta$2-microglobulin, and immunoglobulin (Ig) levels.[17]

We recently performed a prospective, multicenter, follow-up study including 41 pSS patients with early (ranging from 6 to 21 months), active (ESSDAI $\geq$6) disease receiving either RTX or conventional DMARDs plus a stable dose of prednisone.[27] Unlike previous studies, pSS patients included in the RTX arm received six courses of therapy (twice 1 g with an interval of 15 days, every 6 months). We reported a significant improvement in ESSDAI as early as the second course of therapy, which was more pronounced in the RTX arm when compared with the DMARDs arm. This effect was sustained over time and could be observed throughout the study. In particular, this data is partially related to a rapid and consistent score reduction of constitutional, lymphadenopathical, glandular, articular, and cutaneous domains. The response curves for VAS global disease activity, VAS pain, VAS fatigue, and physician global assessment mirrored the pattern of the ESSDAI. Of interest, a significant improvement in objective (unstimulated salivary flow and Schirmer test) and histological (Chisholm and Mason grading and focus score) parameters was also observed in the RTX arm.

## 2.2 Retreatment and Safety

The beneficial effects of RTX in patients with Sjögren's syndrome (SS), when observed, are transient and responders generally experience a disease relapse. These relapses parallel the B-cell repopulation in the PB. Furthermore, the local persistence of clonally related Ig-producing B cells, both in salivary glands and PB, despite RTX treatment, suggests the lack of a full restoration of the B cell repertoire to a predisease state.[37,38] Moreover, the persistence of B-cell clones may explain the occurrence of relapses after treatment, possibly triggered by additional pathological stimuli. In particular, B-cell depletion therapy with RTX is followed by an increase of serum BAFF levels inversely correlated to the B-cell number after repopulation, highlighting the role of BAFF both in B-cell homeostasis and in predicting the duration of B-cell suppression.[21,39] It is worth noting that serum a proliferation-inducing ligand (APRIL) levels seem not to be affected by RTX.[39] This may be explained by the notion that APRIL receptors, TACI and BCMA, are selectively expressed by activated B cells, which generally have a low number in pSS, and by plasma cells, which are unaffected by RTX.

On these bases, it may be suggested that pSS patients should be treated either at fixed time points or, alternatively, according to the circulating B-cell number. Recently, we demonstrated a sustained clinical response and a good safety profile during six courses of RTX (given every 24 weeks) in 19 pSS patients with early and active disease.[27] Meiners et al., analyzing data of 15 pSS patients retreated with RTX after recurrence of symptoms, found beneficial effects comparable with the initial treatment evaluated by ESSDAI and other objective parameters, whereas the positive effects on patient-reported parameters were less pronounced.[40]

The main goals of retreatment should include both the maintenance of efficacy and the prevention of disease flare. In this context, further studies are needed to investigate both optimal timing of RTX retreatment in pSS patients and the clinical value of a combination therapy, including different biological agents, in a sequential timing.

Unlike in patients with lymphoma or other hematological malignancies, RTX in patients with autoimmune disease does not increase the risk of serious infection.[16] Hypogammaglobulinemia is more likely associated with repeated courses of RTX treatment, although is still not clearly established if the decrease of Igs, reported in these patients, may be associated with higher risk of infection.[41] We demonstrated that treating our patients for a long period, 120 weeks of RTX administration, in combination with a small and stable dosage of prednisone did not lead to increased adverse events compared with patients treated with DMARDs alone,[27] although acute infusion reactions and serum sickness–like disease have been described in the literature.[29–31]

RTX administration may be associated with general infusion reactions, including fever, chills, and rigors, as well as allergic (type IV) anaphylactoid spectrum reactions such as urticaria, angioedema, and hypotension, typically occurring during infusions. These symptoms are reported to be more common and severe at the first infusion of the drug, and seem to be more common in patients with hematological malignancies than in those with autoimmune diseases.[42] A lower infusion rate and/or the concurrent administration of corticosteroids and antihistamines decrease the occurrence of these infusion reactions. Because these reactions often occur with the first dose, it has been hypothesized that these are caused by complement activation and mast cell degranulation in the setting of rapid cell lysis rather than preformed IgE against the molecule.[43]

In contrast to the infusion reactions described, serum sickness (or type III) hypersensitivity reactions are the result of immune activation against the infused agent, and take a significantly longer time (1 to 3 weeks) to mobilize. Symptoms include fever, rash, and polyarthralgia or arthritis, mimicking the disease that they are used to treat. Serum sickness reactions typically represent host immune responses mediated through complement-fixing IgM and IgG antibodies directed toward an immunogenic portion of a drug.[44] In this context, the reexposure can result in recurrent and more severe manifestations. Recently, a systematic review on RTX-induced serum sickness analyzing 33 cases from 25 articles showed that the majority of cases were associated with an underlying rheumatological condition ($n=17$, 51.5%), most commonly Sjögren's syndrome ($n=8$, 44.4%).[43] The time to resolution was significantly greater for rheumatological versus hematological indications (mean time 2.50 vs. 1.00 days, $P=0.035$) and corticosteroids were the most commonly used treatment, with all cases reporting a complete resolution of symptoms in a few days. Although various factors, including reduced clearance of immune complexes, elevated levels of RF, human antichimeric antibodies, and hypergammaglobulinemia, have been implicated, the reason it tends to be more common in patients with SS is unclear.

Finally, biological therapies, including RTX, are also potentially associated with an increased risk of progressive multifocal leukoencephalopathy.[45] This is a rare, fatal, central nervous system demyelinating disease that results from reactivation of the JC virus, which usually occurs in immunosuppressed hosts. Although progressive multifocal leukoencephalopathy is rare, the risk of developing this complication must be considered in the decision to use biological treatments in pSS.

## 2.3 What Have We Learned About Rituximab From Clinical Trials in pSS?

B-cell depletion therapy with RTX in pSS has shown conflicting but promising results in clinical trials. The heterogeneity of both primary outcomes and selected patients probably accounts for the variability in the results of randomized trials and open-label studies. Moreover, the failure to achieve consistent clinical benefits with B-cell depletion therapy in some patients may be the result of non-B immune abnormalities, an imbalance in T-cell subsets, and/or a depletion of regulatory B cells. Although data present in literature do not allow the drawing of definitive conclusions on the efficacy of RTX, B-cell depletion may be considered a therapeutic option for selected pSS patients. In particular, RTX treatment seems to be effective in glandular swelling, in some systemic manifestations, and in early and active disease. The debate about the real effectiveness of RTX in pSS underscores that the development of sensitive and reproducible outcome measures for pSS is a strong unmet need, as are further studies on B-cell depletion regimens. To date, the ideal primary end point to assess treatment efficacy in pSS remains unknown. Although the ESSDAI includes different domains related to the large variability of clinical and laboratory aspects of the disease, it does not incorporate assessments of dryness and has not been extensively validated in controlled trials. Moreover, it should be kept in mind that although patients included in clinical trials might display the same scores, this does not reflect an overlapping clinical and serological picture. Furthermore, the VAS improvement derived from expert opinion is based on subjective measures and may contribute to the variability of the results. Finally, the optimal RTX regimen required to reach disease improvement in pSS, is still unclear.

## 3. EPRATUZUMAB, AN ANTI-CD22 ANTIBODY IN pSS TREATMENT

Epratuzumab is an mAb directed against another B-cell–specific transmembrane protein, CD22, which functions primarily as a negative regulator of the B-cell receptor. Moreover, CD22, acting as a homing receptor, may play a role in the entry of B cells into the target tissues of pSS patients. This humanized IgG1 anti-CD22 seems to modulate B-cell activity more than B-cell depletion in the circulation.[46]

In an open-label study, 16 pSS patients received epratuzumab infusions ($360\,mg/m^2$) at 2-week intervals.[47] Fourteen patients received all four infusions without any significant adverse reaction, one received three infusions, and one experienced a mild acute reaction to the first infusion that led to discontinuation of the study protocol. Interestingly, human antihuman antibodies were found in three patients but were not associated with adverse events. A composite end point involving the Schirmer test, nonstimulated whole salivary flow, fatigue, ESR, and IgG level was devised to assess the clinical response, defined as a 20% or greater improvement in at least two parameters. Schirmer test, nonstimulated whole salivary flow, and VAS fatigue score were the most commonly improved parameters. A clinical response was noted in 53% of patients at 6 weeks and 67% at 32 weeks. Unlike RTX, this anti–B-cell antibody leads to only partial B-cell depletion. Although epratuzumab holds promise for the treatment of pSS, randomized placebo-controlled trials are needed.

## 4. ANTI–B LYMPHOCYTE STIMULATOR THERAPY IN pSS

Another biological approach to deplete pathogenic B lymphocytes may be the targeting of soluble factors involved in their survival, activation, and expansion. Important cytokines involved in B-cell survival and activation of B cells are BAFF and APRIL, both belonging to the TNF family. BAFF, also named B-lymphocyte stimulator (BlyS), is involved in B-cell survival and humoral immune responses, playing a critical role in B-cell homeostasis. Produced by multiple cellular types, including epithelial cells and T and B lymphocytes, BAFF overexpression rescues autoreactive cells from depletion in periphery, leading to a higher number of mature autoreactive B cells.[48] BAFF, but not APRIL, binds to BAFF receptor, which is widely expressed by human peripheral B cells except for BM plasma cells.[49] BAFF and APRIL may also activate B cells by interaction with the receptor TACI (a transmembrane activator and calcium-modulating and cyclophilin ligand–interacting protein), predominantly expressed on human CD27+ memory B cells, activated B cells, and plasma cells.

Patients with pSS display elevated levels of BAFF and APRIL in serum, saliva, and salivary glands.[50–52] In the sera, BAFF levels correlate with gamma-globulin levels and anti-Ro/SSA and/or anti-La/SSB antibodies. Furthermore, higher BAFF levels are observed in patients with GCs in salivary glands.[53,54] However, BAFF is a very complex cytokine which appears in multiple forms and variants, displaying different effects and making the interpretation of these observations difficult.[55] The pathogenic role of BAFF in pSS-associated lymphoproliferation has been demonstrated in both the prelymphomatous stage and mucosa-associated lymphoid tissue (MALT) lymphomas,[56] and pSS patients coaffected by severe clinical manifestations associated with B-cell lymphoproliferation have higher BAFF serum levels than patients without comorbidities.[57] Finally, B-cell depletion therapy with RTX in pSS patients results in a rise in serum BAFF levels, which decreases again when B cells start to reappear.[39] By contrast, serum APRIL levels are not affected by B-cell depletion therapy.

In this context, BAFF-blocking agents were proposed as potentially effective therapeutic targets in SS.

### 4.1 Belimumab

The Belimumab in Sjögren's Syndrome trial is the first open-label phase II study conducted in pSS patients for investigating the efficacy and safety of belimumab, a human mAb-neutralizing soluble BAFF.[58] The patients received belimumab, 10 mg/kg, at weeks 0, 2, and 4 and then every 4 weeks to week 24. Although the authors failed to observe an improvement of objective measures of salivary and lacrimal secretion, more than half of the patients achieved improvements in subjective symptoms of dryness, fatigue, and pain; in objective activity scores; and/or in laboratory markers of disease-related immune system dysregulation, including serum levels of free light chains of Ig, $\beta$2-microglobulin, monoclonal component, and C4 levels. In addition, the mean ESSDAI and ESSPRI scores significantly decreased and the safety profile was good.

Subsequently, 19 patients terminated the 52-week study with a response rate of 86.7%.[59] The improvement in ESSDAI and ESSPRI scores observed at week 28 showed a trend to further improvement at week 52. The decrease in biomarkers of B-cell activation observed at week 28 persisted unchanged until week 52. However, salivary flow, the Schirmer test, and the focus score of salivary biopsy did not change. Furthermore, the safety of treatment was confirmed.

On these bases, randomized, double-blind, controlled studies for the use of belimumab in larger pSS populations are encouraged.

As mentioned, a number of patients with MALT lymphoma, mainly of parotid gland, experience a treatment failure when RTX monotherapy is employed. This issue has been recently addressed by Quartuccio et al., and they have provided evidence for the involvement of BAFF.[60] In particular, it appeared that the lack of response to RTX may arise from both tissue and systemic overexpression of this B-cell–related cytokine. In fact, despite B-cell depletion, the microenvironment which is able to promote their repopulation remained stable over time. This intriguing evidence may provide the rationale to combine direct B-cell depletion induced by RTX and indirect B-cell targeting employing anti-BAFF antibodies.[61] In addition, this novel approach may also replace chemotherapy in combination with RTX, thereby reducing the burden of adverse events.

## 5. FUTURE PERSPECTIVES AND PERSONALIZED THERAPY

Although the local production of cytokines such as BAFF and the formation of ectopic lymphoid structures promote the differentiation of B cells into antibody-producing plasma cells, the selective forces driving B-cell selection and proliferation in pSS remain unclear. B-cell survival factors such as BAFF, APRIL, and IL-6, B-cell and plasma cell–attracting chemokines such as CXCL13, CXCL12, and molecules involved in the ectopic lymphoneogenesis such as LTs, and lymphoid chemokines CXCL12, CXCL13, CCL19, and CCL21 certainly play a central role in pSS pathogenesis, thus representing possible new targeted molecules.[2,62,63]

### 5.1 Inhibition of Lymphotoxin-β

More efficacious strategies to block ectopic lymphoneogenesis are under investigation, including blockade of LTβ receptor signaling by the decoy receptor baminercept. Treatment with baminercept, a LTβ receptor–Ig fusion protein, showed a dramatic effect in reducing salivary B-cell infiltrates in nonobese diabetic mice.[64] Its utility in pSS is currently under investigation in a placebo-controlled trial in the United States (A Randomized, Double-Blind, Placebo-Controlled Phase II Clinical Trial of Baminercept, an LTβ Receptor Fusion Protein, for the Treatment of Primary Sjögren's Syndrome, NCT01552681).

## 5.2 Interleukin-6 Inhibition

Il-6 is an important mediator of the acute phase response, activating both T and B cells, and playing a very important role in the balance among regulatory T cells, T helper (Th) 17 cells, and follicular helper T cells.[65] Many cell types may produce this cytokine, although the primary sources of IL-6 are monocytes/macrophages at sites of inflammation. In patients with pSS, IL-6 is overexpressed, promoting the IL-21–mediated plasma cell differentiation. Although IL-21 is clearly derived from CD4+ T cells, it has been shown that an alternative source of IL-6 might be activated B cells.[66] IL-6–producing B cells have been observed in labial salivary glands of pSS patients, and the increased serum levels of IL-6 drop after B-cell depletion therapy of pSS patients with RTX but not after placebo treatment.[25] These observations suggest that in pSS patients, B cells are an important source for IL-6. Moreover, several studies identified increased IL-6 levels in the serum, saliva, and tears of patients with pSS,[67,68] suggesting that the inhibition of IL-6 might be of interest in pSS therapy. A French multicenter randomized placebo-controlled trial of tocilizumab, a humanized anti–IL-6 receptor monoclonal antibody is ongoing (A Randomized, Double-blind, Parallel, Placebo-Controlled Trial to Evaluate the Efficacy of Tocilizumab for the Treatment of Primary Sjögren's Syndrome, NCT01782235). This study includes patients with systemic disease activity (ESSDAI ≥5), and the primary outcome is based on the change in the ESSDAI score (decrease of at least three points of the initial ESSDAI score).

## 5.3 B-/T-Cell Cooperation Interference

B cells may also be hampered indirectly by targeting membrane-bound and soluble molecules involved in disease pathogenesis via the B/T cells' cooperation. In this setting, interference with cell-to-cell cooperation represents a line of investigation worth pursuing for therapeutic purposes. For example, the targeting of T-cell costimulatory molecules, aimed at preventing their antigen-driven activation and expansion, may further impair B cells' activities. A recent trial evaluating the CTLA-4 Ig abatacept revealed that besides its clinical efficacy, a reduction of both CD3+ T lymphocytes and CD20+ B cells may be observed in MSGs.[69] A prospective, single-center pilot study with a similar design recruited 15 patients with pSS.[70] After eight infusions, abatacept was effective, safe, and well-tolerated, improving the disease activity, laboratory parameters, fatigue level, and health-related quality of life in patients with early and active pSS.

## 5.4 Potential Therapies Not Investigated in pSS

Given all the previous discussion, we may suggest that the more B-cell–driven pathogenic mechanisms are unmasked, the more potential therapeutic targets become worth evaluating. Indeed, a further intriguing aspect that could be investigated for therapeutic purposes includes some human protein kinases, namely "the human kinome" associated with pSS manifestations or complications. In fact, serum fms-like tyrosine kinase 3 ligand, a transmembrane protein with a role in stimulating the growth of progenitor cells in BM and blood, has been recently identified as a potential biological marker of lymphoma in pSS and a therapeutic target.[71]

Another reason for variable efficacy of B-cell depletion is the persistence of long-lived CD20 negative plasma cells and pathogenic autoantibodies. This observation has raised interest in targeting the plasma cell compartment. Bortezomib is a proteasome inhibitor that effectively depletes long-lived plasma cells, showing efficacy in the treatment of murine lupus,[72] and it has been recently reported to have beneficial effects in a small open-label trial in human SLE.[73]

Up-regulation of Toll-like receptors (TLRs), which is known to be implicated in the initiation of both innate and adaptive immune responses, is believed to contribute to salivary gland inflammation. TLR-9 overexpression has been identified in the salivary glands of pSS patients and animal models, and might have a role in the aberrant B-cell differentiation.[74]

## 6. CONCLUSIONS

Although the use of biological therapy in pSS is rapidly expanding with new evidence regarding potential therapeutic targets, the identification of which patients will respond and benefit from these treatments remains difficult. Moreover, biological therapies are expensive and weighted by potential risk.

pSS encompasses several subsets of patients with different genetic backgrounds, pathophysiological pathways, demographic features, responses to proposed therapies, and prognoses. Despite the acknowledged role of B cells in pSS, mechanisms leading to their abnormal activation and their contribution to pSS pathogenesis are not fully elucidated. In this setting, in order to develop a "treat-to-target" strategy in pSS, we still need to identify those molecular mechanisms, thus explaining the clinical and pathological differences observed among patients. A great effort should be made in order to define practical tools to recognize these different subsets of patients, as well as to be able to identify the most effective best treatments in each individual situation. In this setting, it must be pointed out that, at present, B-cell targeting may be considered a therapeutic option for selected patients with pSS, and the conflicting results published until now underscore the need to develop more sensitive and reproducible outcome measures for pSS.

## REFERENCES

1. Kroese FG, Abdulahad WH, Haacke E, Bos NA, Vissink A, Bootsma H. B-cell hyperactivity in primary Sjögren's syndrome. *Expert Rev Clin Immunol* 2014;**10**:483–99.
2. Carubbi F, Alunno A, Cipriani P, Di Bendetto P, Ruscitti P, Berardicurti O, et al. Is minor salivary gland biopsy more than a diagnostic tool in primary Sjögren's s syndrome? Association between clinical, histopathological, and molecular features: a retrospective study. *Semin Arthritis Rheum* 2014;**4**:314–24.
3. Voulgarelis M, Tzioufas AG. Pathogenetic mechanisms in the initiation and perpetuation of Sjögren's syndrome. *Nat Rev Rheumatol* 2010;**6**:529–37.

4. Nocturne G, Mariette X. Advances in understanding the pathogenesis of primary Sjögren's syndrome. *Nat Rev Rheumatol* 2013;**9**:544–56.

5. Ioannidis JP, Vassiliou VA, Moutsopoulos HM. Long-term risk of mortality and lymphoproliferative disease and predictive classification of primary Sjögren's syndrome. *Arthritis Rheum* 2002;**46**:741–7.

6. Baldini C, Pepe P, Quartuccio L, Priori R, Bartoloni E, Alunno A, et al. Primary Sjögren's syndrome as a multi-organ disease: impact of the serological profile on the clinical presentation of the disease in a large cohort of Italian patients. *Rheumatol Oxf* 2014;**53**:839–44.

7. Quartuccio L, Isola M, Baldini C, Priori R, Bartoloni Bocci E, Carubbi F, et al. Biomarkers of lymphoma in Sjögren's syndrome and evaluation of the lymphoma risk in prelymphomatous conditions: results of a multicenter study. *J Autoimmun* 2014;**51**:75–80.

8. Ramos-Casals M, Tzioufas AG, Stone JH, Sisó A, Bosch X. Treatment of primary Sjögren syndrome: a systematic review. *JAMA* 2010;**304**:452–60.

9. Ramos-Casals M, Brito-Zerón P, Sisó-Almirall A, Bosch X, Tzioufas AG. Topical and systemic medications for the treatment of primary Sjögren's syndrome. *Nat Rev Rheumatol* 2012;**8**(7):399–411.

10. Mavragani CP, Nezos A, Moutsopoulos HM. New advances in the classification, pathogenesis and treatment of Sjögren's syndrome. *Curr Opin Rheumatol* 2013;**25**:623–9.

11. Brito-Zerón P, Sisó-Almirall A, Bové A, Kostov BA, Ramos-Casals M. Primary Sjögren syndrome: an update on current pharmacotherapy options and future directions. *Expert Opin Pharmacother* 2013;**14**(3):279–89.

12. Fazaa A, Bourcier T, Chatelus E, Sordet C, Theulin A, Sibilia J, et al. Classification criteria and treatment modalities in primary Sjögren's syndrome. *Expert Rev Clin Immunol* 2014;**10**(4):543–51.

13. Cornec D, Saraux A, Devauchelle-Pensec V, Clodic C, Pers J-O. The future of B cell-targeted therapies in Sjögren's syndrome. *Immunotherapy* 2013;**5**(6):639–46.

14. Pescovitz MD. Rituximab, an anti-CD20 monoclonal antibody: history and mechanism of action. *Am J Transpl* 2006;**6**:859–66.

15. Kuijpers TW, Bende RJ, Baars PA, Grummels A, Derks IA, Dolman KM, et al. CD20 deficiency in humans results in impaired T cell–independent antibody responses. *J Clin Invest* 2010;**120**(1):214–22.

16. Chen S, Liu Y, Shi G. Anti-CD20 antibody in primary Sjögren's syndrome management. *Curr Pharm Biotechnol* 2014;**15**:535–41.

17. Carubbi F, Alunno A, Cipriani P, Bartoloni E, Ciccia F, Triolo G, et al. Rituximab in primary Sjögren's syndrome: a ten-year journey. *Lupus* 2014;**23**:1337–49.

18. Perosa F, Prete M, Racanelli V, Dammacco F. CD20-depleting therapy in autoimmune diseases: from basic research to the clinic. *J Intern Med* 2010;**267**:260–77.

19. Devauchelle-Pensec V, Pennec Y, Morvan J, Pers JO, Daridon C, Jousse-Joulin S, et al. Improvement of Sjögren's syndrome after two infusions of rituximab (anti-CD20). *Arthritis Rheum* 2007;**57**(2):310–7.

20. Pijpe J, Meijer JM, Bootsma H, van der Wal JE, Spijkervet FK, Kallenberg CG, et al. Clinical and histologic evidence of salivary gland restoration supports the efficacy of rituximab treatment in Sjögren's syndrome. *Arthritis Rheum* 2009;**60**(11):3251–6.

21. Pers JO, Devauchelle V, Daridon C, Bendaoud B, Le Berre R, Bordron A, et al. BAFF-modulated repopulation of B lymphocytes in the blood and salivary glands of rituximab-treated patients with Sjögren's syndrome. *Arthritis Rheum* 2007;**56**:1464–77.

22. Abdulahad WH, Meijer JM, Kroese FG, Meiners PM, Vissink A, Spijkervet FK, et al. B cell reconstitution and T helper cell balance after rituximab treatment of active primary Sjögren's syndrome: a double-blind, placebo-controlled study. *Arthritis Rheum* 2011;**63**(4):1116–23.

23. Ciccia F, Giardina A, Rizzo A, Guggino G, Cipriani P, Carubbi F, et al. Rituximab modulates the expression of IL-22 in the salivary glands of patients with primary Sjögren's syndrome. *Ann Rheum Dis* 2013;**72**:782–3.

24. Ciccia F, Guggino G, Rizzo A, Alessandro R, Carubbi F, Giardina A, et al. Rituximab modulates IL-17 expression in the salivary glands of patients with primary Sjögren's syndrome. *Rheum Oxf* 2014;**53**:1313–20.

25. Pollard RP, Abdulahad WH, Bootsma H, Meiners PM, Spijkervet FK, Huitema MG, et al. Predominantly proinflammatory cytokines decrease after B cell depletion therapy in patients with primary Sjögren's syndrome. *Ann Rheum Dis* 2013;**72**:2028–50.

26. Lisi S, Sisto M, D'Amore M, Lofrumento DD. Co-culture system of human salivary gland epithelial cells and immune cells from primary Sjögren's syndrome patients: an in vitro approach to study the effects of rituximab on the activation of the Raf-1/ERK1/2 pathway. *Int Immunol* 2015;**27**:183–94.

27. Carubbi F, Cipriani P, Marrelli A, Di Bendetto P, Ruscitti P, Berardicurti O, et al. Efficacy and safety of rituximab treatment in early primary Sjögren's syndrome: a prospective, multicenter, follow-up study. *Arthritis Res Ther* 2013;**15**:R172.

28. St Clair EW, Levesque MC, Prak ET, Vivino FB, Alappatt CJ, Spychala ME, et al. Rituximab therapy for primary Sjögren's syndrome: an open-label clinical trial and mechanistic analysis. *Arthritis Rheum* 2013;**65**:1097–106.

29. Dass S, Bowman SJ, Vital EM, Ikeda K, Pease CT, Hamburger J, et al. Reduction of fatigue in Sjögren's syndrome with rituximab: results of a randomised, double-blind, placebo-controlled pilot study. *Ann Rheum Dis* 2008;**67**:1541–4.

30. Meijer JM, Meiners PM, Vissink A, Spijkervet FK, Abdulahad W, Kamminga N, et al. Effectiveness of rituximab treatment in primary Sjögren's syndrome: a randomized, double-blind, placebo-controlled trial. *Arthritis Rheum* 2010;**62**:960–8.

31. Devauchelle-Pensec V, Mariette X, Jousse-Joulin S, Berthelot JM, Perdriger A, Puéchal X, et al. Treatment of primary Sjögren's syndrome with rituximab: a randomized trial. *Ann Intern Med* 2014;**160**:233–42.

32. Brown S, Navarro Coy N, Pitzalis C, Emery P, Pavitt S, Gray J, et al. The TRACTISS protocol: a randomized double blind placebo controlled clinical trial of anti-B–cell therapy in patients with primary Sjögren's Syndrome. *BMC Musculoskelet Disord* 2014;**17**(15):21.

33. Gottenberg JE, Cinquetti G, Larroche C, Combe B, Hachulla E, Meyer O, et al. Efficacy of rituximab in systemic manifestations of primary Sjögren's syndrome: results in 78 patients of the autoimmune and rituximab registry. *Ann Rheum Dis* 2013;**72**:1026–31.

34. Mekinian A, Ravaud P, Hatron PY, Larroche C, Leone J, Gombert B, et al. Efficacy of rituximab in primary Sjögren's syndrome with peripheral nervous system involvement: results from the AIR registry. *Ann Rheum Dis* 2012;**71**:84–7.

35. Meiners PM, Arends S, Brouwer E, Spijkervet FK, Vissink A, Bootsma H. Responsiveness of disease activity indices ESSPRI and ESSDAI in patients with primary Sjögren's syndrome treated with rituximab. *Ann Rheum Dis* 2012;**71**:1297–302.

36. Seror R, Sordet C, Guillevin L, Hachulla E, Masson C, Ittah M, et al. Tolerance and efficacy of rituximab and changes in serum B cell biomarkers in patients with systemic complications of primary Sjögren's syndrome. *Ann Rheum Dis* 2007;**66**(3):351–7.

37. Hamza N, Bootsma H, Yuvaraj S, Spijkervet FK, Haacke EA, Pollard RP, et al. Persistence of immunoglobulin-producing cells in parotid salivary glands of patients with primary Sjögren's syndrome after B cell depletion therapy. *Ann Rheum Dis* 2012;**71**:1881–7.

38. Hershberg U, Meng W, Zhang B, Haff N, St Clair EW, Cohen PL, et al. Persistence and selection of an expanded B cell clone in the setting of rituximab therapy for Sjögren's syndrome. *Arthritis Res Ther* 2014;**16**:R51.

39. Pollard RP, Abdulahad WH, Vissink A, Hamza N, Burgerhof JG, Meijer JM, et al. Serum levels of BAFF, but not APRIL, are increased after rituximab treatment in patients with primary Sjögren's syndrome: data from a placebo-controlled clinical trial. *Ann Rheum Dis* 2013;**72**:146–8.

40. Meiners PM, Arends S, Meijer JM, Moerman RV, Spijkervet FK, Vissink A, et al. Efficacy of retreatment with rituximab in patients with primary Sjögren's syndrome. *Clin Exp Rheumatol* 2015;**33**(3):443–4.

41. Bowman S, Barone F. Biologic treatments in Sjögren's syndrome. *Presse Med* 2012;**41**:e495–509.

42. Kumar A, Khamkar K, Gopal H. Serum sickness and severe angioedema following rituximab therapy in RA. *Int J Rheum Dis* 2012;**15**:e6–7.

43. Karmacharya P, Poudel DR, Pathak R, Donato AA, Ghimire S, et al. Rituximab-induced serum sickness: a systematic review. *Semin Arthritis Rheum* June 26, 2015;**45**(3):334–40.

44. Le Guenno G, Ruivard M, Charra L, Philippe P. Rituximab-induced serum sickness in refractory immune thrombocytopenic purpura. *Intern Med J* 2011;**41**:202–5.

45. Bharat A, Xie F, Baddley JW, Beukelman T, Chen L, Calabrese L, et al. Incidence and risk factors for progressive multifocal leukoencephalopathy among patients with selected rheumatic diseases. *Arthritis Care Res* 2012;**64**:612–5.

46. Haas KM, Sen S, Sanford IG, Miller AS, Peo JC, Tedder TF. CD22 ligand binding regulates normal and malignant B lymphocyte survival in vivo. *J Immunol* 2006;**177**:3063–73.

47. Steinfeld SD, Tant L, Burmester GR, Teoh NKW, Wegener WA, Goldenberg DM, et al. Epratuzumab (humanised anti-CD22 antibody) in primary Sjögren's syndrome: an open-label phase I/II study. *Arthritis Res Ther* 2006;**8**(4):R129.

48. Thien M, Phan TG, Gardam S. Excess BAFF rescues self-reactive B cells from peripheral deletion and allows them to enter forbidden follicular and marginal zone niches. *Immunity* 2004;**20**:785–98.

49. Mackay F, Schneider P. Cracking the BAFF code. *Nat Rev Immunol* 2009;**9**(7):491–502.

50. Groom J, Kalled SL, Cutler AH. Association of BAFF/BLyS overexpression and altered B cell differentiation with Sjögren's syndrome. *J Clin Invest* 2002;**109**:59–68.

51. Lavie F, Miceli-Richard C, Quillard J. Expression of BAFF (BLyS) in T cells infiltrating labial salivary glands from patients with Sjögren's syndrome. *J Pathol* 2004;**202**:496–502.

52. Pers JO, Daridon C, Devauchelle V. BAFF overexpression is associated with autoantibody production in autoimmune diseases. *Ann N Y Acad Sci* 2005;**1050**:34–9.

53. Mariette X, Roux S, Zhang J. The level of BLyS (BAFF) correlates with the titre of autoantibodies in human Sjögren's syndrome. *Ann Rheum Dis* 2003;**62**:168–71.

54. Szodoray P, Alex P, Jonsson MV. Distinct profiles of Sjögren's syndrome patients with ectopic salivary gland germinal centers revealed by serum cytokines and BAFF. *Clin Immunol* 2005;**117**:168–76.

55. Lahiri A, Pochard P, Le Pottier L, Tobón GJ, Bendaoud B, Youinou P, et al. The complexity of the BAFF TNF-family members: implications for autoimmunity. *J Autoimmun* 2012;**39**(3):189–98.

56. De Vita S, Boiocchi M, Sorrentino D, Carbone A, Avellini C, Dolcetti R, et al. Characterization of prelymphomatous stages of B cell lymphoproliferation in Sjögren's syndrome. *Arthritis Rheum* 1997;**40**:31831.

57. Quartuccio L, Salvin S, Fabris M, Maset M, Pontarini E, Isola M, et al. BLyS upregulation in Sjögren's syndrome associated with lymphoproliferative disorders, higher ESSDAI score and B-cell clonal expansion in the salivary glands. *Rheumatology* 2013;**52**:276–81.

58. Mariette X, Seror R, Quartuccio L, Maset M, Pontarini E, Isola M, et al. Efficacy and safety of belimumab in primary Sjögren's syndrome: results of the BELISS open-label phase II study. *Ann Rheum Dis* 2015;**74**:526–31.

59. De Vita S, Quartuccio L, Seror R, Salvin S, Ravaud P, Fabris M, et al. Efficacy and safety of belimumab given for 12 months in primary Sjögren's syndrome: the BELISS open-label phase II study. *Rheumatol Oxf* August 4, 2015;**54**(12):2249–56. pii: kev257.

60. Quartuccio L, Fabris M, Moretti M, Barone F, Bombardieri M, Rupolo M, et al. Resistance to rituximab therapy and local BAFF overexpression in Sjögren's syndrome-related myoepithelial sialadenitis and low-grade parotid B-cell lymphoma. *Open Rheumatol J* 2008;**2**:38–43.

61. De Vita S, Quartuccio L, Salvin S, Picco L, Scott CA, Rupolo M, et al. Sequential therapy with belimumab followed by rituximab in Sjögren's syndrome associated with B-cell lymphoproliferation and overexpression of BAFF: evidence for long-term efficacy. *Clin Exp Rheumatol* 2014;**32**:490–4.

62. Bombardieri M, Pitzalis C. Ectopic lymphoid neogenesis and lymphoid chemokines in Sjögren's syndrome: at the interplay between chronic inflammation, autoimmunity and lymphomagenesis. *Curr Pharm Biotechnol* 2012;**13**:1989–96.

63. Luciano N, Valentini V, Calabrò A, Elefante E, Vitale A, Baldini C, et al. One year in review 2015: Sjögren's syndrome. *Clin Exp Rheumatol* 2015;**33**(2):259–71.

64. Gatumu MK, Skarstein K, Papandile A, Browning JL, Fava RA, Bolstad AI. Blockade of lymphotoxin-beta receptor signaling reduces aspects of Sjögren's syndrome in salivary glands of non-obese diabetic mice. *Arthritis Res Ther* 2009;**11**(1):R24.

65. Youinou P, Jamin C. The weight of interleukin-6 in B cell-related autoimmune disorders. *J Autoimmun* 2009;**32**:206–10.

66. Daridon C, Guerrier T, Devauchelle V, Saraux A, Pers JO, Youinou P. Polarization of B effector cells in Sjögren's syndrome. *Autoimmun Rev* 2007;**6**(7):427–31.

67. Grisius MM, Bermudez DK, Fox PC. Salivary and serum interleukin 6 in primary Sjögren's syndrome. *J Rheumatol* 1997;**24**:1089–91.

68. Halse A, Tengnér P, Wahren-Herlenius M, Haga H, Jonsson R. Increased frequency of cells secreting interleukin-6 and interleukin-10 in peripheral blood of patients with primary Sjögren's syndrome. *Scand J Immunol* 1999;**49**:533–8.

69. Adler S, Körner M, Förger F, Huscher D, Caversaccio MD, Villiger PM. Evaluation of histological, serological and clinical changes in response to abatacept treatment of primary Sjögren's syndrome: a pilot study. *Arthritis Care Res* 2013;**65**:1862–8.

70. Meiners PM, Vissink A, Kroese FGM, Spijkervet FK, Smitt-Kamminga NS, Abdulahad WH, et al. Abatacept treatment reduces disease activity in early primary Sjögren's syndrome (open-label proof of concept ASAP study). *Ann Rheum Dis* 2014;**73**:1393–6.

71. Tobon GJ, Saraux A, Gottenberg JE. Role of fms-like tyrosine kinase 3 ligand as a potential biologic marker of lymphoma in primary Sjögren's syndrome. *Arthritis Rheum* 2013;**65**:3218–27.

72. Neubert K, Meister S, Moser K, Weisel F, Maseda D, Amann K, et al. The proteasome inhibitor bortezomib depletes plasma cells and protects mice with lupus-like disease from nephritis. *Nat Med* 2008;**14**:748–55.

73. Alexander T, Sarfert R, Klotsche J, Kühl AA, Rubbert-Roth A, Lorenz HM, et al. The proteasome inhibitor bortezomib depletes plasma cells and ameliorates clinical manifestations of refractory systemic lupus erythematosus. *Ann Rheum Dis* 2015;**74**(7):1474–8.

74. Shi H, Yu CQ, Xie LS. Activation of TLR9-dependent p38MAPK pathway in the pathogenesis of primary Sjögren's syndrome in NOD/Ltj mouse. *J Oral Pathol Med* 2014;**43**:785–91.

Chapter 19

# Novel Therapeutic Strategies in Sjögren's Syndrome: T-Cell Targeting

**V.C. Kyttaris, G.C. Tsokos**

*Harvard Medical School, Boston, MA, United States*

In the past decade, the treatment of autoimmune diseases [such as rheumatoid arthritis (RA) and Crohn disease] has fundamentally changed with the introduction of targeted therapies. On the contrary, the treatment of Sjögren's syndrome (SS) and especially the eye and mouth dryness that are its main manifestations has remained purely symptomatic and the systemic effects, such as inflammatory arthritis continue to be treated with nonspecific immunosuppressive medications. As our understanding of the pathophysiology has improved and new measures of disease activity have been designed, SS is poised to enter the era of biological therapies.

One of the most striking pathophysiological features of SS is the infiltration of tissues such as salivary glands with lymphocytes, both B and T cells. The CD4+ but also CD4–CD8–T cells promote local inflammation by producing proinflammatory cytokines such as interferon-γ and interleukin (IL) 17.[1] Moreover, follicular T helper cells (Tfhs) help organize locally secondary lymphoid structures and promote B-cell activation.[2] Although the initiating factor(s) and exact mechanisms are still unclear, T cells are attracted to the salivary glands by chemokines and encounter a locally activated epithelium that can further promote their activation. Moreover, imbalance between effector and regulatory T (Treg) cell activity may also contribute to both the local and systemic manifestations of the disease, making T cells prime therapeutic targets (Fig. 19.1).

## 1. COSTIMULATION

T cells bind to antigen-presenting cells (APCs), such as dendritic cells and B cells through a cognate interaction but rely on a second signal to stabilize and enhance the rather weak T-cell receptor (TCR) antigen–major histocompatibility complex (MHC) interaction. This second costimulatory signal is absolutely

*Sjögren's Syndrome.* http://dx.doi.org/10.1016/B978-0-12-803604-4.00019-8
**291**

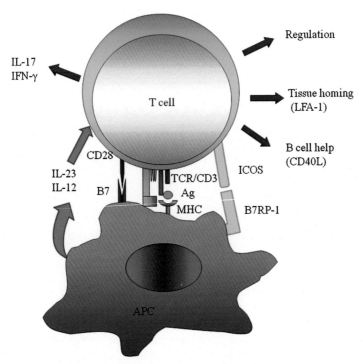

**FIGURE 19.1** The T-cell receptor *(TCR)* recognizes antigens that are presented by antigen presenting cells *(APCs)* in the context of major histocompatibility complex *(MHC)*. This interaction is enhanced and stabilized by the costimulatory pairs ICOS-B7RP1, CD28-B7. Upon the T-cell–APC interaction, T cells get activated, produce cytokines, home to target tissues, differentiate into regulatory T cells, or provide help to B cells. Moreover, APCs control T-cell activation by producing cytokines such as interleukin *(IL)* 23, which leads to production of IL-17 and IL-12, which promotes interferon γ *(IFN-γ)* production. *Ag*, antigen; *B7RP1*, B7-related peptide 1; *CD40L*, CD40 ligand; *ICOS*, inducible T-cell costimulator; *LFA-1*, lymphocyte function–associated antigen 1.

necessary for a productive immune response and can readily be targeted using monoclonal antibodies and soluble receptors. In the following sections, we describe the main pathways that have been targeted in SS.

## 1.1 CD28–B7

One of the main costimulatory molecules that delivers this second signal to T cells is CD28. CD28 binds to its ligand B7 (CD80 or CD86) on APC and enhances the TCR-initiated T-cell activation. Then after this initial activation phase, T cells express in lieu of CD28, CTLA4 that also binds to B7 but delivers an inhibitory signal to T cells, effectively ending activation. In SS, salivary gland epithelial cells also express B7 molecules that show an increased affinity for CD28 and decrease binding for CTLA4.[3] Capitalizing on this naturally occurring phenomenon, the antirheumatic drug abatacept was engineered. Abatacept is a fusion molecule of CTLA4 and immunoglobulin that can effectively interrupt T-cell activation and is proven to be an effective treatment for RA.

As RA patients often have secondary SS, the effect of abatacept was evaluated in 32 patients with RA and secondary SS in an open-label 1-year pilot study.[4] Abatacept had a modest effect, primarily on eye dryness (increase in the Schirmer test result from $3.6 \pm 4.6$ mm/5 min at 0 weeks to $5.5 \pm 7.1$ mm/5 min at 24 weeks of treatment) and less on oral sicca symptoms. Interestingly, abatacept decreased the levels of rheumatoid factor (RF) and total immunoglobulin (Ig) G, but had no effect on the levels of Ro/SSA.

In a small, open label study in primary SS patients, abatacept was given subcutaneously to 15 patients for 24 weeks.[5] The primary endpoint was the European League Against Rheumatism (EULAR) Sjögren Syndrome Disease Activity Index (ESSDAI). ESSDAI significantly decreased while the patients were receiving treatment, only to increase back to baseline 24 weeks after treatment ended. The salivary and lacrimal flows did not change significantly as in the aforementioned secondary SS study, but the RF and total IgG did decrease.

In yet another study, 11 patients with primary SS received eight doses of abatacept.[6] Abatacept treatment led to modest decrease in salivary gland inflammation as measured by the number of lymphocytic foci. Saliva production increased modestly, with this increase being statistically significant only when adjusted for disease duration. Serum IgG decreased slightly after treatment.

Overall, these small studies showed that CD28–B7 interaction might be an important pathway for intervention in primary SS. A large, placebo control phase III clinical trial in patients with primary SS of less than 7 years' duration is currently underway. The primary outcome of the blinded study is ESSDAI at 24 weeks, with an open label extension for another 24 weeks.

## 1.2 ICOS-B7RP1

Upon activation, T cells express the inducible costimulator that binds to its ligand [or inducible T-cell costimulator ligand (ICOSL), also called *B7-related peptide 1 (B7RP1)*] on a variety of cells, such as APCs and B cells. The ICOS-B7RP1 binding is important for both T and B cells, because it promotes T-cell activation and differentiation to Tfh as well B-cell maturation and antibody production. In SS-activated epithelial cells, expressing B7RP may induce Tfh generation from naive CD4+ T cells.[7] AMG-557 is a human IgG2 antibody against B7RP1 that has been shown to be safe in phase I trial systemic lupus erythematosus (SLE) patients. Importantly, it blocked the production of antibodies to the neoantigen keyhole limpet hemocyanin that was injected to the subjects receiving AMG-557. It is currently undergoing a phase IIa clinical trial in subjects with SS as well as in patients with SLE arthritis and subacute cutaneous lupus (a disease linked to Ro/SSA antibodies). The primary outcome is ESSDAI at day 99 of therapy.

## 1.3 CD154–CD40

CD154 [also called *CD40 ligand (CD40L)*] is expressed on T cells shortly after activation. It engages CD40 on B cells, driving B-cell activation and maturation. T cells upregulate CD154 on their surface after activation in a calcium-dependent manner. In autoimmune diseases, such as SLE, T-cell calcium influx is up-regulated, leading to increased and sustained expression of CD154.[8,9] CD154–CD40 interaction is one of the most important checkpoints in the production of high-affinity IgG antibodies and has therefore been an early therapeutic target in diseases that are characterized by increased Ig production such as SLE.[10] Patients with SS have elevated serum levels of CD154[11] and often do have hypergammaglobulinemia, including high titers of various autoantibodies, highlighting the importance of CD154–CD40 interaction as a therapeutic target. Because this first generation of anti-CD154 antibodies was associated with thrombotic events, CD40 was targeted instead with a human Fc-silent antibody, CFZ533. This antibody blocks CD40–CD154 interaction without depleting the B cells, and in preliminary trials was efficacious in prolonging renal allograft survival.[12] It is currently undergoing an early phase double-blind placebo control trial in patients with primary SS focusing on safety and pharmacokinetics. The endpoint is ESSDAI at 12 weeks.

## 2. T-CELL TRAFFICKING

The influx of T cells in salivary glands of patients with SS is thought to be key for local inflammation and secondary destruction of the glands. For the successful tissue migration, T cells bind to endothelial cells through interaction of lymphocyte function–associated antigen 1 (LFA-1) on T cells with intercellular adhesion molecule 1 on endothelial cells. Efalizumab, an antibody that binds to the CD11a chain of LFA-1, was effective in the treatment of psoriasis[13] and a clinical trial in SS patients was designed. The medication was withdrawn because of increased incidence of progressive multifocal leukoencephalopathy (PML), a potentially fatal disease attributed to reactivation of John Cunningham (JC) virus.[14] Importantly, the risk of PML is also increased in patients treated with another T-cell trafficking blocker, natalizumab. This antibody blocks α4 integrins and, although efficacious in Crohn disease[15] and multiple sclerosis,[16] its use is limited because of the significant risk of JC reactivation. More recently, fingolimod, a sphigosine-1 phosphate receptor analog was shown to be effective in relapsing remitting multiple sclerosis.[17] Fingolimod is a small molecule that prevents T-cell trafficking and sequesters them in the lymph nodes. In an interesting case of concomitant SS and multiple sclerosis,[18] fingolimod was found to be effective in treating the central nervous system disease but also decreased the level of Ro/SSA antibodies, suggesting that blocking lymphocyte trafficking may have an effect on the systemic autoimmunity associated with SS.

## 3. CYTOKINES

Several studies over the past decade suggested that T cells expressing the proinflammatory cytokine IL-17 [T helper (Th) 17] are important in the pathogenesis of primary SS.[19] This is in keeping with several studies in autoimmune mouse models showing that Th17 cells are present in areas of inflammation as well as in secondary lymphoid organs.[20,21] Importantly, a transgenic mouse that overexpresses the Th17 signature transcription factor ROR-γt develops profound sialadenitis, mimicking the human disease.[22] Surprisingly IL-17A was dispensable for the development of sialadenitis in this mouse, suggesting that other mechanisms may be playing a role. Indeed, these mice had reduced numbers of Treg cells, which contributed to the development of the disease. In a different mouse model however, in which sialadenitis was induced by injecting salivary gland proteins, IL-17 played an indispensable role in the development of the disease.[23]

IL-17 and IL-23, the cytokine that in part drives IL-17 production, have been targeted in a variety of autoimmune diseases. Ustekinumab is an antibody that blocks the p40 subunit that is shared by IL-12 and IL-23 and is effective in the treatment of psoriasis and psoriatic arthritis.[24] Anti–IL-17 antibodies secukinumab and brodalumab are also effective in psoriatic arthritis[25,26] but not as effective in RA.[27,28] In addition, in murine lupus, anti–IL-23 treatment results in amelioration of nephritis,[29] whereas anti–IL-17A treatment is not as effective.[30] This discrepancy may be caused by expression of other cytokines such as IL-17F or by decreased production of IL-2, which would lead to decreased Treg function. Indeed, infusion of an IL-2–expressing viral vector in lupus-prone mice ameliorated nephritis by boosting Treg function while decreasing the expansion of CD4−CD8− IL-17 + T cells.[31] This strategy was also efficacious in patients with graft-versus-host disease, whereas low-dose IL-2 infusions[32] resulted in increased Treg activity and eventually in disease amelioration. Based on these preclinical studies, a successful strategy in complex autoimmune diseases such as SLE[33] or SS should aim at restoring the balance between proinflammatory and counterinflammatory cytokines rather than just blocking an individual cytokine.

## 4. CONCLUSION

Targeted therapies for SS are still in their infancy. The first large trial of abatacept opens the gates for more large clinical trials that should eventually help change the current paradigm that is based on nonspecific immunosuppression. Eventually the goal should be not just to suppress the immune system but also to restore the balance between proinflammatory and counterinflammatory pathways.

# REFERENCES

1. Alunno A, Bistoni O, Bartoloni Bocci E, Caterbi S, Bigerna B, Pucciarini A, et al. IL-17–producing double-negative T cells are expanded in the peripheral blood, infiltrate the salivary gland and are partially resistant to corticosteroid therapy in patients with Sjögren's syndrome. *Rheumatism* 2013;**65**:192–8.

2. Maehara T, Moriyama M, Hayashida JN, Tanaka A, Shinozaki S, Kubo Y, et al. Selective localization of T helper subsets in labial salivary glands from primary Sjögren's syndrome patients. *Clin Exp Immunol* 2012;**169**:89–99.

3. Kapsogeorgou EK, Moutsopoulos HM, Manoussakis MN. Functional expression of a costimulatory B7.2 (CD86) protein on human salivary gland epithelial cells that interacts with the CD28 receptor, but has reduced binding to CTLA4. *J Immunol* 2001;**166**:3107–13.

4. Tsuboi H, Matsumoto I, Hagiwara S, Hirota T, Takahashi H, Ebe H, et al. Efficacy and safety of abatacept for patients with Sjögren's syndrome associated with rheumatoid arthritis: Rheumatoid Arthritis with Orencia Trial Toward Sjögren's Syndrome Endocrinopathy (ROSE) trial: an open-label, one-year, prospective study, interim analysis of 32 patients for 24 weeks. *Mod Rheumatol* 2015;**25**:187–93.

5. Meiners PM, Vissink A, Kroese FG, Spijkervet FK, Smitt-Kamminga NS, Abdulahad WH, et al. Abatacept treatment reduces disease activity in early primary Sjögren's syndrome (open-label proof of concept ASAP study). *Ann Rheum Dis* 2014;**73**:1393–6.

6. Adler S, Korner M, Forger F, Huscher D, Caversaccio MD, Villiger PM. Evaluation of histologic, serologic, and clinical changes in response to abatacept treatment of primary Sjögren's syndrome: a pilot study. *Arthritis Care Res* 2013;**65**:1862–8.

7. Gong YZ, Nititham J, Taylor K, Miceli-Richard C, Sordet C, Wachsmann D, et al. Differentiation of follicular helper T cells by salivary gland epithelial cells in primary Sjögren's syndrome. *J Autoimmun* 2014;**5**:57–66.

8. Kyttaris VC, Zhang Z, Kampagianni O, Tsokos GC. Calcium signaling in systemic lupus erythematosus T cells: a treatment target. *Arthritis Rheum* 2011;**63**:2058–66.

9. Kyttaris VC, Wang Y, Juang YT, Weinstein A, Tsokos GC. Increased levels of NF-ATc2 differentially regulate CD154 and IL-2 genes in T cells from patients with systemic lupus erythematosus. *J Immunol* 2007;**178**:1960–6.

10. Boumpas DT, Furie R, Manzi S, Illei GG, Wallace DJ, Balow JE, et al. A short course of BG9588 (anti-CD40 ligand antibody) improves serologic activity and decreases hematuria in patients with proliferative lupus glomerulonephritis. *Arthritis Rheum* 2003;**48**:719–27.

11. Goules A, Tzioufas AG, Manousakis MN, Kirou KA, Crow MK, Routsias JG. Elevated levels of soluble CD40 ligand (sCD40L) in serum of patients with systemic autoimmune diseases. *J Autoimmun* 2006;**26**:165–71.

12. Cordoba F, Wieczorek G, Audet M, Roth L, Schneider MA, Kunkler A, et al. A novel, blocking, Fc-silent anti-CD40 monoclonal antibody prolongs nonhuman primate renal allograft survival in the absence of B cell depletion. *Am J Transpl* 2015;**15**(11):2825–36.

13. Gordon KB, Papp KA, Hamilton TK, Walicke PA, Dummer W, Li N, et al. Efalizumab for patients with moderate to severe plaque psoriasis: a randomized controlled trial. *JAMA* 2003;**290**:3073–80.

14. Molloy ES, Calabrese LH. Therapy: targeted but not trouble-free—efalizumab and PML. *Nat Rev Rheumatol* 2009;**5**:418–9.

15. Ghosh S, Goldin E, Gordon FH, Malchow A, Rask-Madsen J, Rutgeerts P, et al. Natalizumab for active Crohn's disease. *N Engl J Med* 2003;**348**:24–32.

16. Miller DH, Khan OA, Sheremata WA, Blumhardt LD, Rice GP, Libonati MA, et al. A controlled trial of natalizumab for relapsing multiple sclerosis. *N Engl J Med* 2003;**348**:15–23.

17. Kappos L, Radue EW, O'Connor P, Polman C, Hohfeld R, Calabresi P, et al. A placebo-controlled trial of oral fingolimod in relapsing multiple sclerosis. *N Engl J Med* 2010;**362**: 387–401.

18. Signoriello E, Sagliocchi A, Fratta M, Lus G. Fingolimod efficacy in multiple sclerosis associated with Sjögren syndrome. *Acta Neuro Scand* 2015;**131**:140–3.

19. Nguyen CQ, Hu MH, Li Y, Stewart C, Peck AB. Salivary gland tissue expression of interleukin-23 and interleukin-17 in Sjögren's syndrome: findings in humans and mice. *Arthritis Rheum* 2008;**58**:734–43.

20. Crispin JC, Oukka M, Bayliss G, Cohen RA, Van Beek CA, Stillman IE, et al. Expanded double negative T cells in patients with systemic lupus erythematosus produce IL-17 and infiltrate the kidneys. *J Immunol* 2008;**181**:8761–6.

21. Zhang Z, Kyttaris VC, Tsokos GC. The role of IL-23/IL-17 axis in lupus nephritis. *J Immunol* 2009;**183**:3160–9.

22. Iizuka M, Tsuboi H, Matsuo N, Asashima H, Hirota T, Kondo Y, et al. A crucial role of RORγt in the development of spontaneous sialadenitis-like Sjögren's syndrome. *J Immunol* 2015;**194**:56–67.

23. Lin X, Rui K, Deng J, Tian JJ, Wang S, Ko KH, et al. Th17 cells play a critical role in the development of experimental Sjögren's syndrome. *Ann Rheum Dis* 2015;**74**:1302–10.

24. Ritchlin C, Rahman P, Kavanaugh A, McInnes IB, Puig L, Li S, et al. Efficacy and safety of the anti-IL-12/23 p40 monoclonal antibody, ustekinumab, in patients with active psoriatic arthritis despite conventional non-biological and biological anti-tumour necrosis factor therapy: 6-month and 1-year results of the phase 3, multicentre, double-blind, placebo-controlled, randomised PSUMMIT 2 trial. *Ann Rheum Dis* 2014;**73**:990–9.

25. McInnes IB, Mease PJ, Kirkham B, Kavanaugh A, Ritchlin CT, Rahman P, et al. Secukinumab, a human anti-interleukin-17A monoclonal antibody, in patients with psoriatic arthritis (FUTURE 2): a randomised, double-blind, placebo-controlled, phase 3 trial. *Lancet* 2015;**386**(9999):1137–46.

26. Mease PJ, Genovese MC, Greenwald MW, Ritchlin CT, Beaulieu AD, Deodhar A, et al. Brodalumab, an anti-IL17RA monoclonal antibody, in psoriatic arthritis. *N Engl J Med* 2014;**370**:2295–306.

27. Genovese MC, Durez P, Richards HB, Supronik J, Dokoupilova E, Mazurov V, et al. Efficacy and safety of secukinumab in patients with rheumatoid arthritis: a phase II, dose-finding, double-blind, randomised, placebo controlled study. *Ann Rheum Dis* 2013;**72**:863–9.

28. Pavelka K, Chon Y, Newmark R, Lin SL, Baumgartner S, Erondu N. A study to evaluate the safety, tolerability, and efficacy of brodalumab in subjects with rheumatoid arthritis and an inadequate response to methotrexate. *J Rheumatol* 2015;**42**:912–9.

29. Kyttaris VC, Kampagianni O, Tsokos GC. Treatment with anti-interleukin 23 antibody ameliorates disease in lupus-prone mice. *Biomed Res Int* 2013;**2013**:861028.

30. Schmidt T, Paust HJ, Krebs CF, Turner JE, Kaffke A, Bennstein SB, et al. Function of the Th17/interleukin-17A immune response in murine lupus nephritis. *Arthritis Rheum* 2015;**67**:475–87.

31. Mizui M, Koga T, Lieberman LA, Beltran J, Yoshida N, Johnson MC, et al. IL-2 protects lupus-prone mice from multiple end-organ damage by limiting CD4−CD8− IL-17-producing T cells. *J Immunol* 2014;**193**:2168–77.

32. Koreth J, Matsuoka K, Kim HT, McDonough SM, Bindra B, Alyea 3rd EP, et al. Interleukin-2 and regulatory T cells in graft-versus-host disease. *N Engl J Med* 2011;**365**:2055–66.

33. Tsokos GC. Systemic lupus erythematosus. *N Engl J Med* 2011;**365**:2110–21.

Chapter 20

# New Biological Avenues for Sjögren's Syndrome

**R. Priori, S. Colafrancesco, G. Valesini**
Sapienza University of Rome, Rome, Italy

**F. Barone**
University of Birmingham, Birmingham, United Kingdom

The introduction of biological treatments that target leukocytes and their cytokine products has led to a major change in the management of immune-mediated inflammatory diseases, among them Sjögren's syndrome (SS). The recent improved understanding of the mechanisms involved in SS pathogenesis and persistence has prompted the development of new classes of drugs aimed at blocking or interfering with these pathways. This chapter aims to review the evidence in support of these drugs in SS and, where available, will highlight the clinical attempts to translate these compounds into clinical treatment. B cell–targeting therapies will be discussed elsewhere.

## 1. NEW BIOLOGICAL TREATMENTS FOR AUTOIMMUNE DISEASE

SS is characterized by loss of function of the exocrine glands (sicca syndrome) and systemic manifestations caused by B cell hyperactivation and autoantibody production. One-third of the patients present signs of extraglandular involvement that extend from cutaneous vasculitis to peripheral neuropathy or pulmonary involvement. The remaining two-thirds experience mainly dryness-related symptoms. Systemic manifestations are most commonly observed in immunologically active patients and are characterized by high titers of anti-Ro/SSA and anti-La/SSB autoantibodies and rheumatoid factor.[1–3] The major comorbidity in patients with SS is the development of non-Hodgkin lymphoma (NHL) that commonly arises in affected salivary glands (parotids) and confers a higher mortality risk to SS patients, significantly affecting disease prognosis.[4] SS also represents a significant health and economic burden in patients who do not develop NHL.[5–7] Recent data highlight the increased comorbid cardiovascular risk associated with SS,[8] and the

Sjögren's Syndrome. http://dx.doi.org/10.1016/B978-0-12-803604-4.00020-4

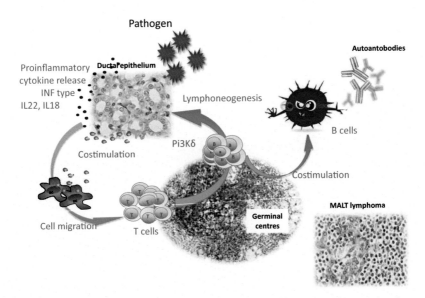

**FIGURE 20.1** Sjögren's syndrome: pathogenesis and targets. *IL*, Interleukin; *INF*, interferon; *MALT*, mucosa-associated lymphoid tissue; *PI3Kδ*, phosphatidylinositol 3–kinase δ isoform.

reduced quality of life of SS patients has also been described.[7,9] To date, there is no approved, specific treatment for the disease. Patients are managed with a combination of immunosuppressive drugs and, in some cases, systemic disease is treated with steroids. A general consensus among SS experts is that biological therapies will play a key role in the management of subsets of SS patients, but it remains unclear what the most appropriate targets might be.[10] Great efforts have been made in the United Kingdom[11] and in the international community to better define subtypes of patients with SS and refine tools to measure disease activity and outcome in clinical trials.[12,13] It appears that a better definition of *biological* as well as *clinical* measures of outcome will be required in the phase of the design of clinical trials.

SS pathogenesis is complex and as such provides a series of potential therapeutic targets that range from inflammatory cytokines to costimulatory molecules or cellular target therapies (Fig. 20.1). SS treatment will mainly involve the repurposing of strategies used to tackle more complex and life-threatening autoimmune diseases. However, the possibility to define SS-specific targets should also be also considered, with the final aim to provide patients with SS with valuable therapeutic possibilities.

## 2. THE INTERFERON SIGNATURE

In 1994, Moutsopoulos first described SS as "autoimmune epithelitis"[14] with the aim at highlighting the key role played by epithelium in the regulation of local inflammatory responses at salivary glands level. Twenty years later, it is well accepted that "activated" epithelial cells play a functional role in SS development, and in maintenance and progression of the local autoimmune inflammatory responses. Latent viral infections of the epithelium have been causally implicated in the epithelial activation, with Epstein-Barr virus, cytomegalovirus, retroviral elements, human herpes virus type 6, human T lymphotropic virus type I, human herpes virus type 8, and Coxsackie virus having been suggested at different stages as inducing or contributing to the activated state of the epithelial compartment.[15] Although no convincing evidence has supported the causative role of any of those pathogens, the hypothetical role of a viral infection before the aberrant activation of the resident epithelium is widely accepted. More intriguingly, the persistence of viral genetic material within the epithelial cytoplasm has been suggested,[16] which would be able to alter the biological properties of the cell and support the ongoing aberrant immune response. Supporting evidence for a viral involvement in SS pathogenesis is provided by the aberrant immune responses characterized by the type I interferon (IFN) signature.[17] Type I IFNs are proteins able to trigger the induction of hundreds of genes implicated in antiviral response, including the B cell activating factor *(BAFF)* and the IFN-induced transmembrane protein 1.[18] A prominent type I IFN signature in patients with SS has been shown both in the gene expression profile within the minor salivary glands (MSGs)[19] and in peripheral blood cells.[20] Moreover, plasmacytoid dendritic cells (DCs), which represent the main source of type I IFN, also accumulate in the MSGs.[21] Despite playing an important antiviral role, type I INF appears to be responsible for the fatigue and malaise often observed in SS patients. Currently there are no clinical trials exploring the use of anti-IFN I agents in SS patients; however, some evidence derives from patients with systemic lupus erythematosus (SLE). Blocking the interferon pathway with rontalizumab, a humanized immunoglobulin (Ig) G1 anti-IFNα monoclonal antibody, in patients with moderate to severe SLE has been associated with improvements in disease activity, reduced flares, and decreased steroid use in patients with low IFN signature metric (ISM) scores. However, there has been a failure to meet the primary endpoint in patients with high ISM scores.[22] Use of another anti-IFNα monoclonal antibody, sifalimumab, has also showed safety/tolerability in SLE patients and a partial improvement in clinical activity profile was shown.[23] The use of compounds interfering with the IFN cascade might represent a potential target for SS.

## 3. INNATE INFLAMMATORY CYTOKINES

High expression of several inflammatory cytokines belonging to the innate arm of the immune system has been found in MSG inflammatory infiltrates. Despite being highly expressed in SS salivary glands anti–tumor necrosis factor (TNF)α blocking strategies have not been proved efficacious in SS. The use of both etanercept and infliximab has not been associated to significant, clinical or histological (decrease in the focus score) improvement.[24] Indeed, in an animal model transgenic for the B cell survival factor *BAFF*, TNFα was shown to provide a protective role toward the potential lymphomatous transformation of the reactive B cell infiltrate.[25]

Interleukin (IL) 6 levels are significantly increased in the blood and salivary glands of SS patients. The pathogenic role of IL-6 in fatigue is also well known,[26] thus supporting the use of anti–IL-6 therapies in SS. A large randomized, placebo-controlled study focused on this compound is currently recruiting in France (https://clinicaltrials.gov).

In 2004, Bombardieri et al. provided the first evidence of increased circulating levels and salivary gland expression of IL-18 in patients with SS that correlated with the serum titers of anti-Ro/SSA and anti-La/SSB antibodies.[27] Although targeting IL-18 has not been considered, an attempt to target IL-1, which belongs to the same family as IL-18 and is found upregulated in SS salivary glands on infiltrating and epithelial cells, using anakinra has shown some improvement on fatigue.[28]

Ciccia et al. identified the presence of IL-22 overexpression both at IL-22 protein and messenger (mRNA) in inflamed salivary glands. According to this finding, T helper (Th) 17 and natural killer (NK) p44(+) NK cells were both found to produce IL-22.[29] Interestingly, IL-18 levels correlate with the levels of IL-22 receptor 1 both in tissues and in circulating myeloid cells from patients with SS and in macrophages of SS non-Hodgkin lymphoid tissues, thus suggesting a potential link between these two cytokines.[30] Recently, a novel role of IL-22 has been described in the induction of CXCL13, a chemokine required for germinal center (GC) organization and formation of tertiary lymphoid organs (TLOs).[31] Treatment of an inducible model of SS with anti–IL-22 blocking antibodies significantly impacts CXCL13 release and B cell recruitment into the glands, inducing disaggregation of the aggregates and a significant decrease in autoantibody production.[31]

## 4. T CELL TARGETING

T cells play a key pathogenic role in SS. T cells provide antigen-specific stimulation and cytokines that are required for the aggregate maintenance, sustaining B cell activation and survival within the glands.

Interfering with T cell migration into the target organs of autoimmune diseases has been considered in the treatment of rheumatological conditions. In SS patients, the use of the monoclonal antibodies efalizumab, which binds to CD11a (a subunit of lymphocyte function–associated antigen 1) and inhibits its interaction with intercellular adhesion molecule 1 on tissue cells, and natalizumab, a monoclonal antibody that targets the cellular adhesion molecule α4 integrin, have been associated to the development of progressive multifocal leukoencephalopathy and consequently abandoned.[32]

The use of the oral sphingosine-1-phosphate inhibitor fingolimod (FTY720) appears more promising. FTY720, which was approved as the first oral treatment for relapsing forms of multiple sclerosis (MS) in 2010, revealed its ability to cause substantial lymphopenia and prolonged allograft survival in various animal models.[33] The S1P receptor (S1PR) signaling is associated with vascular development, central nervous system homeostasis, and lymphocyte recirculation. FTY720, a compound generated by chemical modification of the fungal derivative myriocin that is able to down-modulate S1P1 receptors on lymphocytes, causes substantial lymphopenia and prolonged allograft survival by interfering with lymphocyte egress from lymphoid tissue and into the periphery.[33] FTY720 has been proposed as a valid therapeutic option for several inflammatory-mediated diseases, including psoriasis and MS. FTY720 initially acts as an agonist of the S1P1 receptor and then becomes a highly potent functional antagonist, leading to internalization of S1P1 receptors on lymph-node T cells. As a result, autoreactive naive and central memory T cells are confined to the secondary lymphoid organs while the functionality and frequency of circulating effector T memory cells is enhanced. Moreover, regulatory T (Treg) cell increase and the overall Th17 polarization is reduced.[34] The expression of S1P1 within the cytoplasm of inflammatory mononuclear cells, vascular endothelial cells, and salivary gland epithelial cells in patients with SS has been demonstrated, where its expression is increased in correlation with disease stage.[35] Preliminary evidence showing efficacy of FTY720 in reducing salivary gland infiltrates and increasing salivary flow in a mouse model of SS was presented at the 12th International Symposium on SS held in Japan in November 2013 (Cohen PL). More recently, a good response to treatment with FTY720 has been described in a single, isolated case report for both SS and MS.[36]

T cell homeostasis can be also be disturbed by interfering with cytokines involved in its regulation. IL-7 is a non–hematopoietic-derived cytokine that is involved in T cell proliferation, survival, and differentiation, as well as in the activation of DCs and B cells.[37] Excessive IL-7 production results in enhanced T cytotoxic 1 response, which is in turn characterized by IFNγ production.[38] There is evidence of an increased number of IL-7R cells (mainly CD4 and CD8) within the salivary glands of SS patients compared with sicca patients.[39] Furthermore, there is some evidence that the overexpression of IL-7 in the salivary glands directly regulates the Th1/Th17 response. Several studies pointed out that Toll-like receptor ligands might represent possible triggers for IL-7 production.[40,41] As observed in experimental models for autoimmune arthritis and SS, it is reasonable to think that the blockade of the IL-7/IL-7Rα pathway could be an effective treatment in autoimmune disorders.[42] A randomized, double-blind, placebo-controlled phase 1 study to evaluate the safety, tolerability, pharmacokinetics, pharmacodynamics, and immunogenicity of single ascending doses of a fully humanized anti–IL-7Rα monoclonal antibody has been recently completed in healthy volunteers and its transfer to SS is awaited in 2016.

Serum IL-21 levels are higher in SS patients compared with controls and correlate with IgG1 levels and anti-Ro/SSA antibody titers. In physiological conditions, IL-21 is produced by activated CD4+ T cells, whereas the IL-21 receptor (IL-21R) is expressed on hematopoietic as well as nonhematopoietic cells (T cells, NK cells, B cells, DCs, macrophages, keratinocytes, fibroblasts). This cytokine moderates T cell function; it increases the proliferation of T cells, facilitates the differentiation of Th17 cells induced by IL-23, and inhibits the Treg cells. IL-21 acts also on B cells, where it induces plasma cell differentiation and GC formation. Interestingly, in the salivary glands, IL-21 expression colocalizes with CXCR5 (the ligand for CXCL13), which is a chemokine receptor involved in GC formation. Within the salivary gland infiltrates, the expression of IL-21 correlates with the degree of lymphocytic infiltration.[43] IL-21 is also an excellent marker of follicular T helper (Tfh) cells, a subset of T cells that expresses CXCR5 and is specialized in providing B cell help.[44] In SS patients, an increased number of circulating and salivary gland Tfh cells has been observed[45] that correlates with the number of memory B cells and plasma cells. The blocking of IL-21 activity in SS could represent an additional therapeutic approach as proposed for other autoimmune diseases. Indeed, a monoclonal antibody made by a fusion of the IL-21R extracellular domain to the Fc portion of murine IgG and able to neutralize IL-21 in vitro has been demonstrated to reduce disease activity in murine models of SLE, rheumatoid arthritis, and inflammatory bowel disease (IBD).[46-48]

## 5. TERTIARY LYMPHOID ORGAN DEVELOPMENT AND THE ROLE OF CHEMOKINES

TLOs are accumulations of lymphoid cells within nonlymphoid organs that share the cellular compartments (T cell/B cell segregation), spatial organization, vasculature, chemokines, and function with secondary lymphoid organs and depend on the expression of lymphotoxin α and β. Salivary gland TLOs are characterized by the presence of T cell/B cell compartments, follicular DC networks within the GC,[49] and local expression of activation-induced cytidine deaminase, the enzyme instrumental for B cell affinity maturation.[50] In SS and rheumatoid arthritis, a correlation has been established between TLO formation, autoantibody serum levels, and disease severity, thus suggesting that the presence of TLOs is associated with disease progression rather than resolution.[51-58] TLO-associated B cell activation is a recognized mechanism of lymphoma progression in the salivary glands of patients with SS and in the gastric mucosa of patients with *Helicobacter pylori* gastritis.[59-62] In fact, in SS the identification of ectopic TLOs with fully formed GCs within the MSGs biopsy is currently used as histological biomarker and prognostic tool for lymphoma development.[63] A randomized, double-blind, placebo-controlled phase II clinical trial is now ongoing concerning the use of baminercept, a lymphotoxin–β receptor fusion protein, for the treatment of SS patients.

Downstream of the lymphotoxin pathway, there is the production of the lymphoid chemokines CCL21, CCL19, CXCL13, and CXCL12 involved in the organization of GCs and TLOs. In 2001, Amft et al.[64] described CXCL13 expression within lymphoid aggregates and endothelial cells in salivary glands of SS patients and of CXCL12 on ductal epithelial cells. Given its overexpression in serum and saliva from patients with SS, CXCL13 has been proposed as a biomarker of disease.[65] After administration of an anti-CXCL13 antibody, an improvement in disease has been observed in animal models of SS, providing evidence for a potential therapeutic use of anti-CXCL13 in clinical trials. An indirect effect on CXCL13 expression can also be achieved by interfering with IL-17 production. IL-17 has indeed been demonstrated as being able to directly induce the expression of CXCL13 and CCL21 (alongside CXCL10, CXCL11, and CXCL9),[53] thus directly contributing to lymphoneogenesis. More recently, Kuchroo's group has also demonstrated that Th17 cells are required for the induction of TLOs in the central nervous system in the experimental autoimmune encephalomyelitis mouse model.[66] Although anti–IL-17 therapy is considered in spondyloarthropathies and IBDs, there are no active studies with this compound which are recruiting SS patients. Our group has recently shown that CX3CL1 (known by the name of *fractalkine*) is increased in serum from patients with SS.[67] Fractalkine is present in the CD20+ area of salivary glands and within the GC-like structures.[67] A positive correlation between CX3CL1 serum levels and focus score has been also described. Because the administration of anti-CX3CL1 antibodies induced an improvement in experimental models of rheumatoid arthritis,[68] targeting fractalkine is conceivable in SS.

## 6. GERMINAL CENTERS AND COSTIMULATORY MOLECULES

In secondary and TLOs, upon antigen encounter, B cells upregulate the chemokine receptor CCR7 and congregate at the boundary between B cell and T cell areas in search of T cell help. T cell help is provided upon successful stimulation of T cells with DCs. Cognate encounters of these activated T cells with the B cells specific for the same antigen, at the T–B boundary drive initial B cell proliferation. Ultimately, this process is critically dependent on the presence and efficient activation of the complex costimulatory cascade.[69] Excessive costimulation has been reported in autoimmune conditions and models of autoimmune diseases. Accordingly, targeting costimulatory molecules with the aim of disrupting the cross talk between T and B cells and between T cells and DCs that occurs within secondary lymphoid organs or TLOs is an intriguing possibility to treat autoimmunity.

Abatacept is a fusion protein resulting from the binding of CTLA-4 to the Fc portion of IgG1, able to inhibit T cell activation by interfering with the CD80/ CD86 interaction. Abatacept was first licensed for the treatment of rheumatoid arthritis[70] and in 2014 an open-label study evaluating the efficacy and safety of abatacept was conducted in SS patients with promising results. Fifteen patients with SS (according to the American European Consensus Group Criteria) were treated with eight intravenous abatacept infusions on days 1, 15, and 29 and every 4 weeks thereafter. Abatacept showed itself to be well tolerated by

SS patients. Disease activity, laboratory parameters, and fatigue significantly improved during treatment. More interestingly, whereas abatacept administration was not able to significantly decrease the number of infiltrating T and B cells within the glands, it still succeeds in decreasing the focus score of the aggregates, thus suggesting efficacy in its ability to inhibit the immune cell cross talk and therefore interfering with TLO aggregation.[71] Another study, with the aim of evaluating efficacy and safety of subcutaneous abatacept treatment in SS in a larger and randomized double-blind phase III clinical trial, is currently recruiting patients.

Inducible T-cell costimulator (ICOS) protein is a member of the Ig superfamily of costimulatory molecules and it is a CD28-like molecule that interacts with B7-related peptide 1 (B7RP1). ICOS is upregulated after T cell receptor engagement on activated CD3+ cells and is a critical regulator of the GC reaction.[69,72] There is evidence that mice which are deficient in ICOS or its ligand have impaired GC formation and isotype switching.[72] Moreover, ICOS blockade prevents the development of spontaneous disease in prediabetic nonobese diabetic (NOD) mice.[73] Treatment with an anti-B7RP1 antibody in two mouse models of SLE and collagen-induced arthritis demonstrated efficacy in improving disease manifestation in association with a decrease in the percentage of Tfh cells and GC B cells, as well as a decrease in the frequency of ICOS(+) T cells.[74] A phase IIa, randomized, placebo-controlled clinical trial is now recruiting patients to evaluate the safety and efficacy of a monoclonal antibody directed to B7-related protein in SS.

The interaction between CD40 ligand (CD40L) (on T cells) and CD40 (on antigen-presenting cells and B cells) is another potential target in SS. Treatment with ruplizumab of patients with SLE was proved to reduce anti–double-stranded DNA antibodies, increase C3 serum levels, and decrease hematuria. This trial was discontinued because of the increased risk of thromboembolic events given to the off target of the antibody on platelet-bound CD40.[75] A different anti-CD40L monoclonal antibody (toralizumab) has, however, also been used in SLE patients and demonstrated to be safe and well tolerated. Nonetheless, in this trial a real efficacy of the drug compared with placebo was not demonstrated.[76] A multicenter randomized double-blind placebo-controlled phase II clinical trial is currently recruiting patients with SS in order to assess the safety, tolerability, and pharmacokinetics of multiple doses of subcutaneous injection of a monoclonal antibody directed to CD40.

Recently, the possible role of a different costimulatory molecule known as *OX40* has been described. The axis OX40 ligand (OX40L)–OX40 has been proved to provide a great contribution to the aberrant Tfh response in SLE.[77] Specifically, the frequency of circulating OX40L-expressing myeloid antigen-presenting cells positively correlates with disease activity and the frequency of ICOS(+) blood Tfh cells in SLE.[77] Thus a rationale for the use of therapies targeting the OX40L–OX40 axis in SLE has been provided, suggesting a possible utility of targeting this pathway also in SS patients. The use of monoclonal antibodies targeting OX40 has been described only in phase I and II clinical trials in cancer-affected patients (such as ipilimumab in metastatic melanoma), but discussions to translate this pathway in autoimmunity are ongoing.

## 7. INTRACELLULAR CASCADE TARGETING

A large body of evidence has highlighted the role of shared pathways of intra-cellular activation in SS pathogenesis. The phosphatidylinositol 3–kinase δ isoform (PI3Kδ) belongs to a large class 1 phosphoinositide-3-kinase family of intracellular lipid kinases that regulate metabolism, survival, proliferation, apoptosis, growth, and cell migration.[78] Extensive data indicate that PI3Kδ is a predominant isoform in transducing signals from the B cell receptor as well as from receptors for various cytokines, chemokines, and costimulatory mol-ecules.[79,80] Accordingly, B cells derived from mice which are deficient in PI3Kδ activity or wild-type B cells treated with the PI3Kδ inhibitor all have reduced proliferative ability and increased susceptibility to apoptosis in response to anti-CD40, IL-4, or anti-IgM stimulation. The B cell activating factor *(BAFF)* supported survival of B cells is also mediated by PI3kδ.[81–83] PI3Kδ activation is also important in the antigen-presenting function of B cells. Even though PI3Kδ-deficient B cells can internalize and process antigens normally, they are inefficient in the forming of polarized synapses with the T cells, resulting in defective B cell/T cell activation. Accordingly, T cell–dependent antibody responses are impaired in the absence of PI3kδ isoform.[84,85] B cell chemotaxis to CXCL13 and S1P largely relies on PI3kδ to activate Rap1, a key guanosine triphosphatase in B cell migration.[86,87] In addition to its role in B cells, PI3Kδ is important for the differentiation of T cells into Th cells that are necessary for GC response and antibody production. Memory T cell generation and function is impaired in the absence of PI3Kδ.[85,88,89] The significant role of PI3Kδ in regulating B cell activation, proliferation, and survival led to the development of PI3Kδ inhibitor as a target in B cell malignancies. Recently, the PI3Kδ selective inhibitor idelalisib has received US Food and Drug Administration approval for the treatment of chronic lymphocytic leukemia (CLL) and NHL. The results of an early clinical trial have been very promising and have indicated that idelalisib does inhibit not only B cell survival pathways but also both the production of chemokines and their response to these mediators that serve to retain CLL cells in their protective lymph-node microenvironments.[90] Because of its crucial and nonredundant roles in regulating cellular mechanisms underlying inflammation and successful targeting in lymphoproliferative malignancies, it is an interesting target in diseases caused by dysfunctional immune responses such as SS. The PI3Kδ pathway has been successfully targeted in a mouse model of SLE.[91] In SS there are reports on the involvement of the PI3K–Akt signaling pathway in the regulation of the apoptotic cell death of salivary gland epithelial cells.[92,93]

The epidermal growth factor (EGF)–receptor (EGFR) pathway is believed to be activated as an attempt to preserve salivary gland integrity during the disease.[94]

Indeed, EGFR signaling leads to the activation of the PI3K-Akt and IκB kinase (IKK)–nuclear factor-κB (NF-κB) pathways. By immunohistochemical analysis, Nakamura and colleagues[92] have proved a colocalization of phosphorylated EGFR, phosphorylated Akt, and NF-kB p65 in the salivary glands of SS patients. The same study included the stimulation of salivary epithelial cells in vitro with EGF-induced phosphorylation of the EGFR and Akt, and NF-κB p65 nuclear translocation. The exposure to chemical inhibitors of PI3K significantly reduced Akt phosphorylation, supporting the hypothesis of an EGF/EGFR involvement in antiapoptogenic signals through PI3K-Akt and IKK–NF-κB. A double-blind, placebo-controlled clinical study looking at the safety and efficacy of PI3Kδ blocking in SS is in the pipeline for the beginning of 2016.

## 8. REGENERATIVE MEDICINE FOR SJÖGREN'S SYNDROME

During the last few decades, knowledge of stem cell biology has increasingly opened new avenues to regenerative medicine based on cellular immune-modulatory therapies. Consequently stem cell transplant (SCT) has emerged as a rescue therapy for a widening spectrum of diseases.[95] The majority of SCTs worldwide have utilized hematopoietic stem cells (HSCs) as opposed to mesenchymal stem cells (MSCs). MSCs, a heterogeneous group of progenitor, plastic-adherent cells, are able to self-renew and to differentiate toward many cells of mesodermal lineage but also into other lineages such as ectodermal (epithelial cells and neuroglial-like cells) and endodermal (muscle cells, lung cells, gut epithelial cells, and hepatocyte-like cells) ones.[96,97] MSCs bear stromal surface markers (CD76, CD90, and CD105) and lack hematopoietic cell markers such as CD11a, CD14, CD19, CD34, CD45, and major histocompatibility complex class II.[98] The capacity of differentiating in such a wide array of diverse cells which possibly repair damaged tissues and organs, along with immunomodulatory properties, confers to bone marrow (BM)–derived MSCs a great therapeutic potential for several disorders including ischemic, neurodegenerative, and autoimmune diseases.[95] Even if the exact molecular mechanism remains unclear, MSCs have been shown to act on different types of cells involved in the immune response, including T cells, B cells, NK cells, and DCs, with an overall immunosuppressive capacity.[99–101] Autologous BM-derived MSCs have been shown to exert an anti-proliferative effect against activated T cells derived either from normal subjects or from patients with rheumatoid arthritis, systemic sclerosis (SSc), and SLE.[102] MSCs are able to influence T cell plasticity and favor the generation of cells with regulatory activity. Because of their low expression of human leukocyte antigen (HLA) class I and negligible expression of HLA class II, MSCs present an immunologically privileged phenotype which, unlike HSC transplantation, makes a conditioning regimen unnecessary before use. MSCs have been successfully used in graft-versus-host disease,[103] Crohn disease,[104] SLE,[105] polymyositis and dermatomyositis,[106] SSc,[107] and type I diabetes mellitus.[108] However, the potential cancer-related risks of MSC infusion should be carefully considered.[109]

In SS the salivary gland function is compromised, and among the current pharmacological approaches to restore, or at least ameliorate it, there is the attempt to increase the secretory capacity of the acinar cells. The potential use of BM-derived cells (BMDCs) to repair oral tissues and restore salivation has been widely reviewed by Maria et al.[110] In co-culture experiments performed with human parotid or submandibular gland biopsy specimens, human MSCs have been demonstrated to be able to differentiate into salivary gland exocrine cells.[111] BMDCs and peripheral blood stem cells from healthy male donors are able to differentiate into buccal (oral) epithelial cells of female transplant recipients and donor cell microchimerism can be found in salivary glands after allogeneic BMDC or peripheral blood stem cell transplantation.[112] These preliminary observations led to the development of some interesting experimental mouse models, which produced some promising data on the use of MSC in SS. The combined use of MSC and complete Freund's adjuvant has proved to be effective in both preventing loss of saliva secretion and in reducing lymphocytic infiltration in the salivary glands of NOD mice. In particular, MSC infusion appears to decrease the number of T and B lymphocytes in the inflammatory aggregates and to increase the frequency of Foxp3+ Treg cells.[113] Treatment of allogeneic MSCs prevented and suppressed experimental SS-like diseases in an experimental murine model, reducing the salivary gland damage and improving salivary gland function in NOD/Ltj mice.[114] The same authors demonstrated the efficacy of MSCs in alleviating symptoms in SS patients. Such beneficial effects were attributed to the immunoregulatory activity of MSC that favors the development of Treg and a Th2 switch while inhibiting Th17 and Tfh differentiation. The use of MSC for the treatment of SS is further supported by the evidence of an impressive amelioration of hyposalivation of radiation-damaged rat salivary glands by human salivary gland stem cells which restore acinar and duct cell structure, and decrease the amount of apoptotic cells.[115] Interestingly, a fundamental role of the stromal cell–derived factor 1–CXCR4 axis in directing MSC trafficking toward inflammation has been demonstrated.[116] Salivary gland expression of CXCL12 during SS would therefore support the use of these cells in this context. If MSCs can be considered as a helpful candidate for partial salivary gland tissue repair, a further step to the medicine of the future is whole salivary gland replacement therapy, which may become the "next-generation organ regenerative treatment." In this context, the complete functional regeneration of ectodermal organs such as the teeth, hair follicles, salivary glands, and lacrimal glands using "organ germ methods," that involve epithelial and mesenchymal stem cell manipulation techniques to induce the organ germ formation has been demonstrated.[117–121]

## 9. CONCLUSIONS

The novel interest of pharmaceutical companies in the market of SS has provided a large range of potential treatments for this orphan disease. Nonetheless, SS pathogenesis is still unclear and it is not known how different patients will respond to different treatments. There is enough evidence to support the principle that SS patients could be stratified either on the basis of their histopathology or response to treatment. The collection of biomarkers in blood, saliva, or tissue will potentially provide a critical tool for this process and support the future personalized medicine approach to SS.

## ACKNOWLEDGMENT

We thank Dott Antonina Minniti for her help in preparing the manuscript.

## REFERENCES

1. Anaya JM, Delgado-Vega AM, Castiblanco J. Genetic basis of Sjögren's syndrome: how strong is the evidence? *Clin Dev Immunol* 2006;**13**:209–22.
2. Brito-Zeron SN, Muñoz S, Bové A, Akasbi M, Belenguer R, et al. Prevalence and clinical relevance of autoimmune neutropenia in patients with primary Sjögren's syndrome. *Semin Arthritis Rheum* 2009;**38**:389–95.
3. Brito-Zeron P, Ramos-Casals M. Prognosis of patients with primary Sjögren's syndrome. *Med Clin Barc* 2008;**130**:109–15.
4. Moutsopoulos HM, Manoussakis MN. Lumping or splitting autoimmune rheumatic disorders? Lessons from Sjögren's syndrome. *Br J Rheumatol* 1998;**37**:1263–4.
5. Callaghan R, Prabu A, Allan RB, Clarke AE, Sutcliffe N, Pierre YS, et al. Direct healthcare costs and predictors of costs in patients with primary Sjögren's syndrome. *Rheumatology (Oxford)* 2007;**46**:105–11.
6. Bowman SJ, St Pierre Y, Sutcliffe N, Isenberg DA, Goldblatt F, Price E, et al. Estimating indirect costs in primary Sjögren's syndrome. *J Rheumatol* 2010;**37**:1010–5.
7. Lendrem D, Mitchell S, McMeekin P, Bowman S, Price E, Pease CT, et al. Health-related utility values of patients with primary Sjögren's syndrome and its predictors. *Ann Rheum Dis* 2014;**73**:1362–8.
8. Juarez M, Toms TE, de Pablo P, Mitchell S, Bowman S, Nightingale P, et al. Cardiovascular risk factors in women with primary Sjögren's syndrome: United Kingdom primary Sjögren's syndrome registry results. *Arthritis Care Res (Hoboken)* 2014;**66**:757–64.
9. Kotsis K, Voulgari PV, Tsifetaki N, Drosos AA, Carvalho AF, Hyphantis T. Illness perceptions and psychological distress associated with physical health-related quality of life in primary Sjögren's syndrome compared to systemic lupus erythematosus and rheumatoid arthritis. *Rheumatol Int* 2014;**34**:1671–81.
10. Bowman S, Barone F. Biologic treatments in Sjögren's syndrome. *Presse Med* 2012;**41**:495–509.
11. Ng WF, Bowman SJ, Griffiths B. United Kingdom Primary Sjögren's Syndrome Registry–a united effort to tackle an orphan rheumatic disease. *Rheumatology (Oxford)* 2011;**50**:32–9.
12. Seror R, Mariette X, Bowman S, Baron G, Gottenberg JE, Bootsma H, et al. Accurate detection of changes in disease activity in primary Sjögren's syndrome by the European League Against Rheumatism Sjögren's Syndrome Disease Activity Index. *Arthritis Care Res (Hoboken)* 2010;**62**:551–8.
13. Seror R, Ravaud P, Bowman SJ, Baron G, Tzioufas A, Theander E, et al. EULAR Sjögren's syndrome disease activity index: development of a consensus systemic disease activity index for primary Sjögren's syndrome. *Ann Rheum Dis* 2010;**69**:1103–9.

14. Skopouli FN, Moutsopoulos HM. Autoimmune epitheliitis: Sjögren's syndrome. *Clin Exp Rheumatol* 1994;**12**(Suppl. 11):S9–11.
15. Kivity S, Arango MT, Ehrenfeld M, Tehori O, Shoenfeld Y, Anaya JM, et al. Infection and autoimmunity in Sjögren's syndrome: a clinical study and comprehensive review. *J Autoimmun* 2014;**51**:17–22.
16. Croia C, Astorri E, Murray-Brown W, Willis A, Brokstad KA, Sutcliffe N, et al. Implication of Epstein–Barr virus infection in disease-specific autoreactive B cell activation in ectopic lymphoid structures of Sjögren's syndrome. *Arthritis Rheumatol* 2014;**66**:2545–57.
17. Gottenberg JE, Astorri E, Murray-Brown W, Willis A, Brokstad KA, Sutcliffe N, et al. Activation of IFN pathways and plasmacytoid dendritic cell recruitment in target organs of primary Sjögren's syndrome. *Proc Natl Acad Sci USA* 2006;**103**:2770–5.
18. Mavragani CP, Moutsopoulos HM. The geoepidemiology of Sjögren's syndrome. *Autoimmun Rev* 2010;**9**:305–10.
19. Hjelmervik TO, Petersen K, Jonassen I, Jonsson R, Bolstad AI. Gene expression profiling of minor salivary glands clearly distinguishes primary Sjögren's syndrome patients from healthy control subjects. *Arthritis Rheum* 2005;**52**:1534–44.
20. Emamian ES, Leon JM, Lessard CJ, Grandits M, Baechler EC, Gaffney PM, et al. Peripheral blood gene expression profiling in Sjögren's syndrome. *Genes Immun* 2009;**10**:285–96.
21. Wildenberg ME, van Helden-Meeuwsen CG, van de Merwe JP, Drexhage HA, Versnel MA. Systemic increase in type I interferon activity in Sjögren's syndrome: a putative role for plasmacytoid dendritic cells. *Eur J Immunol* 2008;**38**:2024–33.
22. Kalunian KC, Merrill JT, Maciuca R, McBride JM, Townsend MJ, Wei X, et al. A phase II study of the efficacy and safety of rontalizumab (rhuMAb interferon-α) in patients with systemic lupus erythematosus (ROSE). *Ann Rheum Dis* 2015;**75**(1):196–202. pii: annrheumdis-2014–206090.
23. Petri M, Wallace DJ, Spindler A, Chindalore V, Kalunian K, Mysler E, et al. Sifalimumab, a human anti-interferon-α monoclonal antibody, in systemic lupus erythematosus: a phase I randomized, controlled, dose-escalation study. *Arthritis Rheum* 2013;**65**:1011–21.
24. Sankar V, et al. Etanercept in Sjögren's syndrome: a twelve-week randomized, double-blind, placebo-controlled pilot clinical trial. *Arthritis Rheum* 2004;**50**:2240–5.
25. Batten M, Brennan MT, Kok MR, Leakan RA, Smith JA, Manny J, et al. TNF deficiency fails to protect BAFF transgenic mice against autoimmunity and reveals a predisposition to B cell lymphoma. *J Immunol* 2004;**172**:812–22.
26. d'Elia HF, Bjurman C, Rehnberg E, Kvist G, Konttinen YT. Interleukin 6 and its soluble receptor in a central role at the neuroimmunoendocrine interface in Sjögren syndrome: an explanatory interventional study. *Ann Rheum Dis* 2009;**68**:285–6.
27. Bombardieri M, Barone F, Pittoni V, Alessandri C, Conigliaro P, Blades MC, et al. Increased circulating levels and salivary gland expression of interleukin-18 in patients with Sjögren's syndrome: relationship with autoantibody production and lymphoid organization of the periductal inflammatory infiltrate. *Arthritis Res Ther* 2004;**6**:447–56.
28. Norheim KB, Harboe E, Gøransson LG, Omdal R. Interleukin-1 inhibition and fatigue in primary Sjögren's syndrome: a double blind, randomised clinical trial. *PLoS One* 2012;**7**:30123.
29. Ciccia F, Accardo-Palumbo A, Alessandro R, Rizzo A, Principe S, Peralta S, et al. Interleukin-22 and interleukin-22-producing NKp44+ natural killer cells in subclinical gut inflammation in ankylosing spondylitis. *Arthritis Rheum* 2012;**64**:1869–78.
30. Ciccia F, Guggino G, Rizzo A, Bombardieri M, Raimondo S, Carubbi F, et al. Interleukin (IL)-22 receptor 1 is over-expressed in primary Sjögren's syndrome and Sjögren-associated non-Hodgkin lymphomas and is regulated by IL-18. *Clin Exp Immunol* 2015;**181**:219–29.

31. Barone F, Nayar S, Campos J, Cloake T, Withers DR, Toellner KM, et al. IL-22 regulates lymphoid chemokine production and assembly of tertiary lymphoid organs. *Proc Natl Acad Sci USA* 2015;**112**:11024–9.

32. Keene DL, Legare C, Taylor E, Gallivan J, Cawthorn GM, Vu D. Monoclonal antibodies and progressive multifocal leukoencephalopathy. *Can J Neurol Sci* 2011;**38**:565–71.

33. Pelletier D, Hafler DA. Fingolimod for multiple sclerosis. *N Engl J Med* 2012;**366**:339–47.

34. Garris CS, Blaho VA, Hla T, Han MH. Sphingosine-1-phosphate receptor 1 signalling in T cells: trafficking and beyond. *Immunology* 2014;**142**:347–53.

35. Sekiguchi M, Iwasaki T, Kitano M, Kuno H, Hashimoto N, Kawahito Y, et al. Role of sphingosine 1-phosphate in the pathogenesis of Sjögren's syndrome. *J Immunol* 2008;**180**:1921–8.

36. Signoriello E, Sagliocchi A, Fratta M, Lus G. Fingolimod efficacy in multiple sclerosis associated with Sjögren syndrome. *Acta Neurol Scand* 2015;**131**:140–3.

37. Sprent J, Surh CD. Normal T cell homeostasis: the conversion of naive cells into memory-phenotype cells. *Nat Immunol* 2011;**12**:478–84.

38. Lee H, Park HJ, Sohn HJ, Kim JM, Kim SJ. Combinatorial therapy for liver metastatic colon cancer: dendritic cell vaccine and low-dose agonistic anti-4-1BB antibody co-stimulatory signal. *J Surg Res* 2011;**169**:43–50.

39. Bikker A, Kruize AA, Wenting M, Versnel MA, Bijlsma JW, Lafeber FP, et al. Increased interleukin (IL)-7Ralpha expression in salivary glands of patients with primary Sjögren's syndrome is restricted to T cells and correlates with IL-7 expression, lymphocyte numbers and activity. *Ann Rheum Dis* 2012;**71**:1027–33.

40. Jin JO, Kawai T, Cha S, Yu Q. Interleukin-7 enhances the Th1 response to promote the development of Sjögren's syndrome-like autoimmune exocrinopathy in mice. *Arthritis Rheum* 2013;**65**:2132–42.

41. Jin JO, Shinohara Y, Yu Q. Innate immune signaling induces interleukin-7 production from salivary gland cells and accelerates the development of primary Sjögren's syndrome in a mouse model. *PLoS One* 2013;**8**:77605.

42. Hartgring SA, Willis CR, Alcorn D, Nelson LJ, Bijlsma JW, Lafeber FP, et al. Blockade of the interleukin-7 receptor inhibits collagen-induced arthritis and is associated with reduction of T cell activity and proinflammatory mediators. *Arthritis Rheum* 2010;**62**:2716–25.

43. Kang KY, Kim HO, Kwok SK, Ju JH, Park KS, Sun DI, et al. Impact of interleukin-21 in the pathogenesis of primary Sjögren's syndrome: increased serum levels of interleukin-21 and its expression in the labial salivary glands. *Arthritis Res Ther* 2011;**13**:179.

44. Breitfeld D, Ohl L, Kremmer E, Ellwart J, Sallusto F, Lipp M. Follicular B helper T cells express CXC chemokine receptor 5, localize to B cell follicles, and support immunoglobulin production. *J Exp Med* 2000;**192**:1545–52.

45. Jin L, Yu D, Li X, Yu N, Li X, Wang Y, et al. CD4+CXCR5+ follicular helper T cells in salivary gland promote B cells maturation in patients with primary Sjögren's syndrome. *Int J Clin Exp Pathol* 2014;**7**:1988–96.

46. Bubier JA, Bennett SM, Sproule TJ, Lyons BL, Olland S, Young DA, et al. Treatment of BXSB-Yaa mice with IL-21R-Fc fusion protein minimally attenuates systemic lupus erythematosus. *Ann N Y Acad Sci* 2007;**1110**:590–601.

47. Herber D, Brown TP, Liang S, Young DA, Collins M, Dunussi-Joannopoulos K. IL-21 has a pathogenic role in a lupus-prone mouse model and its blockade with IL-21R.Fc reduces disease progression. *J Immunol* 2007;**178**:3822–30.

48. Young DA, Hegen M, Ma HL, Whitters MJ, Albert LM, Lowe L, et al. Blockade of the interleukin-21/interleukin-21 receptor pathway ameliorates disease in animal models of rheumatoid arthritis. *Arthritis Rheum* 2007;**56**:1152–63.

49. Salomonsson S, Jonsson MV, Skarstein K, Brokstad KA, Hjelmström P, Wahren-Herlenius M, et al. Cellular basis of ectopic germinal center formation and autoantibody production in the target organ of patients with Sjögren's syndrome. *Arthritis Rheum* 2003;**48**:3187–201.

50. Bombardieri M, Barone F, Humby F, Kelly S, McGurk M, Morgan P, et al. Activation-induced cytidine deaminase expression in follicular dendritic cell networks and interfollicular large B cells supports functionality of ectopic lymphoid neogenesis in autoimmune sialoadenitis and MALT lymphoma in Sjögren's syndrome. *J Immunol* 2007;**179**:4929–38.

51. Salomonsson S, Larsson P, Tengnér P, Mellquist E, Hjelmström P, Wahren-Herlenius M. Expression of the B cell-attracting chemokine CXCL13 in the target organ and autoantibody production in ectopic lymphoid tissue in the chronic inflammatory disease Sjögren's syndrome. *Scand J Immunol* 2002;**55**:336–42.

52. Astorri E, Bombardieri M, Gabba S, Peakman M, Pozzilli P, Pitzalis C. Evolution of ectopic lymphoid neogenesis and in situ autoantibody production in autoimmune nonobese diabetic mice: cellular and molecular characterization of tertiary lymphoid structures in pancreatic islets. *J Immunol* 2010;**185**:3359–68.

53. Rangel-Moreno J, Carragher DM, de la Luz Garcia-Hernandez M, Hwang JY, Kusser K, Hartson L, et al. The development of inducible bronchus-associated lymphoid tissue depends on IL-17. *Nat Immunol* 2011;**12**:639–46.

54. Weyand CM, Klimiuk PA, Goronzy JJ. Heterogeneity of rheumatoid arthritis: from phenotypes to genotypes. *Springer Semin Immunopathol* 1998;**20**:5–22.

55. Takemura S, Braun A, Crowson C, Kurtin PJ, Cofield RH, O'Fallon WM, et al. Lymphoid neogenesis in rheumatoid synovitis. *J Immunol* 2001;**167**:1072–80.

56. Weyand CM, Goronzy JJ. Ectopic germinal center formation in rheumatoid synovitis. *Ann N Y Acad Sci* 2003;**987**:140–9.

57. Bugatti S, Manzo A, Caporali R, Montecucco C. Assessment of synovitis to predict bone erosions in rheumatoid arthritis. *Ther Adv Musculoskelet Dis* 2012;**4**:235–44.

58. Bugatti S, Caporali R, Manzo A, Vitolo B, Pitzalis C, Montecucco C. Involvement of subchondral bone marrow in rheumatoid arthritis: lymphoid neogenesis and in situ relationship to subchondral bone marrow osteoclast recruitment. *Arthritis Rheum* 2005;**52**:3448–59.

59. Hallas C, Greiner A, Peters K, Müller-Hermelink HK. Immunoglobulin VH genes of high-grade mucosa-associated lymphoid tissue lymphomas show a high load of somatic mutations and evidence of antigen-dependent affinity maturation. *Lab Invest* 1998;**78**:277–87.

60. Qin Y, Greiner A, Hallas C, Haedicke W, Müller-Hermelink HK. Intraclonal offspring expansion of gastric low-grade MALT-type lymphoma: evidence for the role of antigen-driven high-affinity mutation in lymphomagenesis. *Lab Invest* 1997;**76**:477–85.

61. Barone F, Nayar S, Buckley CD. The role of non-hematopoietic stromal cells in the persistence of inflammation. *Front Immunol* 2012;**3**:416.

62. Barone F, Bombardieri M, Rosado MM, Morgan PR, Challacombe SJ, De Vita S, et al. CXCL13, CCL21, and CXCL12 expression in salivary glands of patients with Sjögren's syndrome and MALT lymphoma: association with reactive and malignant areas of lymphoid organization. *J Immunol* 2008;**180**:5130–40.

63. Theander E, Vasaitis L, Baecklund E, Nordmark G, Warfvinge G, Liedholm R, et al. Lymphoid organisation in labial salivary gland biopsies is a possible predictor for the development of malignant lymphoma in primary Sjögren's syndrome. *Ann Rheum Dis* 2011;**70**:1363–8.

64. Amft N, Curnow SJ, Scheel-Toellner D, Devadas A, Oates J, Crocker J, et al. Ectopic expression of the B cell-attracting chemokine BCA-1 (CXCL13) on endothelial cells and within lymphoid follicles contributes to the establishment of germinal center-like structures in Sjögren's syndrome. *Arthritis Rheum* 2001;**44**:2633–41.

65. Kramer JM, Klimatcheva E, Rothstein TL. CXCL13 is elevated in Sjögren's syndrome in mice and humans and is implicated in disease pathogenesis. *J Leukoc Biol* 2013;**94**:1079–89.

66. Peters A, Pitcher LA, Sullivan JM, Mitsdoerffer M, Acton SE, Franz B, et al. Th17 cells induce ectopic lymphoid follicles in central nervous system tissue inflammation. *Immunity* 2011;**35**:986–96.

67. Astorri E, Scrivo R, Bombardieri M, Picarelli G, Pecorella I, Porzia A, et al. CX3CL1 and CX3CR1 expression in tertiary lymphoid structures in salivary gland infiltrates: fractalkine contribution to lymphoid neogenesis in Sjögren's syndrome. *Rheumatology (Oxford)* 2014;**53**:611–20.

68. Nanki T, Urasaki Y, Imai T, Nishimura M, Muramoto K, Kubota T, et al. Inhibition of fractalkine ameliorates murine collagen-induced arthritis. *J Immunol* 2004;**173**:7010–6.

69. Wolniak KL, Shinall SM, Waldschmidt TJ. The germinal center response. *Crit Rev Immunol* 2004;**24**:39–65.

70. Westhovens R, Kremer JM, Moreland LW, Emery P, Russell AS, Li T, et al. Safety and efficacy of the selective costimulation modulator abatacept in patients with rheumatoid arthritis receiving background methotrexate: a 5-year extended phase IIB study. *J Rheumatol* 2009;**36**:736–42.

71. Meiners PM, Vissink A, Kroese FG, Spijkervet FK, Smitt-Kamminga NS, Abdulahad WH, et al. Abatacept treatment reduces disease activity in early primary Sjögren's syndrome (open-label proof of concept ASAP study). *Ann Rheum Dis* 2014;**73**:1393–6.

72. Gatto D, Brink R. The germinal center reaction. *J Allergy Clin Immunol* 2010;**126**:898–907.

73. Bozulic LD, Huang Y, Xu H, Wen Y, Ildstad ST. Differential outcomes in prediabetic vs. overtly diabetic NOD mice nonmyeloablatively conditioned with costimulatory blockade. *Exp Hematol* 2011;**39**:977–85.

74. Hu YL, Metz DP, Chung J, Siu G, Zhang M. B7RP-1 blockade ameliorates autoimmunity through regulation of follicular helper T cells. *J Immunol* 2009;**182**:1421–8.

75. Boumpas DT, Furie R, Manzi S, Illei GG, Wallace DJ, Balow JE, et al. A short course of BG9588 (anti-CD40 ligand antibody) improves serologic activity and decreases hematuria in patients with proliferative lupus glomerulonephritis. *Arthritis Rheum* 2003;**48**:719–27.

76. Kalunian KC, Davis Jr JC, Merrill JT, Totoritis MC, Wofsy D. IDEC-131 Lupus Study Group. Treatment of systemic lupus erythematosus by inhibition of T cell costimulation with anti-CD154: a randomized, double-blind, placebo-controlled trial. *Arthritis Rheum* 2002;**46**:3251–8.

77. Jacquemin C, Schmitt N, Contin-Bordes C, Liu Y, Narayanan P, Seneschal J, et al. OX40 ligand contributes to human lupus pathogenesis by promoting T follicular helper response. *Immunity* 2015;**42**:1159–70.

78. Stephens L, Hawkins P. Signalling via class IA PI3Ks. *Adv Enzyme Regul* 2011;**51**:27–36.

79. Okkenhaug K, Bilancio A, Emery JL, Vanhaesebroeck B. Phosphoinositide 3-kinase in T cell activation and survival. *Biochem Soc Trans* 2004;**32**:332–5.

80. Jou ST, Carpino N, Takahashi Y, Piekorz R, Chao JR, Carpino N, et al. Essential, nonredundant role for the phosphoinositide 3-kinase p110delta in signaling by the B-cell receptor complex. *Mol Cell Biol* 2002;**22**:8580–91.

81. Okkenhaug K, Bilancio A, Farjot G, Priddle H, Sancho S, Peskett E, et al. Impaired B and T cell antigen receptor signaling in p110delta PI 3-kinase mutant mice. *Science* 2002;**297**:1031–4.

82. Bilancio A, Okkenhaug K, Camps M, Emery JL, Ruckle T, Rommel C, et al. Key role of the p110delta isoform of PI3K in B-cell antigen and IL-4 receptor signaling: comparative analysis of genetic and pharmacologic interference with p110delta function in B cells. *Blood* 2006;**107**:642–50.

83. Clayton E, Bardi G, Bell SE, Chantry D, Downes CP, Gray A, et al. A crucial role for the p110delta subunit of phosphatidylinositol 3-kinase in B cell development and activation. *J Exp Med* 2002;**196**:753–63.

84. Al-Alwan MM, Okkenhaug K, Vanhaesebroeck B, Hayflick JS, Marshall AJ. Requirement for phosphoinositide 3-kinase p110delta signaling in B cell antigen receptor-mediated antigen presentation. *J Immunol* 2007;**178**:2328–35.

85. Hawkins PT, Stephens LR. PI3K signalling in inflammation. *Biochim Biophys Acta* 2015;**1851**:882–97.

86. Durand CA, Hartvigsen K, Fogelstrand L, Kim S, Iritani S, Vanhaesebroeck B, et al. Phosphoinositide 3-kinase p110 delta regulates natural antibody production, marginal zone and B-1 B cell function, and autoantibody responses. *J Immunol* 2009;**183**:5673–84.

87. Reif K, Okkenhaug K, Sasaki T, Penninger JM, Vanhaesebroeck B, Cyster JG. Cutting edge: differential roles for phosphoinositide 3-kinases, p110gamma and p110delta, in lymphocyte chemotaxis and homing. *J Immunol* 2004;**173**:2236–40.

88. Rolf J, Bell SE, Kovesdi D, Janas ML, Soond DR, Webb LM, et al. Phosphoinositide 3-kinase activity in T cells regulates the magnitude of the germinal center reaction. *J Immunol* 2010;**185**:4042–52.

89. Venable JD, Ameriks MK, Blevitt JM, Thurmond RL, Fung-Leung WP. Phosphoinositide 3-kinase gamma (PI3Kgamma) inhibitors for the treatment of inflammation and autoimmune disease. *Recent Pat Inflamm Allergy Drug Discov* 2010;**4**:1–15.

90. Okkenhaug K, Fruman DA. PI3Ks in lymphocyte signaling and development. *Curr Top Microbiol Immunol* 2010;**346**:57–85.

91. Maxwell MJ, Tsantikos E, Kong AM, Vanhaesebroeck B, Tarlinton DM, Hibbs ML. Attenuation of phosphoinositide 3-kinase δ signaling restrains autoimmune disease. *J Autoimmun* 2012;**38**:381–91.

92. Nakamura H, Kawakami A, Ida H, Koji T, Eguchi K. Epidermal growth factor inhibits Fas-mediated apoptosis in salivary epithelial cells of patients with primary Sjögren's syndrome. *Clin Exp Rheumatol* 2007;**25**:831–7.

93. Nakamura H, Horai Y, Suzuki T, Okada A, Ichinose K, Yamasaki S, et al. TLR3-mediated apoptosis and activation of phosphorylated Akt in the salivary gland epithelial cells of primary Sjögren's syndrome patients. *Rheumatol Int* 2013;**33**:441–50.

94. Gorgoulis V, Giatromanolaki A, Iliopoulos A, Kanavaros P, Aninos D, Ioakeimidis D, et al. EGF and EGF-r immunoexpression in Sjögren's syndrome secondary to rheumatoid arthritis: correlation with EBV expression? *Clin Exp Rheumatol* 1993;**11**:623–7.

95. Cipriani P, Carubbi F, Liakouli V, Marrelli A, Perricone C, Perricone R, et al. Stem cells in autoimmune diseases: implications for pathogenesis and future trends in therapy. *Autoimmun Rev* 2013;**12**:709–16.

96. Pittenger MF, Mackay AM, Beck SC, Jaiswal RK, Douglas R, Mosca JD, et al. Multilineage potential of adult human mesenchymal stem cells. *Science* 1999;**284**:143–7.

97. Kopen GC, Prockop DJ, Phinney DG. Marrow stromal cells migrate throughout forebrain and cerebellum, and they differentiate into astrocytes after injection into neonatal mouse brains. *Proc Natl Acad Sci USA* 1999;**96**:10711–6.

98. Dominici M, Le Blanc K, Mueller I, Slaper-Cortenbach I, Marini F, Krause D, et al. Minimal criteria for defining multipotent mesenchymal stromal cells: the International Society for Cellular Therapy position statement. *Cytotherapy* 2006;**8**:315–7.

99. Tse WT, Pendleton JD, Beyer WM, Egalka MC, Guinan EC. Suppression of allogeneic T-cell proliferation by human marrow stromal cells: implications in transplantation. *Transplantation* 2003;**75**:389–97.

100. Fibbe WE, Nauta AJ, Roelofs H. Modulation of immune responses by mesenchymal stem cells. *Ann N Y Acad Sci* 2007;**1106**:272–8.

101. Sotiropoulou PA, Perez SA, Salagianni M, Baxevanis CN, Papamichail M. Cell culture medium composition and translational adult bone marrow-derived stem cell research. *Stem Cells* 2006;**24**:1409–10.

102. Bocelli-Tyndall C, Bracci L, Spagnoli G, Braccini A, Bouchenaki M, Ceredig R, et al. Bone marrow mesenchymal stromal cells (BM-MSCs) from healthy donors and auto-immune disease patients reduce the proliferation of autologous- and allogeneic-stimulated lymphocytes in vitro. *Rheumatology (Oxford)* 2007;**46**:403–8.

103. Le Blanc K, Frassoni F, Ball L, Locatelli F, Roelofs H, Lewis I, et al. Mesenchymal stem cells for treatment of steroid-resistant, severe, acute graft-versus-host disease: a phase II study. *Lancet* 2008;**371**:1579–86.

104. Duijvestein M, Vos AC, Roelofs H, Wildenberg ME, Wendrich BB, Verspaget HW, et al. Autologous bone marrow-derived mesenchymal stromal cell treatment for refractory luminal Crohn's disease: results of a phase I study. *Gut* 2010;**59**:1662–9.

105. Sun L. Stem cell transplantation: progress in Asia. *Lupus* 2010;**19**:1468–73.

106. Wang D, Zhang H, Cao M, Tang Y, Liang J, Feng X, et al. Efficacy of allogeneic mesenchymal stem cell transplantation in patients with drug-resistant polymyositis and dermatomyositis. *Ann Rheum Dis* 2011;**70**:1285–8.

107. Christopeit M, Schendel M, Föll J, Müller LP, Keysser G, Behre G. Marked improvement of severe progressive systemic sclerosis after transplantation of mesenchymal stem cells from an allogeneic haploidentical-related donor mediated by ligation of CD137L. *Leukemia* 2008;**22**:1062–4.

108. Ezquer FE, Ezquer ME, Parrau DB, Carpio D, Yañez AJ, Conget PA. Systemic administration of multipotent mesenchymal stromal cells reverts hyperglycemia and prevents nephropathy in type 1 diabetic mice. *Biol Blood Marrow Transpl* 2008;**14**:631–40.

109. Bocelli-Tyndall C, Bracci L, Schaeren S, Feder-Mengus C, Barbero A, Tyndall A. Human bone marrow mesenchymal stem cells and chondrocytes promote and/or suppress the in vitro proliferation of lymphocytes stimulated by interleukins 2, 7 and 15. *Ann Rheum Dis* 2009;**68**:1352–9.

110. Maria OM, Khosravi R, Mezey E, Tran SD. Cells from bone marrow that evolve into oral tissues and their clinical applications. *Oral Dis* 2007;**13**:11–6.

111. Maria OM, Tran SD. Human mesenchymal stem cells cultured with salivary gland biopsies adopt an epithelial phenotype. *Stem Cells Dev* 2011;**20**:959–67.

112. Tran SD, Redman RS, Barrett AJ, Pavletic SZ, Key S, Liu Y, et al. Microchimerism in salivary glands after blood- and marrow-derived stem cell transplantation. *Biol Blood Marrow Transpl* 2011;**17**:429–33.

113. Khalili S, Liu Y, Kornete M, Roescher N, Kodama S, Peterson A, et al. Mesenchymal stromal cells improve salivary function and reduce lymphocytic infiltrates in mice with Sjögren's-like disease. *PLoS One* 2012;**7**:e38615.

114. Xu J, Wang D, Liu D, Fan Z, Zhang H, Liu O, et al. Allogeneic mesenchymal stem cell treatment alleviates experimental and clinical Sjögren syndrome. *Blood* October 11, 2012;**120**(15):3142–3151.

115. Jeong J, Baek H, Kim YJ, Choi Y, Lee H, Lee E, et al. Human salivary gland stem cells ameliorate hyposalivation of radiation-damaged rat salivary glands. *Exp Mol Med* 2013;**45**:58.

116. Xu X, Zhu F, Zhang M, Zeng D, Luo D, Liu G, et al. Stromal cell-derived factor-1 enhances wound healing through recruiting bone marrow-derived mesenchymal stem cells to the wound area and promoting neovascularization. *Cells Tissues Organs* 2013;**197**:103–13.

117. Nakao K, Morita R, Saji Y, Ishida K, Tomita Y, Ogawa M, et al. The development of a bioengineered organ germ method. *Nat Methods* 2007;**4**:227–30.

118. Ogawa M, Oshima M, Imamura A, Sekine Y, Ishida K, Yamashita K, et al. Functional salivary gland regeneration by transplantation of a bioengineered organ germ. *Nat Commun* 2013;**4**:2498.
119. Hirayama M, Oshima M, Tsuji T. Development and prospects of organ replacement regenerative therapy. *Cornea* 2013;**32**:S13–21.
120. Ogawa M, Tsuji T. Functional salivary gland regeneration as the next generation of organ replacement regenerative therapy. *Odontology* 2015;**103**:248–57.
121. Ogawa M, Tsuji T. Reconstitution of a bioengineered salivary gland using a three-dimensional cell manipulation method. *Curr Protoc Cell Biol* 2015;**66**:19 17 1–3.

# Index

Printed in the United States
By Bookmasters